This significant new publication on genomic or parental imprinting has been prepared by an outstanding team of international authorities and supported by the distinguished Nobel foundation. Genomic imprinting results in the preferential expression of one allele, depending on the parent of origin. It is associated with several disease syndromes in humans. Interest in this area has expanded rapidly from the time when it was first recognized that some aspects of inheritance were not adequately explained by the Mendelian laws.

The chapters cover a wealth of material to help explain not only the mechanisms of genomic imprinting but also its biological and medical consequences. This interdisciplinary volume encompasses clinical genetics, pathology, developmental biology, evolution and genetics. It will be an essential resource for all scientists and clinicians working in these areas.

Genomic imprinting

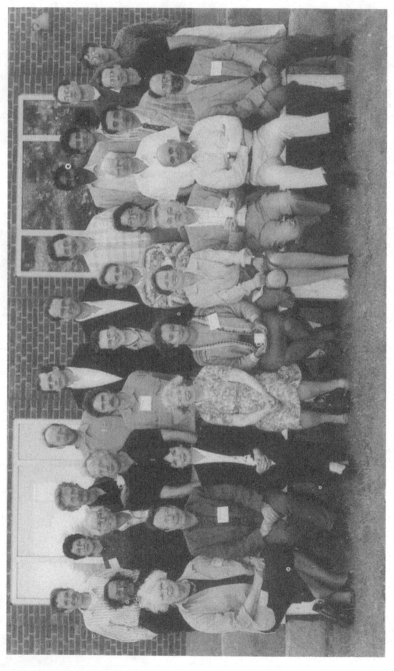

Participants in the 1994 Nobel symposium, Stockholm, which gave rise to this volume.
Back row, from left: Howard Cedar, Denise Barlow, Rudolf Jaenisch, David Haig, Timothy Bestor, Alan Wolffe, Andrew Feinberg, Tharappel James, Robert Nicholls, Kevin Davies (editor, *Nature Genetics*), Rory Howlett (assistant editor, *Nature*).
Middle row, from left: Azim Surani, Martin Ritzen, Davor Solter, Bernhardt Horsthemke, Rolf Ohlsson, Marcel Mannens, Wolf Reik, Bruce Cattanach, Tsunehiro Mukai, Benjamin Tycko.
Front row, from left: Kerstin Hall, Anthony Reeve, Sinead Jones (formerly acting editor, *Trends in Genetics*), Mary Lyon, Uta Francke, Shirley Tilghman, Jiří Forejt, D. R. Tata, Gilbert Côté.

Genomic imprinting
causes and consequences

Edited by

R. OHLSSON, K. HALL *and* M. RITZEN

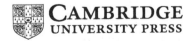

CAMBRIDGE
UNIVERSITY PRESS

CAMBRIDGE UNIVERSITY PRESS
Cambridge, New York, Melbourne, Madrid, Cape Town, Singapore,
São Paulo, Delhi, Dubai, Tokyo, Mexico City

Cambridge University Press
The Edinburgh Building, Cambridge CB2 8RU, UK

Published in the United States of America by Cambridge University Press, New York

www.cambridge.org
Information on this title: www.cambridge.org/9780521179997

First published 1995
Reprinted 1997
First paperback edition 2010

A catalogue record for this publication is available from the British Library

Library of Congress Cataloguing in Publication data

Genomic imprinting: causes and consequences / edited by R. Ohlsson,
K. Hall, and M. Ritzen.
p. cm.
ISBN 0 521 47243 1 hardback
1. Genomic imprinting. 2. Genetic diseases. 1. Ohlsson, R.
(Rolf) II. Hall, K. III. Ritzen, Martin, 1937–
QH450.G467 1995
575.2 – dc20 95–4982 CIP

ISBN 978-0-521-47243-2 Hardback
ISBN 978-0-521-17999-7 Paperback

Contents

Contributors   xi

I   *Genomic imprinting in mammals*   1

1   The role of imprinting in early mammalian development
     A. GILLIGAN AND D. SOLTER   3

2   The evolution of parental imprinting: a review of hypotheses
     D. HAIG AND R. TRIVERS   17

3   Genetic variations in parental imprinting on mouse
     chromosome 17   J. FOREJT, S. GREGOROVÁ, M. LANDÍKOVÁ,
     J. ČAPKOVÁ AND L. M. SILVER   29

II   *Chromatin structure and DNA modifications*   47

4   Epigenetic inheritance: the chromatin connection
     A. P. WOLFFE   49

5   Chromobox genes and the molecular mechanisms of cellular
     determination   P. B. SINGH AND T. C. JAMES   71

6   The biochemical basis of allele-specific gene expression in
     genomic imprinting and X inactivation   T. H. BESTOR   109

7   DNA methylation and mammalian development
     R. JAENISCH, C. BEARD AND E. LI   118

III   *Mechanisms of imprinting*   127

8   X chromosome inactivation and imprinting   M. F. LYON   129

9   Imprinting of *H19* and *Xist* in uniparental embryos
     M. A. SURANI, A. C. FERGUSON-SMITH, H. SASAKI AND
     S. C. BARTON   142

10   Imprinted genes, allelic methylation, and imprinted modifiers
     of methylation   W. REIK, R. FEIL, N. D. ALLEN,
     T. F. MOORE AND J. WALTER   157

11 Genomic imprinting of the *H19* and *Igf2* genes in the mouse
S. M. TILGHMAN, M. S. BARTOLOMEI, A. L. WEBBER, M. E.
BRUNKOW, J. SAAM, P. A. LEIGHTON AND K. PFEIFER 170

12 Plasticity of imprinting R. OHLSSON, T. EKSTRÖM,
G. FRANKLIN, S. PFEIFER-OHLSSON, H. CUI, S. MILLER,
R. FISHER AND C. WALSH 182

13 Regional regulation of allele-specific gene expression
I. SIMON AND H. CEDAR 195

IV **Genomic imprinting in embryonal tumors and overgrowth disorders** 207

14 Genomic imprinting in embryonal tumors and overgrowth
disorders A. E. REEVE 209

15 Tracking imprinting: the Beckwith–Wiedemann syndrome
M. MANNENS 224

16 Genomic imprinting in Beckwith–Wiedemann syndrome
R. WEKSBERG AND J. SQUIRE 237

17 Mitotic crossing over and the disruption of genomic imprinting
G. B. CÔTÉ 252

18 Evaluating *H19* as an imprinted tumor suppressor gene
B. TYCKO 264

19 A domain of abnormal imprinting in human cancer
A. P. FEINBERG 273

V **Genomic imprinting and the Prader–Willi syndrome** 293

20 Parent-of-origin-specific DNA methylation and imprinting
mutations on human chromosome 15 B. HORSTHEMKE,
B. DITTRICH AND K. BUITING 295

21 The *SNRPN* gene and Prader–Willi syndrome U. FRANCKE,
J. A. KERNS AND J. GIACALONE 309

VI **Imprinting: a search for new genes and unifying principles** 325

22 Use of chromosome rearrangements for investigations into
imprinting in the mouse B. M. CATTANACH, J. BARR AND
J. JONES 327

23   A new imprinted gene, *U2af-related sequence*, isolated by a
      methylation-sensitive genome scanning method   T. MUKAI,
      I. HATADA, T. YAMAOKA, K. KITAGAWA, X.-D. WANG,
      T. SUGAMA, J. MASUDA AND J. OGATA   342

24   The mouse *Igf2/MPR* gene: a model for all gametic imprinted
      genes?   D. P. BARLOW   357

Index   369

Contributors

Nicholas D. Allen
Laboratory of Developmental Genetics and Imprinting, The Babraham Institute, Babraham, Cambridge CB2 4AT, UK

Denise P. Barlow
Research Institute of Molecular Pathology, Dr. Bohr-Gasse 7, A-1030 Vienna, Austria

Marisa S. Bartolomei
Department of Cell and Developmental Biology, University of Pennsylvania School of Medicine, Philadelphia, PA 19104, USA

Jacky Barr
MRC Radiobiology Unit, Chilton, Didcot, Oxon OX11 0RD, UK

Sheila C. Barton
Wellcome/CRC Institute of Cancer and Developmental Biology, Tennis Court Road, Cambridge CB2 1QR, UK

Caroline Beard
Whitehead Institute for Biomedical Research *and* Department of Biology, Massachusetts Institute of Technology, 9 Cambridge Center, Cambridge MA 02142, USA

Timothy H. Bestor
Department of Cell Biology, Harvard Medical School, 25 Shattuck Street, Boston, MA 02115, USA

Mary E. Brunkow
Samuel Lunenfeld Research Institute, Mount Sinai Hospital, Toronto, Ontario, Canada M5G 1X5

Karen Buiting
Institut für Humangenetik, Universitätsklinikum Essen, Hufelandstrasse 55, D-45122 Essen, Germany

Jana Capková
Laboratory of Mammalian Molecular Genetics, Institute of Molecular Genetics, Academy of Sciences of the Czech Republic, Vídeňská 1083, 142 20 Prague 4, Czech Republic

Bruce M. Cattanach
MRC Radiobiology Unit, Chilton, Didcot, Oxon OX11 0RD, UK

Howard Cedar
Department of Cellular Biochemistry, Hebrew University Medical School, PO Box 12272, Jerusalem, Israel

Gilbert B. Côté
Department of Genetics, Sudbury General Hospital, 700 Paris Street, Sudbury, Ontario, Canada P3E 3B5

Hengmi Cui
Department of Animal Development and Genetics, University of Uppsala, Norbyvägen 18 A, S-752 36 Uppsala, Sweden

Bärbel Dittrich
Institut für Humangenetik, Universitätsklinikum Essen, Hufelandstrasse 55, D-45122 Essen, Germany

Thomas Ekström
Department of Clinical Neuroscience, Alcohol and Drug Addiction Research, Karolinska Institute, 171 76 Stockholm, Sweden

Robert Feil
Laboratory of Developmental Genetics and Imprinting, The Babraham Institute, Babraham, Cambridge CB2 4AT, UK

Andrew P. Feinberg
Departments of Medicine *and* Molecular Biology and Genetics, Johns Hopkins University School of Medicine, 1064 Ross, 720 Rutland Avenue, Baltimore, MD 21205, USA

Anne C. Ferguson-Smith
Department of Anatomy, University of Cambridge, Downing Street, Cambridge CB2 3DY, UK

Rosemary Fisher
CRC Laboratories, Department of Medical Oncology, Charing Cross Hospital, Fulham Palace Road, London W6 8RF, UK

Jiří Forejt
Department of Molecular Biology, Lewis Thomas Laboratory, Princeton University, Princeton, NJ 08540, USA

Uta Francke
Departments of Genetics *and* Pediatrics *and* Howard Hughes Medical Institute, Stanford University Medical Center, Beckman Center, Stanford, CA 94305-5428, USA

Gary Franklin
Department of Animal Development and Genetics, University of Uppsala, Norbyvägen 18 A, S-752 36 Uppsala, Sweden

Joseph Giacalone
Department of Genetics, Stanford University Medical Center, Beckman Center, Stanford, CA 94305-5428, USA

A. Gilligan
The Wistar Institute, 3601 Spruce Street, Philadelphia, PA 19104, USA

Soňa Gregorová
Laboratory of Mammalian Molecular Genetics, Institute of Molecular Genetics, Academy of Sciences of the Czech Republic, Vídeňská 1083, 142 20 Prague 4, Czech Repbulic

David Haig
Museum of Comparative Zoology, Harvard University, 26 Oxford Street, Cambridge, MA 02138, USA

Izuho Hatada
National Cardiovascular Center Research Institute, 5-7-1 Fujishiro-dai, Suita, Osaka 565, Japan

Bernhard Horsthemke
Institut für Humangenetik, Universitätsklinikum Essen, Hufelandstrasse 55, D-45122 Essen, Germany

Rudolf Jaenisch
Whitehead Institute for Biomedical Research *and* Department of Biology, Massachusetts Institute of Technology, 9 Cambridge Center, Cambridge MA 02142, USA

Tharappel C. James
Department of Molecular Biology and Biochemistry, Wesleyan University, Middletown, CT 06459-0175, USA (present address: Department of Biology, Fairfield University, Fairfield, CT 06430, USA)

Janet Jones
MRC Radiobiology Unit, Chilton, Didcot, Oxon OX11 0RD, UK

Julie A. Kerns
Howard Hughes Medical Institute, Stanford University Medical Center, Beckman Center, Stanford, CA 94305-5428, USA

Kazunori Kitagawa
National Cardiovascular Center Research Institute, 5-7-1 Fujishiro-dai, Suita, Osaka 565, Japan; *and* Department of Surgery II, Osaka University Medical School, Suita, Osaka 565, Japan

Marta Landíková
Laboratory of Mammalian Molecular Genetics, Institute of Molecular Genetics, Academy of Sciences of the Czech Republic, Vídeňská 1083, 142 20 Prague 4, Czech Republic

Philip A. Leighton
Howard Hughes Medical Institute *and* Department of Molecular Biology, Princeton University, Princeton, NJ 08454, USA

En Li
Massachusetts General Hospital – East, Cardiovascular Research Center, 149 13th Street, 4th floor, Charlestown, MA 02129, USA

Mary F. Lyon
MRC Radiobiology Unit, Chilton, Didcot, Oxon OX11 0RD, UK

Marcel Mannens
Academ Medical Center, Institute of Human Genetics, University of Amsterdam, Meibergdreef 15, 1105 AZ Amsterdam, The Netherlands

Junichi Masuda
National Cardiovascular Center Research Institute, 5-7-1 Fujishiro-dai, Suita, Osaka 565, Japan

Stephen Miller
Department of Animal Development and Genetics, University of Uppsala, Norbyvägen 18 A, S-752 36 Uppsala, Sweden

Thomas F. Moore
Laboratory of Developmental Genetics and Imprinting, The Babraham Institute, Babraham, Cambridge CB2 4AT, UK

Tsunehiro Mukai
National Cardiovascular Center Research Institute, 5-7-1 Fujishiro-dai, Suita, Osaka 565, Japan

Jun Ogata
National Cardiovascular Center Research Institute, 5-7-1 Fujishiro-dai, Suita, Osaka 565, Japan

Rolf Ohlsson
Department of Animal Development and Genetics, University of Uppsala, Norbyvägen 18 A, S-752 36 Uppsala, Sweden

Karl Pfeifer
Howard Hughes Medical Institute *and* Department of Molecular Biology, Princeton University, Princeton, NJ 08454, USA

Susan Pfeifer-Ohlsson
Department of Animal Development and Genetics, University of Uppsala, Norbyvägen 18 A, S-752 36 Uppsala, Sweden

Anthony E. Reeve
Cancer Genetics Laboratory, Department of Biochemistry, University of Otago, PO Box 56, Dunedin, New Zealand

Wolf Reik
Laboratory of Developmental Genetics and Imprinting, The Babraham Institute, Babraham, Cambridge CB2 4AT, UK

Jennifer Saam
Howard Hughes Medical Institute *and* Department of Molecular Biology, Princeton University, Princeton, NJ 08454, USA

Hiroyuki Sasaki
Institute of Genetic Information, Kyushu University, 3-1-1 Maidashi, Higashi-ku, Fukuoka 812, Japan

Lee M. Silver
Department of Molecular Biology, Lewis Thomas Laboratory, Princeton University, Princeton, NJ 08540, USA

Itamar Simon
Department of Cellular Biochemistry, Hebrew University Medical School, PO Box 12272, Jerusalem, Israel

Prim B. Singh
Cell Determination Group, Department of Development and Signalling, The Babraham Institute, Babraham, Cambridge CB2 4AT, UK

Davor Solter
Max-Planck-Institute for Immunobiology, Department of Developmental Biology, Stübeweg 51, 79108 Freiburg, Germany

Jeremy Squire
Department of Pathology, Hospital for Sick Children/University of Toronto, 555 University Avenue, Toronto, Canada M5G 1X8

Takako Sugama
National Cardiovascular Center Research Institute, 5-7-1 Fujishiro-dai, Suita, Osaka 565, Japan

M. Azim Surani
Wellcome/CRC Institute of Cancer and Developmental Biology, Tennis Court Road, Cambridge CB2 1QR, UK

Shirley M. Tilghman
Howard Hughes Medical Institute *and* Department of Molecular Biology, Princeton University, Princeton, NJ 08454, USA

Robert Trivers
Department of Anthropology, Rutgers University, New Brunswick, NJ 08903, USA

Benjamin Tycko
Department of Pathology, Columbia University College of Physicians and Surgeons, 630 W168th Street, New York, NY 10032, USA

Colum Walsh
Department of Animal Development and Genetics, University of Uppsala, Norbyvägen 18 A, S-752 36 Uppsala, Sweden

Jörn Walter
Max-Planck-Institute of Molecular Genetics, Ihnestrasse 73, Berlin, Germany

Xu-Dong Wang
National Cardiovascular Center Research Institute, 5-7-1 Fujishiro-dai, Suita, Osaka 565, Japan

Andrea L. Webber
Howard Hughes Medical Institute *and* Department of Molecular Biology, Princeton University, Princeton, NJ 08454, USA

Rosanna Weksberg
Department of Pediatrics and Genetics, Hospital for Sick Children/University of Toronto, 555 University Avenue, Toronto, Canada M5G 1X8

Alan P. Wolffe
Laboratory of Molecular Embryology, National Institute of Child Health and Human Development, National Institutes of Health, Bethesda, MD 20892, USA

Tetsuji Yamaoka
National Cardiovascular Center Research Institute, 5-7-1 Fujishiro-dai, Suita, Osaka 565, Japan; *and* Department of Polymer Science and Engineering, Kyoto Institute of Technology, Matsugasaki, Kyoto 606, Japan

I

Genomic imprinting in mammals

1

The role of imprinting in early mammalian development

A. GILLIGAN AND D. SOLTER

Introduction

Nuclear transfer experiments (McGrath & Solter, 1984) and the analysis of various chromosomal abnormalities (Cattanach & Kirk, 1985) have clearly demonstrated that maternal and paternal genomes as gametic contributions are functionally not identical and that both are essential for normal development. Functional differences are likely to be imposed during gametogenesis. This phenomenon acquired the name *imprinting*, with various adjective modifiers (genomic, parental, etc.). The possible role of imprinting in normal development and in numerous inherited disease states generated considerable interest in the subject, this book being one of the examples. One also has the impression that imprinting is one of the rare biological subjects having more reviews than original articles devoted to it. Among the many reviews one, our own (Solter, 1988), covers reasonably well the early part of the story; Efstratiadis (1994) deals in detail (also with substantial flair) with the more recent developments. Among the many and various aspects of imprinting, we here restrict our attention to the possible role of imprinted genes in preimplantation mouse development and explore the available evidence for the existence of imprinting-related events during that period.

Effect of imprinting on preimplantation development

Androgenetic and gynogenetic/pathenogenetic embryos can develop to blastocysts *in vitro* (Latham & Solter, 1991; McGrath & Solter, 1984; Surani *et al.*, 1986). The question arises as to whether the development is comparable to the development of control, nuclear transfer embryos containing both the male and female pronucleus. It is somewhat difficult to draw completely unambiguous conclusions on the basis of the available data. In some cases control embryos

3

Table 1.1. *Development (in percentage) to blastocyst of androgenetic, gynogenetic and control embryos* in vitro

Embryos	Series				
	1	2	3	4[a]	5
Control unmanipulated	93	87	95	84	ND
Control manipulated	100	ND	ND	73	87
Gynogenones	73	61	ND	75–93[b]	ND
Androgenones	53	22	19	46–55[b]	35–48[c]

[a] The effect of egg cytoplasm on the development of androgenones is described in this work. Results in this table refer only to the use of cytoplasts that support a high degree of development. For details see text.
[b] Values obtained with different cytoplast–karyoplast combinations.
[c] Values obtained using three different mouse strains (129/Sv, BALB/c and outbred CD-1).
Sources of series: 1, McGrath & Solter (1984); 2, Surani *et al.* (1986); 3, Hagemann & First (1992); 4, Latham & Solter (1991); 5, Mann & Stewart (1991).

were not manipulated; this is acceptable provided the laboratory demonstrated that in their hands control non-manipulated and nuclear transfer embryos developed equally well, as indeed they should (McGrath & Solter, 1984). With this caveat it appears that gynogenones/parthenogenones develop as well as controls or only slightly worse; however, androgenones develop considerably worse (Table 1.1). Since Y–Y androgenetic embryos cannot develop to the blastocyst stage, the expected development of androgenones should be about 75% of the development of gynogenones. In some experimental series (Table 1.1) the development of androgenones is, however, substantially reduced, the values being about one third of those obtained for the development of gynogenones and/or controls.

At the present time it is unclear what causes the differences in the development of androgenones in different experimental series from different laboratories. Technical problems could be part of the answer, although this is unlikely. We recently showed that egg cytoplasm from different mouse strains differs substantially in its ability to support androgenetic development (Latham & Solter, 1991). However, in the majority of series studied (Table 1.1) the egg cytoplasm was derived from mice of strain C57BL/6 or their F1 hybrids; this cytoplasm supports a high level of development. An additional reason for this discrepancy could be the differences in the criteria used to determine what is to be called expanded blastocyst and what is not.

It is important to resolve the issue of the development of androgenones: we have to know whether their development is impaired or not before embarking on an extensive search for the causes of impaired development. It has been reported (Hagemann & First, 1992) that poor development of androgenones can be improved by injecting 4-cell androgenetic embryos with cellular extracts or mRNA isolated from normal or parthenogenetic morulae. These results would indicate the existence of genes that are expressed during preimplantation development when inherited maternally but not paternally. This is a conceptually important result. However, the improvement in development (from 19 to 47%) might be questioned: other workers (McGrath & Solter, 1984), using the same or other (Mann & Stewart, 1991) mouse strains, reported 50% development of androgenones without any cytoplasmic additives. Once the androgenetic embryo reaches the blastocyst stage (regardless of the percentage), the developmental quality of such a blastocyst should be assessed. This assessment poses additional problems, because all androgenetic embryos fail very soon after implantation. The scant information available suggests that androgenetic blastocysts are not normal, as their cell number is substantially reduced (Latham & Solter, 1991).

The problem of the preimplantation development of androgenetic embryos is further compounded by the observation that certain nuclear and cytoplasmic combinations are particularly detrimental for development (Latham & Solter, 1991). Briefly, DBA/2 egg cytoplasm supports the development of androgenones rather poorly when compared with C57BL/6 cytoplasm, especially in combination with C57BL/6 male pronuclei. Complex nuclear–cytoplasmic interactions are probably involved: even brief exposure of male C57BL/6 pronuclei to DBA/2 cytoplasm before returning them to C57BL/6 cytoplasm substantially reduces their developmental potential. It is at present unclear to what extent these and other nucleocytoplasmic incompatibilities (Renard *et al.*, 1994) are related to the imprinting phenomenon.

In summary, although androgenetic and gynogenetic embryos can reach the blastocyst stage and implant, impaired development of androgenones suggests that some of the imprinted genes might be relevant for preimplantation development.

Expression of imprinted genes during preimplantation development

The study of the phenotype of androgenetic and gynogenetic embryos as they progressively fail in development should provide us with some idea of the number and nature of the genes involved. Because the period between first observable abnormalities and the death of the most advanced uniparental embryos is rather long (3–4 days), either the control of expression of imprinted genes is quite leaky or embryonic failure is due to the cumulative effect of the absence of products of numerous genes: death by a thousand cuts.

Androgenetic and gynogenetic preimplantation embryos are remarkably similar to each other and to control embryos in their overall pattern of protein synthesis (Latham & Solter, 1991), so there are no massive differences in gene expression during that time. It is very likely that some of the genes that are crucial during the peri- and early postimplantation period are imprinted. Inner cell mass (ICM) derivatives develop very poorly in androgenetic embryos but the development of the trophoblast is essentially normal; the opposite is true for gynogenetic embryos (Surani *et al.*, 1986). Although imprinting probably does not play a role in the initial allocation of cells to inner cell mass and trophoblast, gynogenetic cells allocated to the trophoblast ultimately fail to thrive (McGrath & Solter, 1986; Surani *et al.*, 1986; Thomson & Solter, 1988, 1989) as do androgenetic cells allocated to ICM. Whether one can conclude from these phenotypic observations that some of the imprinted genes are essential for the early differentiation of cell lineage in mammalian embryos remains to be seen.

As of now about a dozen or so genes are known to be imprinted in the mouse (Efstratiadis, 1994); most of them are also imprinted in humans. The expression of some of them in preimplantation embryos has been investigated; the results are somewhat controversial in terms of expression itself and in terms of expression regulated by imprinting. The insulin-like growth factor II gene (*Igf2*) is expressed from the paternal allele in practically all fetal tissues but both paternal and maternal alleles are expressed in the adult brain, specifically in the leptomeninges and choroid plexus (DeChiara *et al.*, 1991). Expression in blastocysts was not observed using *in situ* hybridization (Lee *et al.*, 1990); however, expression was detected in normal but not parthenogenetic blastocysts by using reverse transcription–polymerase chain reaction (RT–PCR) (Rappolee *et al.*, 1992), later results suggesting that the effect of imprinting is already present in preimplantation embryos. These results were not confirmed by Latham *et al.* (1994) using the same technique: this group observed the expression of *Igf2* in both parthenogenetic cleavage-stage embryos and blastocysts, suggesting that the imprinting may not affect *Igf2* gene expression at this developmental period.

The physiological effects of insulin-like growth factor II (IGF-II) are mediated by the IGF-I receptor (IGF1R) protein and the IGF-II receptor (IGF2R) protein, both of which IGF-II binds with high affinity. The IGF-II receptor gene (*Igf2r*) is also imprinted, although in this case expression from the paternal allele is repressed while expression from the maternal allele is apparently induced by a maternal-specific methylation imprinting signal (Stöger *et al.*, 1993). However, the expression of *Igf2r* is not regulated by imprinting in preimplantation mouse embryos: the gene is expressed in androgenetic blastocysts (Latham *et al.*, 1994).

It is interesting that *Igf2r* in humans is not imprinted (Kalscheuer *et al.*, 1993) or imprinted only in some individuals (Xu *et al.*, 1993). The preponderance of data suggest that *Igf1r* is not imprinted (Liu *et al.* 1993); however, Rappolee *et al.* (1992) report that *Igf1r* is not expressed in parthenogenetic blastocysts although it is expressed in control embryos. This repression of *Igf1r* expression from the maternal allele represents the sole evidence that this gene is imprinted. Because operation of this growth factor circuit is so profoundly affected by genomic imprinting and because of the controversial data in the literature as mentioned above, we decided to reexamine the expression of *Igf2* and *Igf1r* in parthenogenetic and control preimplantation mouse embryos.

Expression of *Igf2* and *Igf1r* in parthenogenetic and control embryos

An *Igf2* band of the appropriate size (255 bp) was observed in the PCR products of both control and parthenogenetic blastocysts after moderate amplification (32 cycles; Fig. 1.1A). The absence of this band in the minus reverse transcriptase controls and in the embryo lysis buffer controls strongly indicates that the RT–PCR protocol specifically amplified mRNA sequences. Genomic DNA should not be amplified using this primer pair, because the amplified sequence contains introns (Dull *et al.*, 1984; Telford *et al.*, 1990). An equivalent number of oocytes did not initially generate a signal, although reamplification of oocyte aliquots generated a strong signal (Fig. 1.1B). In experiments where more oocytes or more cycles were included in the initial amplification, an oocyte *Igf2* signal was observed but of weaker intensity than those observed for control and parthenogenetic blastocysts (data not shown). The identity of the 255 bp band was confirmed by *Sac*II digestion: treated samples yielded a band migrating close to the expected 189 bp (Fig. 1.1C). Additionally, probing blots of *Igf2* gels with [^{32}P]*Igf2* cDNA yielded strong hybridization signals at the 255 bp band (data not shown).

A band migrating in the region (354 bp) expected for the *Igf1r* PCR product was observed in oocytes and in control and parthenogenetic blastocysts (Fig. 1.2). Maternal versus zygotic transcription contribution to the blastocyst signal could not be distinguished by this expression pattern. The absence of signal in the minus reverse transcriptase controls and in embryo lysis buffer controls shows that the 354 bp band reflects mRNA content and not contaminating DNA. This observation is especially important for the *Igf1r* analysis as, unlike the PCR product for *Igf2*, the region of the *Igf1r* being amplified does not contain an intron. Restriction enzyme analysis of the PCR products by digestion with *Hinc*II did not affect their electrophoretic profile (data not shown) and suggest that this primer pair is specifically amplifying IGF-I receptor cDNA and not the homologous insulin receptor cDNA (Telford *et al.*, 1990).

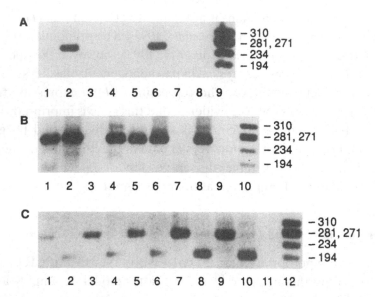

Fig. 1.1. Expression of *Igf2* in oocytes and in control and parthenogenetic blastocysts. C57BL/6 female mice, 6–10 wk old, were superovulated, mated overnight with C57BL/6 × DBA/2 F1 (B6D2) males, checked for vaginal plugs the next morning (day of plug is day 0.5), and zygotes collected (Hogan *et al.*, 1986). Oocytes were collected from unmated females on day 0.5 and subjected to parthenogenetic activation by incubation of cumulus masses in 7% ethanol in HEPES-buffered modified Whitten's (Rothstein *et al.*, 1992) medium for 5 min at room temperature, digestion in hyaluronidase, and incubation of the activated oocytes in cytochalasin B for 5–6 h at 37 °C (Hogan *et al.*, 1986). Non-activated oocytes to be extracted for RNA were incubated in modified Whitten's medium for 3–5 h and RNA prepared by incubation in embryo lysis buffer containing proteinase K and SDS, followed by a series of phenol–chloroform extractions (Rothstein *et al.*, 1992). Parthenogenetic and control embryos were cultured to blastocysts (day 5–5.5) in modified Whitten's medium and extracted for RNA as above.

Embryonic RNA (isolated from 50–200 embryos) was DNased, divided into plus and minus reverse transcriptase samples, and reverse transcribed using oligo d(T) priming and Superscript reverse transcriptase (Boehringer Mannheim) for 1 h at 42 °C. These samples were amplified by PCR using primers specific for a mouse *Igf2* sequence (Telford, 1990). The program used for *Igf2* sequence amplification was: 1 min at 94 °C, 1.5 min 62 °C, 1.5 min 72 °C, 32–40 cycles. The product was identified by size (255 base pairs) on ethidium-bromide-stained 1.5 or 2% agarose gels. Additionally, gels were blotted onto nylon membranes and probed with ^{32}P-labeled pIGF-2/8-1 (ATCC#57483) (Dull *et al.*, 1984). *Igf2* PCR samples were also subjected to *Sac*II enzyme digestion to yield a diagnostic band at 189 bp (Telford *et al.*, 1990).

(A) Lane 1, 96 B6D2 oocytes RT−; lane 2, 98 B6D2 blastocysts RT+; lane 3, 98 B6D2 blastocysts RT−; lane 4, embryo lysis buffer RT+; lane 5, embryo lysis buffer RT−; lane 6, 100 parthenogenetic blastocysts RT+; lane 7, 100 parthenogenetic blastocysts RT−; lane 8, empty; lane 9, PhiX174 DNA markers. One quarter of the 50 μl PCR reaction was loaded onto a 2% agarose gel containing 0.5

This study provides evidence that *Igf2*, which behaves unequivocally like an imprinted gene in the postimplantation embryo, where it is transcribed from the paternal allele only (DeChiara *et al.*, 1991), is transcribed from the maternal allele during preimplantation development, thus confirming previously reported data (Latham *et al.*, 1994). This conclusion is based on the observation that *Igf2* mRNA is present in parthenogenetic blastocysts at concentrations which exceed those observed in oocytes. These results do not rule out a partial contribution of a very stable maternal message to the blastocyst *Igf2* mRNA pool. However, the concentration of *Igf2* mRNA present in oocytes, as determined by the band intensities of ethidium-bromide-stained PCR gels and Southern blots of these gels, was always substantially lower than in either control or parthenogenetic blastocysts (4/4 experiments) when equal numbers of embryos were analyzed. The same was true when comparing 2-cell embryos and blastocysts (data not shown). Zygotic transcription of the *Igf2* maternal allele must, therefore, contribute to the *Igf2* mRNA pool in parthenogenetic blastocysts. This result is significant for two reasons. First, it corrects the previously published data of Rappolee *et al.* (1992) which showed, also using RT–PCR, that *Igf2* mRNA was not detectable in either oocytes or parthenogenetic blastocysts. More importantly, this work shows that the parental genomic imprint, a marking of the maternal or paternal genome which is probably made during gametogenesis, does not affect *Igf2* expression in the same way during the preimplantation stage of development as in the postimplantation stage. One hypothesis to explain this difference is that the imprint is neutral until transcription factors are synthesized which recognize that specific genomic marking. Similar temporally controlled recognition and readout of the previously existing imprint may control the

Caption for Figure 1.1 (*cont.*).
µg ml⁻¹ ethidium bromide and run for 2 h at 100 V. The reverse negatives of the ethidium-bromide-stained bands are shown.

(B) Two microliter (lanes 1–4) and 10 µl (lanes 5–8) aliquots of the oocytes RT+ (lanes 1 and 5), the B6D2 blastocyst RT+ (lanes 2 and 6), and embryo lysis buffer RT+ (lanes 3 and 7), and the parthenogenetic blastocyst RT+ (lanes 4 and 8) from the PCR reactions in (A) were reamplified by PCR for 35 cycles and products analyzed by ethidium bromide–agarose gel electrophoresis as above.

(C) Positive PCR samples were incubated with (lanes 2, 4, 6, 8, 10) and without (lanes 1, 3, 5, 7, 9) *Sac* II and the products analyzed by ethidium bromide – agarose gel electrophoresis. Lanes 1 and 2, B6D2 blastocyst RT+ from (A); lanes 3 and 4, parthenogenetic blastocysts RT+ from (A); lanes 5 and 6, reamplified oocyte RT+ from (B); lanes 7 and 8, reamplified B6D2 blastocysts from (B); lanes 9 and 10, reamplified parthenogenetic blastocysts from (B); lane 12, PhiX174 DNA markers.

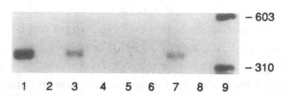

Fig. 1.2. Expression of IGF-1 receptor in oocytes and in control and parthenogenetic blastocysts. For methods of embryo treatment, RNA isolation and
RT–PCR, see Fig. 1.1. Mouse *Igf1r*-specific primer sequences were as described
by Telford *et al.* (1990) and conditions for *Igf1r* sequence amplification were:
1 min at 94 °C, 1.5 min 58 °C, 1.5 min 72 °C, 35–40 cycles. IGFI receptor PCR
samples were subjected to *Hinc*II restriction enzyme analysis. IGFI receptor
bands should be resistant to this enzyme, but bands resulting from amplification
of the homologous insulin receptor will be digested to fragments of 255 bp and
69 bp (Telford *et al.*, 1990).

   Lane 1, 110 oocytes RT+; lane 2, 110 oocytes RT−; lane 3, 67 B6D2
blastocysts RT+; lane 4, 67 B6D2 RT+; lane 5, embryo lysis buffer RT+; lane 6,
embryo lysis buffer RT−; lane 7, 67 parthenogenetic blastocysts RT+; lane 8, 67
parthenogenetic blastocysts RT−; lane 9, PhiX174 DNA markers. One fourth of
the 50 µl PCR product was analyzed by electrophoresis on a 1.5% agarose gel,
containing 0.5 µl ml^{-1} of ethidium bromide, for 2 h at 100 V.

expression of *Xist* and the preferential inactivation of the paternal X chromosome in the trophectoderm (Kay *et al.*, 1993; Norris *et al.*, 1994).

   The expression of *Igf2* exclusively from the paternal allele in most tissues of the
postimplantation embryo (DeChiara *et al.*, 1991) could result from repression at
maternally imprinted loci or from induction at paternally imprinted loci. The
present results show that, in the preimplantation embryo, *Igf2* expression does
not require a paternally imprinted transcription activation signal. The semiquan-
titative nature of this RT–PCR protocol leaves open the possibility that *Igf2*
expression is partly repressed in parthenogenetic blastocysts. Parthenogenetic
embryos at embryonic day 10 do express about 5–8% of the amount of *Igf2*
mRNA as seen in control embryos (Sasaki *et al.*, 1992). Nevertheless, the
observation that the maternal imprint has not completely repressed zygotic
transcription during preimplantation development confirms the hypothesis that
the effects of genomic imprinting on gene expression vary with the stage of
development. If preimplantation expression of other imprinted genes does not
exhibit the pattern predicted by the imprint, the functional effects of imprinting
are likely to be manifested at the postimplantation stages of development.

   Gene targeting experiments have shown that *Igf1r* expression is not regulated
by parental genomic imprinting in postimplantation embryos (Liu *et al.*, 1993).
The observation that *Igf1r* mRNA is present in parthenogenetic blastocysts
refutes the single piece of evidence supporting the conflicting view that this gene

is maternally imprinted (Rappolee *et al.*, 1992). In the absence of other evidence, the question of whether *Igf1r* expression is affected by genomic imprinting during preimplantation development remains open.

The exact meaning and significance of biallelic expression of otherwise imprinted genes during preimplantation development is not completely clear. There is little doubt that mRNA for *Igf2* and *Igf1r* is present in parthenogenetic blastocysts and mRNA for *Igf2r* is found in androgenetic blastocysts. Does that mean that the allele supposed to be silent (owing to the imprinting) is active? In the case of *Igf2* and *Igf2r* this is very likely, since there is a substantial increase in RT–PCR products during preimplantation development, suggesting the activity of embryonic genes.

An alternative explanation of these results would require the presence of very stable oocyte mRNAs, which become progressively more amenable to isolation and/or reverse transcription. No evidence for such a possibility exists and it would be really unlikely for two imprinted genes to be so affected. Nevertheless these data should be explored and improved upon by examining the expression in normal and not gynogenetic and androgenetic embryos to eliminate the possibility that, in the latter, recognition of imprinting for those specific genes is incomplete. In addition, a precise determination of the number of mRNA molecules would be important. Zygotes lacking *Igf2*, *Igf2r* and *Igf1r* genes owing to experimentally induced or natural mutation nevertheless develop into normal blastocysts, so these genes are unlikely to play a crucial role in preimplantation development. Thus in the absence of an obvious function the extent of their expression at that time should be addressed. Regardless of the level of expression, the available data (Latham *et al.*, 1994; this chapter) suggest that at least in some imprinted genes the presence of an imprint does not automatically affect function. We have to assume that the imprint is imposed during gametogenesis, when the maternal and paternal genomes are separated. In order to explain equal expression from both alleles during preimplantation development and expression of only one allele later on, the simplest mechanism would be the existence of an imprint reader, which can activate or inactivate the imprinted gene. Such a reader would be synthesized at the specific time point following fertilization in all or only some of the tissues. Whether every imprinted gene has a specific reader, or whether there is a reader for groups of imprinted genes or for all paternally–maternally imprinted genes, remains to be determined.

Imprinting: who needs it?

No self-respecting scholar of imprinting can write anything on the subject without at least making a token attempt to come up with a theory of imprinting and its purpose and origin. Theories range from vague educated guesses to detailed, imaginative and elaborate structures; their very presence and profusion indicate that we probably do not know nearly enough about the phenomenon. Theory-making is also hampered (or stimulated) by our inability to precisely define the phenomenon and to decide whether the gamete-of-origin- or allele-specific transcriptional regulation observed for some mammalian genes is identical to or different from various other DNA and chromosome-modifying events which are epigenetic and gamete-of-origin-specific. It is our impression that the majority of current theories imply the existence of mammalian-specific imprinting. This is also our view (obviously not supported by facts). Before any imprinted gene was identified, everybody hoped that once they became known the reason for their imprinting would become obvious. As one by one imprinted genes were identified, theories designed to fit those known at the time followed. By now about a dozen imprinted genes have been identified and it is difficult to come up with a unifying theme for all of them; thus the concept of imprinting of innocent bystanders emerged (Varmuza & Mann, 1994). This concept suggests that genes might be imprinted accidentally just because they share target sequences for imprinting with genes that must be imprinted, but the innocent bystander concept is somewhat of an intellectual cop-out and maybe we should keep trying to come up with a unifying theory of imprinting.

Most of the current theories ascribe to imprinting a combative or protective role. It has been suggested that imprinting is derived from the ancestral use of methylation as a device to protect unicellular organisms from invasion of foreign DNA (Barlow, 1993). This is a possible and actually likely explanation for the 'imprinting' behavior of numerous transgenes as suggested previously (Solter, 1988). As a general explanation it suffers from the already mentioned problem that either imprinting is universal or mammals need special protection.

Recent theories restrict imprinting to mammals, either as a device to mediate competition between mother and fetus (Haig, 1992; Haig & Graham, 1991) or to protect females from malignant trophoblastic tumors derived from parthenogenetically activated eggs (Varmuza & Mann, 1994).

The parent–offspring conflict theory (Haig, 1992) proposes that the paternal genome in self-interest would try to promote the growth of the fetus while the maternal genome would try to prevent excessive growth of any single fetus, thus ensuring the success of numerous fetuses and its own dissemination. This theory in the best tradition of the Oxford school of molecular selfishness was nicely aided by the perfect fit of the two imprinted genes first described, *Igf2* and *Igf2r*. Additional imprinted genes do not fit quite so well (but remember the innocent bystanders); however, the major problem with the theory is the absence of imprinting of *Igf2r* in the majority of humans. In addition, if the reciprocal imprinting of *Igf2* and *Igf2r* was necessary to strike the balance between the demands of fetus and mother, the same balance would have been achieved if neither of these genes nor any other gene were to be imprinted.

The theory that visualizes imprinting as a device for protecting 'female mammals from the potential ravages of ovarian trophoblast disease' (Varmuza & Mann, 1994) is rather ingenious and explains several features of imprinting, although innocent bystanders are still necessary. Briefly, the theory states that the occurrence of parthenogenetic activation of eggs in the ovary leading to ovarian tumors, is quite common in humans and in the absence of imprinting the growth of trophoblast (remember that the paternal genome is absolutely essential for trophectoderm differentiation and proliferation) would turn an otherwise benign dermoid cyst into a lethal choriocarcinoma. As long as the genes necessary for trophoblast growth are imprinted (inactivated) in the ovary, this danger is efficiently eliminated. The problem (maybe not insurmountable) with this theory is that it is quite anthropocentric (also feminist, but this is fine; it would be interesting to see whether the personality of scientists often affects the nature of their theories). Spontaneous ovarian teratoma and dermoid cysts derived from parthenogenetic embryos are rather common in humans but are extremely rare in other mammals (with the exception of the LT mouse strain). In addition, the peak incidence of these tumors is between 30 and 35 years of age, which is maybe the prime reproductive age for today's women, but certainly was not prime reproductive age in the time of Lucy. This theory supposes the occurrence of a novel allele, which increases fitness by protecting against trophoblastic disease and thus spreads quickly throughout the population. In view of the virtual absence of the relevant ovarian tumor in non-human mammals and the relatively late onset of the disease in humans, it is difficult to see what could drive the necessary evolutionary change.

The problem with other theories (Efstratiadis, 1994; Solter, 1988) is that, though more encompassing, they are by necessity rather vague and lack predictive tests. The need for precise transcriptional regulation enabling the two-fold differences in gene expression for some specific genes neatly encompasses all imprinting in mammals, but why in that case are both maternal *and* paternal imprinting necessary? The same could easily be achieved if imprinting happened only during oogenesis or only during spermatogenesis except if (as suggested by Rosa Beddington to Davor Solter) some imprinted genes must be expressed in oocyte and some in haploid sperm.

As stated before, there is probably mammalian-specific imprinting, and instead of trying to seek its narrow protective role we should try to see if imprinting was not a *sine qua non* of the emergence of viviparous mammals with the concomitant need for precisely allocating blastomeres to two unique mammalian lineages, inner cell mass and trophectoderm. Genes that regulate this first developmental decision are yet unknown, but if they prove to be imprinted our understanding of the imprinting mechanism and its role will be substantially completed.

Acknowledgments

The technical support of Gustava Black is gratefully acknowledged. The original work was supported by NIH grants HD23291 and HD21355.

References

Barlow, D. P. (1993). Methylation and imprinting: from host defence to gene regulation? *Science* **260**, 309–10.

Cattanach, B. M. & Kirk, M. (1985). Differential activity of maternally and paternally derived chromosome regions in mice. *Nature* **315**, 496–8.

DeChiara, T. M., Robertson, E. J. & Efstratiadis, A. (1991). Parental imprinting of the mouse insulin-like growth factor II gene. *Cell* **64**, 849–59.

Dull, T. J., Gray, A., Hayflick, J. S. & Ullrich, A. (1984). Insulin-like growth factor II precursor gene organization in relation to insulin gene family. *Nature* **310**, 777–81.

Efstratiadis, A. (1994). Parental imprinting of autosomal mammalian genes. *Curr. Opin. Genet. Devel.* **4**, 265–80.

Hagemann, L. J. & First, N. L. (1992). Embryonic cytoplasmic extracts rescue murine androgenones to the blastocyst stage. *Development* **114**, 997–1001.

Haig, D. (1992). Genomic imprinting and the theory of parent–offspring conflict. *Semin. devel. Biol.* **3**, 152–60.

Haig, D. & Graham, C. (1991). Genomic imprinting and the strange case of the insulin-like growth factor II receptor. *Cell* **64**, 1045–6.

Hogan, B., Costantini, F. & Lacy, E. (1986). *Manipulating the Mouse Embryo*. Cold Spring Harbor: Cold Spring Harbor Laboratory.

Kalscheuer, V. M., Mariman, E. C., Schepens, M. T., Rehder, H. & Ropers, H.-H. (1993). The insulin-like growth factor type-2 receptor gene is imprinted in the mouse but not in humans. *Nature Genet.* **5**, 74–8.

Kay, G. F., Penny, G. D., Patel, D., Ashworth, A., Brockdorff, N. & Rastan, S. (1993). Expression of Xist during mouse development suggests a role in the initiation of X chromosome inactivation. *Cell* **72**, 171–82.

Latham, K. E., Doherty, A. S., Scott, C. D. & Schultz, R. M. (1994). *Igf2r* and *Igf2* gene expression in androgenetic, gynogenetic, and parthenogenetic preimplantation mouse embryos: absence of regulation by genomic imprinting. *Genes Devel.* **8**, 290–9.

Latham, K. E. & Solter, D. (1991). Effect of egg composition on the developmental capacity of androgenetic mouse embryos. *Development* **113**, 561–8.

Lee, J., Pintar, J. & Efstratiadis, A. (1990). Pattern of the insulin-like growth factor II gene expression during early mouse embryogenesis. *Development* **110**, 151–9.

Liu, J.-P., Baker, J., Perkins, A. S., Robertson, E. J. & Efstratiadis, A. (1993). Mice carrying null mutations of the genes encoding insulin-like growth factor I (*Igf1*) and type 1 IGF receptor (*Igf1r*). *Cell* **75**, 59–72.

McGrath, J. & Solter, D. (1984). Completion of mouse embryogenesis requires both the maternal and paternal genomes. *Cell* **37**, 179–83.

McGrath, J. & Solter, D. (1986). Nucleocytoplasmic interactions in the mouse embryo. *J. Embryol. exp. Morphol.* **97**, 277–89.

Mann, J. R. & Stewart, C. L. (1991). Development to term of mouse androgenetic aggregation chimeras. *Development* **113**, 1325–33.

Norris, D. P., Patel, D., Kay, G. F., Penny, G. D., Brockdorff, N., Sheardown, S. A. & Rastan, S. (1994). Evidence that random and imprinted *Xist* expression is controlled by preemptive methylation. *Cell* **77**, 41–51.

Ogawa, O., McNoe, L. A., Eccles, M. R., Morison, I. M. & Reeve, A. E. (1993). Human insulin-like growth factor type I and type II receptors are not imprinted. *Hum. molec. Genet.* **2**, 2163–5.

Rappolee, D. A., Sturm, K. S., Begrendtsen, O., Schultz, G. A., Pedersen, R. A. & Werb, Z. (1992). Insulin-like growth factor II acts through an endogenous growth pathway regulated by imprinting in early mouse embryos. *Genes Devel.* **6**, 939–52.

Renard, J.-P. Baldacci, P., Richoux-Duranthon, V., Pournin, S. & Babinet, C. (1994). A maternal factor affecting mouse blastocyst formation. *Development* **120**, 797–802.

Rothstein, J. L., Johnson, D., DeLoia, J. A., Skowronski, J., Solter, D. & Knowles, B. B. (1992). Gene expression during preimplantation mouse development. *Genes Devel.* **6**, 1190–201.

Sasaki, H., Jones, P. A., Chaillet, J. R., Ferguson-Smith, A. C., Barton, S. C., Reik, W. & Surani, M. A. (1992). Parental imprinting: potentially active chromatin of the repressed maternal allele of the mouse insulin-like growth factor II (*Igf2*) gene. *Genes Devel.* **6**, 1843–56.

Solter, D. (1988). Differential imprinting and expression of maternal and paternal genomes. *A. Rev. Genet.* **22**, 127–46.

Stöger, R., Kubicka, P., Liu, C.-G., Kafri, T., Razin, A., Cedar, H. & Barlow, D. (1993). Maternal-specific methylation of the imprinted mouse *Igf2r* locus identifies the expressed locus as carrying the imprinting signal. *Cell* **73**, 61–71.

Surani, M. A. H., Barton, S. C. & Norris, M. L. (1986). Nuclear transplantation in the mouse: heritable differences between parental genomes after activation of the embryonic genome. *Cell* **45**, 127–36.

Telford, N., Watson, A. & Schultz, G. (1990). Transition from maternal to embryonic control in early mammalian development: a comparison of several species. *Molec. Reproduc. Devel.* **26**, 90–100.

Thomson, J. A. & Solter, D. (1988). The developmental fate of androgenetic, parthenogenetic, and gynogenetic cells in chimeric gastrulating mouse embryos. *Genes Devel.* **2**, 1344–51.

Thomson, J. A. & Solter, D. (1989). Chimeras between parthenogenetic or androgenetic blastomeres and normal embryos: Allocation to the inner cell mass and trophectoderm. *Devel. Biol.* **131**, 580–3.

Varmuza, S. & Mann, M. (1994). Genomic imprinting – defusing the ovarian time bomb. *Trends Genet.* **10**, 118–23.

Xu, Y., Goodyer, C. G., Deal, C. & Polychronakis, C. (1993). Functional polymorphism in the parental imprinting of the human *IGF2R* gene. *Biochem. biophys. Res. Commun.* **197**, 747–54.

2

The evolution of parental imprinting: a review of hypotheses

DAVID HAIG AND ROBERT TRIVERS

Introduction

Parental imprinting has been suggested to be an adaptation for preventing parthenogenetic development (Solter, 1988), an expression of genetic conflicts between maternal and paternal genomes (Haig & Westoby, 1989), an outcome of dominance modification (Sapienza, 1989), a means to restrain the growth of the placenta (Hall, 1990), a mechanism of growth factor regulation (Cattanach, 1991), a consequence of host defense mechanisms (Barlow, 1993), and a device to protect females against malignant germ-cell tumors (Varmuza & Mann, 1994). Are these different hypotheses alternative answers to the same question? If so, does the evidence allow us to choose among them?

The purpose of this paper is to review ideas about the adaptive function (or lack of function) of imprinting. We are not impartial commentators and will defend the genetic-conflict hypothesis against other functional hypotheses. Our discussion will often make a distinction between functions of a DNA sequence and side-effects of the sequence. An *effect* of a sequence is a *function* if it has positively contributed to the spread and present frequency of the sequence. All other effects of the sequence are *side-effects*. The italicized terms are defined with greater precision in the Appendix.

The genetic-conflict hypothesis

Genes that are expressed in an individual's soma do not leave direct descendants but are selected to promote the transmission of copies of themselves via the individual's germline. By extension, a gene in the soma of one individual can be selected to promote the transmission of copies of itself in the germlines of other individuals. Hamilton (1964) showed that a gene from one individual will value the reproduction of another individual in proportion to the probability that this

17

individual carries a copy of the gene by direct descent from a common ancestor. The maternal and paternal genes of the first individual may have different probabilities of being present in the second individual. These different values become a source of conflict when the expression of genes in the first individual benefits the first individual at cost to the second, or the second at cost to the first. In such cases, maternal and paternal alleles can be selected to have different patterns of expression (Haig, 1992a).

One situation in which maternal and paternal alleles come into conflict arises from the interaction between mothers and their offspring. Increased maternal investment in one offspring results, on average, in fewer resources available for other offspring of the same mother (including potential future offspring). Therefore, genes that are expressed in offspring will have been selected to make lesser nutritional demands on mothers when the genes are maternally derived than when the genes are paternally derived. This is because the paternal genes of an offspring will value the mother's other offspring less highly than do the maternal genes of the same offspring, whenever there is some possibility that the mother produces offspring by more than one father (Haig, 1992b, 1993a; Haig & Graham, 1991; Haig & Westoby, 1989, 1991).

Other situations can be imagined in which interactions occur between individuals that differ in their degree of relatedness through the maternal and paternal line. For example, many mammals form matrilineal associations in which daughters breed near their mothers while breeding males are outsiders that temporarily enter the group. Altruistic behaviors that benefit kin (e.g. warning cries, support in fights) would be more strongly favored by maternal genes than by paternal genes. Similarly, neighboring plants may be more closely related through the maternal line than the paternal line if pollen has a greater dispersal distance than seeds. The maximum difference between maternal and paternal relatedness is progressively diminished for relatives at greater and greater remove, and the opportunities for conflict within the genome are similarly reduced.

When there is conflict within the genome, the concept of an adaptation of the organism is ill-defined because a given phenotype can favor the transmission of some of the organism's genes but not others. Thus, an aspect of phenotype that is an effect of more than one gene can be a function of one but a side-effect of another. Sapienza (1989) has emphasized the distinction between imprinted genes and imprinting genes. The parent-specific expression of an imprinted gene is an effect of imprinting genes (if these exist) but is also an effect of the gene that is imprinted if there are sequence elements of the imprinted gene (e.g. an 'imprinting box') that make it susceptible to the action of imprinting genes. This is because one can imagine variant alleles at the imprinted locus that are not subject to modification by the imprinting genes. The genetic-conflict hypothesis proposes that imprinting is a *function* of imprinted genes, but is neutral about whether or not imprinting is a function, rather than a side-effect, of imprinting genes.

The hypothesis has little to say about the mechanisms of imprinting. Rather, it predicts that certain kinds of genes will be imprinted (and not others) in certain kinds of organisms (and not others). These predictions are independent of the precise mechanism of imprinting. If there is only one conceivable way in which imprinting can be achieved, all imprinted genes should be imprinted in the same manner, but, if there are many possible mechanisms of imprinting, the particular mechanism adopted may be idiosyncratic for each imprinted gene.

Taxonomic distribution

The genetic-conflict hypothesis predicts that imprinting will have an important role during embryonic development in viviparous taxa, but will be less important in oviparous taxa. Consistent with these predictions, imprinting has significant effects on development in flowering plants and mammals, but is thought to be less important (or absent) in most non-mammalian vertebrates (Haig & Westoby, 1989). Major developmental effects of imprinting appear to be absent in two well-studied oviparous organisms. In *Caenorhabditis elegans*, maternal and paternal uniparental disomy of each chromosome pair is compatible with normal development (Haack & Hodgkin, 1991); similar data exist for *Drosophila melanogaster* (Lindsley & Grell, 1969). Thus, the taxonomic distribution of parental imprinting provides qualified support for the genetic-conflict hypothesis.

Coccoid scale insects and sciarid flies are an exception to the generalization that imprinting is absent from oviparous taxa. In these insects, paternal chromosomes are eliminated during spermatogenesis so that every sperm carries maternal chromosomes. This is a conflict in which maternal chromosomes are clearly the winners and paternal chromosomes the losers. As one would expect, the elimination of paternal chromosomes is controlled by the maternal genome (Haig, 1993b,c). Parental imprinting has also been predicted to occur in the workers of social insects (Haig, 1992a).

IGF-II and the IGF type 2 receptor

The reciprocal imprinting of *Igf2* and *Igf2r* in the mouse provides strong support for the genetic-conflict hypothesis, because the hypothesis predicts that imprinting will primarily affect genes that influence the cost of an offspring to its mother and that the effects of paternally expressed genes at these loci will increase the cost of an offspring whereas the effects of maternally expressed genes will decrease the cost.

Mice that inherit a disrupted paternal copy of *Igf2* are born small, and remain small into adult life. By contrast, mice that inherit a disrupted maternal copy are normal-sized. The difference in phenotype is explained by the observation that the maternal allele is not transcribed in most tissues that express IGF-II (DeChiara *et al.*, 1990, 1991). The genetic-conflict hypothesis proposes that inactivation of the maternal copy of *Igf2* was initially favored because this enabled mothers to produce larger numbers of offspring over the course of their reproductive lives. Subsequent selection would then have favored higher levels of expression by paternal alleles.

IGF-II binds to two receptors in mammals. The type 1 receptor is responsible for most of the growth-promoting effects of IGF-II. The type 2 receptor, encoded by *Igf2r*, has binding sites for mannose 6-phosphate residues in addition to its binding site for IGF-II (Humbel, 1990). The ancestral role of this molecule appears to be that of a mannose 6-phosphate receptor because the IGF-II binding site is absent from the homologous molecule in chickens and toads (Clairmont & Czech, 1989). The principal function of mannose 6-phosphate receptors is to transport molecules into lysosomes (Kornfeld, 1992).

Igf2r is exclusively expressed from the maternal allele in mice (Barlow *et al.*, 1991). Haig & Graham (1991) proposed that the maternally produced type 2 receptor functions as a 'sink' to internalize and degrade paternally produced IGF-II in lysosomes before the growth factor can bind to its type 1 receptor. At the time of this proposal, some experimental evidence suggested that the type 2 receptor had a role in the degradation of IGF-II (e.g. Oka *et al.*, 1985; Sessions *et al.*, 1987; Nolan *et al.*, 1990). This evidence has been strengthened by subsequent studies (Filson *et al.*, 1993).

Imprinting of IGF-II probably preceded the acquisition of an IGF-binding site by the mannose 6-phosphate receptor because unimprinted genes at different loci expressed in an embryo do not 'disagree' about embryonic growth rates, whereas genes at imprinted loci may disagree with genes at unimprinted loci. In this scenario, the IGF-binding site was favored because it reduced the growth-promoting effects of paternally produced IGF-II. Natural selection would then favor alleles at the receptor locus that were inactive when paternally derived. The mannose 6-phosphate receptor of opossums binds IGF-II (Dahms *et al.*, 1993). If our reasoning is correct, this implies that imprinting of IGF-II evolved before the divergence of marsupials from eutherian mammals.

Future tests

Igf2 and *Igf2r* are probably the best understood imprinted genes. We do not yet know whether the effects of other imprinted loci will conform to the predictions of the genetic-conflict hypothesis. Cattanach *et al.* (1992) identified proximal chromosome 7 and distal chromosome 17 of mice as imprinted regions that provided apparent counterexamples to the hypothesis because a paternal duplication of these regions, with an associated maternal deficiency, is associated with poor postnatal growth. The effects of a paternal chromosome in the absence of a maternal homolog may not accurately reflect the effects of the paternal chromosome in a normal mouse. However, this argument cuts both ways and applies with equal force to imprinted regions that apparently conform to predictions. Final judgment must await further information (such as is available for *Igf2* and *Igf2r*) about the effects of the imprinted genes in these regions.

Other hypotheses

Prevention of parthenogenesis

Mouse embryos without a paternal genome do not complete development. Parental imprinting thus eliminates the possibility of parthenogenetic reproduction (Solter, 1988). If this effect is to be a function rather than a side-effect of imprinting, one must argue that the genes responsible for imprinting have been preferentially replicated *because* they prevent parthenogenesis. It is difficult to see how this could be true. A maternally imprinted gene in a parthenogenetic embryo causes the death of the embryo and thus eliminates itself. Imprinting seemingly could not evolve in the face of a gene causing females to reproduce entirely asexually.

Proponents of this hypothesis must therefore argue that the death of parthenogenetic embryos enhances the fitness of surviving sexual embryos with the imprinted allele. If a female is partly asexual, so presumably are her parthenogenetically produced daughters (and at least some of her sexually produced daughters). Parthenogenesis in one generation then does not preclude sexual reproduction in subsequent generations, and vice versa. The advantages that flow from the death of parthenogenetic embryos become harder and harder to find. These difficulties appear insurmountable when one asks how an imprinted allele could first become established in a population of unimprinted alleles. The imprinted allele would initially be present in heterozygous mothers, and whatever benefits accrued from the death of its parthenogenetic carriers would presumably be shared with the 50% of embryos that inherited the unimprinted allele from their mother. The benefits would need to be implausibly large for imprinting to be favored by natural selection.

Other considerations also argue against parental imprinting being an adaptation to ensure sexual reproduction. All that is needed to prevent parthenogenesis is a single locus at which expression of a paternal allele is essential. The mouse genome contains several imprinted regions, all except one of which would be redundant for this function. Furthermore, the proposed function fails to explain the imprinting of genes, such as *Igf2r*, that are required maternally but not paternally. Finally, imprinting occurs in the endosperm of flowering plants but has not prevented parthenogenetic development because the embryo and endosperm are products of separate fertilizations (Haig & Westoby, 1991).

Placentation

The placenta is the structure through which an embryo obtains nutrients from its mother. The genetic-conflict hypothesis therefore predicts that imprinting will play an important role in placental development. For species with invasive placentation, maternally expressed genes are predicted to restrain – and paternally expressed genes to enhance – the invasive potential of trophoblast (Haig, 1993a). Hall (1990) and Varmuza & Mann (1994) have proposed that an important function of imprinting is to restrain the growth of placental cells. Either hypothesis would be preferable to the genetic-conflict hypothesis if it could explain the same data more simply.

Hall (1990) suggested that imprinting might be a consequence of the evolution of placentation because mammalian mothers have to tolerate the implantation of a foreign conceptus while restraining its growth. She proposed that these conflicting requirements might favor the differential functioning of the maternal and paternal genomes of the embryo and placenta. Presumably, the problem of immunological tolerance could be solved by suppressing the expression of paternal antigens (but see Kanbour-Shakir *et al.*, 1993). However, unlike the genetic-conflict hypothesis, Hall's suggestion does not specify the reasons why placental growth should be subject to imprinting, nor the direction in which placental growth factors should be imprinted.

Varmuza & Mann (1994) proposed that 'imprinting is a device that protects female mammals from the potential ravages of ovarian trophoblast disease'. In this hypothesis, the genes necessary for the development of trophoblast are inactivated in oocytes because this prevents ovarian tumors from producing invasive trophoblast. The capacity to produce trophoblast is retained by the male germline rather than the female germline because germ-cell tumors are much less frequent in males. The death of females from malignant trophoblastic disease is thus seen as the principal selective force in the origin and maintenance of imprinting. The hypothesis does not explain why genes, such as *Igf2r*, should be inactivated paternally. Varmuza & Mann suggest that paternally inactive genes may be 'innocent bystanders' caught up in the imprinting process.

This hypothesis applies at most to those mammals with invasive placentation (including mice and humans), leaving parallel phenonema in plants unexplained. Even within mammals it posits that several paternally and maternally imprinted genes have evolved in order to prevent something that requires only a single, maternally inactive gene operating in the trophoblast alone. Many species of mammals have non-invasive placentas (Mossman, 1987); we expect that imprinting will be found in these mammals as well as mice and humans (*contra* Varmuza & Mann).

Dominance modification

Sapienza (1989) proposed that imprinting was a consequence of a process of dominance modification. He believed that imprinting, by itself, would be selected against because functional hemizygosity at imprinted loci exposes loss-of-function mutants to selection. Therefore, the reason why imprinting alleles 'are maintained and appear to be prevalent in some populations must be due to functions which are independent of the effects they exert on other loci'. In other words, Sapienza believed imprinting to be a *deleterious side-effect* of some more important function of the imprinting locus. He was unclear about what this essential function might be, but suggested it could have something to do with the process of sexual reproduction, such that mutants in which the imprinting gene had been rendered non-functional would be sterile.

In Sapienza's hypothesis, imprinting is an effect of the imprinting locus (by definition). Is imprinting also an effect of the imprinted locus? As we have argued above, the answer is *Yes* if there arc sequence elements of the imprinted locus that make it susceptible to the action of the imprinting locus. In this case, his hypothesis does not explain why unimprinted alleles have not arisen by mutation and spread to fixation. The answer is *No* if the imprinted locus would remain imprinted regardless of what changes were made to its sequence. In this case, his hypothesis denies the occurrence of mutations at the imprinting locus that would uncouple its essential function from its unwanted side-effects.

Host defense

Barlow (1993) suggested that 'imprinting may have evolved in mammalian oocytes as an extension of the host defense role of DNA methylation'. She proposed that the original function of imprinting loci (methyltransferases) was to inactivate foreign DNA. In her model, some host genes became subject to modification by methyltransferases because these genes had acquired sequence elements ('imprinting boxes') that resembled foreign DNA. Parent-specific expression of the newly imprinted genes was a consequence of methylation occurring predominantly in the maternal germline.

Barlow's hypothesis addresses the mechanisms of imprinting and the evolutionary history of these mechanisms, but does not address whether imprinting is a function or a side-effect of the imprinted genes. That is, her model is not concerned with the selective (or non-selective) processes by which imprinted alleles became established and are maintained in a population. Whereas the genetic-conflict hypothesis makes claims about the function of imprinting but is silent about the mechanisms, the host-defense hypothesis is silent about functions but makes claims about mechanisms. The two hypotheses address different questions and the truth of one would not negate the other.

Gene regulation

A number of authors have proposed that the function of imprinting is to regulate gene expression and embryonic development. These proposals explain nothing unless reasons are given why some genes are imprinted but not others, why most organisms regulate development without imprinting, why imprinted genes are not regulated by some other mechanism, and so on. As Varmuza & Mann (1994) have noted, 'much more sensitive and sophisticated regulatory mechanisms have evolved that can adjust levels of gene expression by orders of magnitude, and other vertebrates seem to manage quite nicely without imprinting'.

Overview

Imprinted loci have major effects on early growth. Moreover, imprinted alleles inherited from one sex are transcriptionally inactive and are therefore exposed to negative selection when the transcriptionally active allele is a deleterious mutation. Such fitness effects argue strongly against the idea that imprinting does not require a selective explanation because genes could become imprinted as a mere side-effect of some other process. A clear distinction should be made here between the reasons for the persistence of imprinted genes and the reasons for the persistence of imprinting genes. If imprinting genes have regulatory effects on large parts of the genome, their effects on imprinted genes may indeed be a side-effect of more important functions. However, a functional explanation is still required for why genes at imprinted loci remain susceptible to imprinting. In a sense, imprinted alleles could be considered to exploit imprinting loci for their own purposes.

The genetic-conflict hypothesis proposes that imprinting evolves because of conflicts of interest between the maternal and paternal genes of an individual.

One such conflict arises when an individual's actions have opposite fitness implications for itself and for a maternal half-sib. The individual's maternal genes have a 50% chance of being present in the half-sib. Therefore, maternal genes will be selected to forgo a benefit for their own individual if this benefit is associated with a cost that is more than twice as great for the half-sib. On the other hand, the individual's paternal genes are absent from the half-sib, and will be selected to take the benefit no matter what the cost to the half-sib. During mammalian pregnancy, this conflict is mediated through demands on the mother because resources committed to one offspring become unavailable to the offspring's half-sibs. The potential for conflict is muted, but still present, if the mother's offspring include a proportion of full-sibs.

The hypothesis is compatible with multiple loci being imprinted and with some imprinted genes being maternally inactive and others paternally inactive. The expression of maternally inactive genes is predicted to increase the demands on a mother, whereas the expression of paternally inactive genes is predicted to reduce these demands. By contrast, hypotheses that imprinting has evolved to prevent parthenogenesis or to prevent the development of trophoblast in ovarian carcinomas require no more than a single maternally inactive gene. The argument that parental imprinting has evolved as a mechanism of gene regulation merely redescribes the phenomena to be explained.

The genetic-conflict hypothesis does not address the mechanisms of parental imprinting and its predictions are largely independent of the nature of these mechanisms. This independence of mechanism may be considered either a strength or a weakness of the hypothesis, depending on the question of interest. Clearly, hypotheses about the function of imprinting are not in competition with hypotheses about the mechanisms. Both kinds of hypotheses are necessary for a satisfactory understanding of imprinting.

References

Barlow, D. P. (1993). Methylation and imprinting: from host defense to gene regulation? *Science* **260**, 309–10.

Barlow, D. P., Stöger, R., Herrmann, B. G., Saito, K. & Schweifer, N. (1991). The mouse insulin-like growth factor type-2 receptor is imprinted and closely linked to the *Tme* locus. *Nature* **349**, 84–7.

Cattanach, B. M. (1991). Chromosome imprinting and its significance for mammalian development. In *Genome Analysis*, vol. 2: *Gene Expression and its Control*, ed. K. E. Davies & S. M. Tilghman, pp. 41–71. New York: Cold Spring Harbor Laboratory Press.

Cattanach, B. M., Barr, J. A., Evans, E. P., Burtenshaw, M., Beechey, C. V., Leff, S. E., Brannan, C. I., Copeland, N. G., Jenkins, N. A. & Jones, J. (1992). A candidate mouse model for Prader–Willi syndrome which shows an absence of *Snrpn* expression. *Nature Genet.* **2**, 270–4.

Clairmont, K. B. & Czech, M. P. (1989). Chicken and *Xenopus* mannose 6-phosphate receptors fail to bind insulin-like growth factor II. *J. biol. Chem.* **264**, 16390–2.

Dahms, N. M., Brzycki-Wessell, M. A., Ramanujam, K. S. & Seetharam, B. (1993). Characterization of the mannose 6-phosphate receptors (MPRs) from opossum liver: opossum cation-independent MPR binds insulin-like growth factor-II. *Endocrinology* **133**, 440–6.

DeChiara, T. M., Efstratiadis, A. & Robertson, E. J. (1990). A growth-deficiency phenotype in heterozygous mice carrying an insulin-like growth factor II gene disrupted by targeting. *Nature* **345**, 78–80.

DeChiara, T. M., Robertson, E. J. & Efstratiadis, A. (1991). Parental imprinting of the mouse insulin-like growth factor II gene. *Cell* **64**, 849–59.

Filson, A. J., Louvi, A., Efstratiadis, A. & Robertson, E. J. (1993). Rescue of the T-associated maternal effect in mice carrying null mutations in *Igf-2* and *Igf2r*, two reciprocally imprinted genes. *Development* **118**, 731–6.

Haack, H. & Hodgkin, J. (1991). Tests for parental imprinting in the nematode *Caenorhabditis elegans*. *Molec. gen. Genet.* **228**, 482–5.

Haig, D. (1992a). Intragenomic conflict and the evolution of eusociality. *J. theor. Biol.* **156**, 401–3.

Haig, D. (1992b). Genomic imprinting and the theory of parent–offspring conflict. *Semin. devel. Biol.* **3**, 153–60.

Haig, D. (1993a). Genetic conflicts in human pregnancy. *Q. Rev. Biol.* **68**, 495–532.

Haig, D. (1993b). The evolution of unusual chromosomal systems in sciarid flies: intragenomic conflict and the sex ratio. *J. evol. Biol.* **6**, 249–61.

Haig, D. (1993c). The evolution of unusual chromosomal systems in coccoids: extraordinary sex ratios revisited. *J. evol. Biol.* **6**, 69–77.

Haig, D. & Graham, C. (1991). Genomic imprinting and the strange case of the insulin-like growth factor-II receptor. *Cell* **64**, 1045–6.

Haig, D. & Westoby, M. (1989). Parent-specific gene expression and the triploid endosperm. *Am. Nat.* **134**, 147–55.

Haig, D. & Westoby, M. (1991). Genomic imprinting in endosperm: its effects on seed development in crosses between species and between different ploidies of the same species, and its implications for the evolution of apomixis. *Phil. Trans. R. Soc. Lond.* B **333**, 1–13.

Hall, J. G. (1990). Genomic imprinting: review and relevance to human diseases. *Am. J. hum. Genet.* **46**, 857–73.

Hamilton, W. D. (1964). The genetical evolution of social behaviour. *J. theor. Biol.* **7**, 1–52.

Humbel, R. E. (1990). Insulin-like growth factors I and II. *Eur. J. Biochem.* **190**, 445–62.

Kanbour-Shakir, A., Kunz, H. W. & Gill, T. J. (1993). Differential genomic imprinting of major histocompatibility complex class I antigens in the placenta of the rat. *Biol. Reproduc.* **48**, 977–86.

Kornfeld, S. (1992). Structure and function of the mannose 6-phosphate/insulinlike growth factor II receptors. *A. Rev. Biochem.* **61**, 307–30.

Lindsley, D. L. & Grell, E. H. (1969). Spermiogenesis without chromosomes in *Drosophila melanogaster*. *Genetics* (Suppl.) **61**, 69–78.

Moore, T. & Haig, D. (1991). Genomic imprinting in mammalian development: a parental tug-of-war. *Trends Genet.* **7**, 45–9.

Mossman, H. W. (1987). *Vertebrate Fetal Membranes*. New Brunswick: Rutgers University
   Press.
Nolan, C. M., Kyle, J. W., Watanabe, H. & Sly, W. S. (1990). Binding of insulin-like
   growth factor II (IGF-II) by human cation-independent mannose 6-phosphate
   receptor/IGF-II receptor expressed in receptor-deficient mouse L cells. *Cell Regulation*
   1, 197–213.
Oka, Y., Rozek, L. M. & Czech, M. P. (1985). Direct demonstration of rapid insulin-like
   growth factor II receptor internalization and recycling in rat adipocytes. *J. Biol.
   Chem.* **260**, 9435–42.
Sapienza, C. (1989). Genome imprinting and dominance modification. *Ann. N.Y. Acad.
   Sci.* **564**, 24–38.
Sessions, C. M., Emler, C. A. & Schalch, D. S. (1987). Interaction of insulin-like growth
   factor II with rat chondrocytes: receptor binding, internalization, and degradation.
   Endocrinology **120**, 2108–16.
Solter, D. (1988). Differential imprinting and expression of maternal and paternal
   genomes. *A. Rev. Genet.* **22**, 127–46.
Varmuza, S. & Mann, M. (1994). Genomic imprinting – defusing the ovarian time bomb.
   Trends Genet. **10**, 118–23.

Appendix: functions and side-effects

A DNA sequence may have phenotypic effects, which influence the probability that the
sequence itself will be replicated. Sequences that promote their own replication will be
perpetuated, whereas sequences that are less effective replicators will be eliminated. The
effects of a sequence may thus be included among the *causal* factors that account for the
presence of the sequence in a gene pool. It is this causal feedback between genotype and
phenotype – when combined with a source of genetic novelty (mutation) – that explains how a
purposeless process (natural selection) can produce purposeful structures and functions
(adaptation). The functions of a sequence consist of those of its effects that have contributed,
however indirectly, to the sequence's own transmission from past generations. In so far as the
future repeats the past, such functions will contribute to the sequence's transmission to future
generations.

   All effects of a sequence make up its phenotype, but only those effects that promote the
sequence's replication make up its function. Thus, the phenotypic effects of a sequence can be
classified as either *functions* (effects that are beneficial for the sequence) or *side-effects* (effects
that are neutral or harmful for the sequence). For an effect to qualify as a function, variant
sequences must have been eliminated in the past because they lacked the function. If an effect
is to remain a function, such variant sequences must continue to be eliminated whenever they
arise. Thus, a function is both a cause and an effect of the sequence.

   An effect of a sequence has not yet been defined. An *effect* is simply a difference from what
would be observed in the absence of the sequence or in the presence of a variant sequence,
other things being equal. Thus, the effects of a sequence (and likewise its functions) depend on
the implicit or explicit alternatives with which the sequence is compared. These alternatives
can be narrowly or broadly defined. For example, one could argue that the maternal copy of
the *Igf2* locus is inactive in mice *because* this prevents overproduction of IGF-II. The implicit
comparison is to an unimprinted allele that causes no reduction in paternal expression but

increases maternal expression to the same level. A broader definition of the alternatives would compare the imprinted allele to unimprinted alleles with a range of expression levels. This comparison focuses attention on the question why expression levels are regulated by imprinting rather than by some other mechanism.

3

Genetic variations in parental imprinting on mouse chromosome 17

JIŘÍ FOREJT, SOŇA GREGOROVÁ, MARTA LANDÍKOVÁ, JANA
ČAPKOVÁ AND LEE M. SILVER

Introduction

Parental imprinting can be defined as an allele-specific epigenetic modification, dependent on the parental origin of the allele (Solter, 1988; Sapienza, 1989; Cattanach & Beechey, 1990; Bartolomei & Tilghman, 1992; Barlow, 1993; Efstratiadis, 1994; Varmusa & Mann, 1994). The nature of the epigenetic mark is not fully established, but the modification must be reversible and the primary mark must occur during gametogenesis. Methylation of cytosine residues in CpG dinucleotides has been proposed as a potential primary mark, or at least as a part of mechanism maintaining the imprint (Bartolomei *et al.*, 1993; Brandeis *et al.*, 1993; Stöger *et al.*, 1993) since mice homozygous for a loss-of-function mutation in the gene for DNA methyltransferase (Li *et al.*, 1993) show alterations of imprinting of several genes.

In mammals, some imprinted genes cause the functional inequality of the paternal and maternal contribution to the zygotic genome and are thus responsible for the failure of parthenogenesis. Imprinting at the transcriptional level has been observed in eight mouse and/or human genes. *Insulin-like growth factor 2 (Igf2)* (DeChiara *et al.*, 1991), *Insulin 2* (Giddings *et al.*, 1994) and *Snrpn*, a candidate gene for Prader–Willi syndrome in humans (Leff *et al.*, 1992), all map to mouse chromosome 7 (Chr 7) and are paternally expressed; IGF-II receptor (*Igf2r*) on mouse Chr 17 (Barlow *et al.*, 1991) and the *H19* on mouse Chr 7 (Bartolomei *et al.*, 1991) are maternally expressed. The *Xist* gene, an unusual gene expressed from the inactive Chr X (Kay *et al.*, 1993) is paternally active in extraembryonic mouse tissues. The *Sp2* gene (also termed *U2afbp-rs* (Hayashizaki *et al.*, 1994)) is paternally expressed on Chr 11 (Hatada *et al.*, 1993). All imprinted genes thoroughly tested displayed: (1) monoallelic expression, with the suppressed allele practically completely inactivated; (2) inactivation of the suppressed allele at the transcriptional level; (3) specific DNA methylation of either the inactive or the active allele (for review see Reik & Allen, 1994); (4) asynchronous timing of the DNA replication of the inactive and expressed alleles (Kitsberg *et al.*, 1993).

It can be argued that the present choice of imprinted genes may have been biased by the methods used for their selection. Indeed, it can be expected that genes that would show a quantitative rather than a qualitative difference in expression of their paternal and maternal alleles would probably pass unnoticed in screens based on the detection of monoallelic expression. However, analysis of such genes could be of the utmost importance for our understanding of such genetic phenomena as incomplete penetrance and dominance modification (Sapienza, 1989).

Experiments with *Igf2* and *H19* transgenes indicated that mouse development may not tolerate variations in the gene dosage of the imprinted genes. However, recent results show that at least two human genes, *IGF2R* (Xu *et al.*, 1993) and *WT1* (Jinno *et al.*, 1994), show a polymorphism of imprinting, i.e. biallelic and monoallelic expression of the same gene in different individuals. Such polymorphic variants could enable a genetic approach to seek the *cis*-DNA elements and *trans*-acting genes engaged in the imprinting machinery. The mouse Chr 17 harbors the maternally expressed *Igf2r* gene, a candidate for the *T-associated maternal effect (Tme)* locus (Barlow *et al.*, 1991). It also carries the *Fused* mutation, which shows the phenotype variations expected for an imprinted gene (Ruvinsky & Agulnik, 1990; S. Gregorová & J. Forejt, unpublished results); however, the gene has not yet been cloned. In this study we focus on genetic analysis of three loci on the mouse Chr 17 that could reflect a variation of parental imprinting: the variation of lethality of the maternal *Tme* deletion, the parental effects on the *Brachyury* gene expression, and parental effects on the spermatogenic arrest caused by translocation between Chr 16 and 17, T(16;17)43H.

The *T-associated maternal effect* locus

Two overlapping deletions on mouse Chr 17, *T^hp* and *t^{lub2}* (Fig. 3.1) are lethal when inherited from the female, but viable when of paternal origin (Johnson, 1974; Winking & Silver, 1984). The lethality is caused by the functional nullisomy of the *T-associated maternal effect (Tme)* locus, which is paternally imprinted and resides in the region of overlap of these two deletions. By using the candidate gene approach to clone the *Tme* gene, Barlow and her colleagues (Barlow *et al.*, 1991) asked whether any of the known genes in the 800 kb region was expressed only from the maternal allele. The *Plg, Sod2* and *Tcp1* genes were transcribed from both alleles, but *Insulin-like growth factor type 2 receptor (Igf2r)* was expressed only from the maternal allele. Thus *Igf2r* became the best

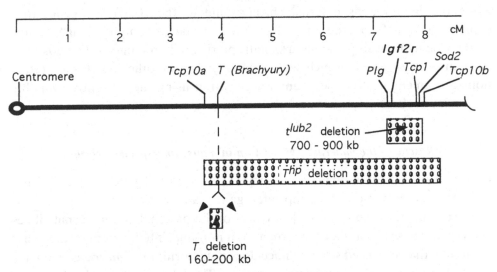

Fig. 3.1. *Thp*, *tlub2*, and *T*-associated deletions on the genetic maps of the mouse Chr 17. The *Tcp10a–Tcp10b* region contains 42 loci on the consensus map of Chr 17 (Himmelbauer *et al.*, 1993); therefore only loci relevant to this study are shown.

candidate gene for the *Tme* locus. Imprinting of the *Igf2r* gene is apparently not evolutionarily conserved: its expression in human embryonic tissues was observed in most cases from both alleles (Kalscheuer *et al.*, 1993; Ogawa *et al.*, 1993) and only in some individuals was the gene imprinted and expressed exclusively from the maternal allele (Xu *et al.*, 1993). If confirmed, this observation may have substantial theoretical consequences as it represents the first evidence for an imprinting polymorphism.

Rescue of the maternal t[lub2] deletion in t[lub2]/Tt[Orl] hybrids

The first successful rescue of the maternal *Tme* deletion was observed in the progeny of the genetic cross *Tt[Orl]/t[lub2]* × *Tt[Orl]/t[ae5]* (Tsai & Silver, 1991). The idea behind this experiment was that by supplying the *t[lub2]* maternal embryo with two doses of the paternal *Tme* (present in both *Tt[Orl]* and *t[ae5]* haplotypes) the dosage effect of the two copies, probably with low basal expression, would overcome the lethality of the maternal *Tme* deletion. The results were striking, as apparently all offspring with maternal *t[lub2]* deletion survived to birth and 16/26 were viable and often fertile. All 16 survivors had short, kinky tails and some of the females revealed abnormalities of the urogenital tract. Those *t[lub2]* heterozygotes who died soon after birth had normal tails. It was speculated that the imprinting machinery could slide in a transvection-like mode from the maternal *Tme* gene along the homologous paternal chromosome to the *Brachyury* gene, thus explaining both effects, the survival and the short tail phenotype (Tsai & Silver, 1991). The hypothesis presumes a somatic pairing of homologous chromosomes early in embryogenesis, which seems unlikely. On the other hand, the predictions are amenable to experimental verification using the currently available molecular probes.

Rescue of the maternal T^{hp} deletion in mouse interspecies hybrids

Deletions of a chromosomal region carrying an imprinted gene, such as T^{hp} and t^{lub2}, or a null mutation of an imprinted gene, can serve as invaluable tool for distinguishing the transcriptional activities of the paternal and maternal alleles and could be used as a selective screen for a non-imprinted variant of the gene. Assuming that an inbred strain of mice does not imprint the *Tme* locus, then in a cross with female mice heterozygous for the T^{hp} deletion, the males from this strain should produce viable offspring heterozygous for the material T^{hp} deletion. We performed such screening and found that although males from five laboratory inbred strains and male mice of *Mus musculus domesticus* did not change the dominant lethal effect of the maternal T^{hp} deletion, the males from PWB, PWD and PWK inbred strains of the mouse subspecies *Mus m. musculus* rescued 70% of the expected offspring with the maternal T^{hp} deletion. The rescued mice with maternal T^{hp} were bigger at birth and were viable and fertile, with the exception of 65% of the female hybrids, who displayed vaginal atresia and enlarged uteri. The loss of lethality of the maternal *Tme* deletion was by definition interpreted as the loss of the *Tme* imprinting (Forejt & Gregorová, 1992). However, this conclusion was complicated by the fact that *Igf2r*, a candidate gene for the *Tme* locus, was normally imprinted in the same hybrid animals that lost the *Tme* imprint. The most parsimonious interpretation of the data was to assume that *Tme* and *Igf2r* were not identical (Forejt & Gregorová, 1992).

Rescue of the maternal t^{lub2} deletion in mouse interspecies hybrids

Recently, we were able to verify the *Tme* rescue by using the t^{lub2} deletion in a cross: ♀129-t^{lub2}/+ × ♂PWD. Although the parents did not carry any *T* mutation, 14 offspring had short, kinky tails and had larger body mass than the remaining 13 normal-tailed animals. Using primers from the *Brachyury* locus, 9 randomly chosen short-tailed and 9 normal-tailed animals were typed for the presence of the t^{lub2} haplotype. All short-tailed mice were t^{lub2}/+ and all normal tailed mice were +/+. The results indicate that the rescue from the *Tme* lethality caused by the deletion of its maternal allele was complete. Incomplete rescue of the maternal T^{hp} deletion could be due to its large size and to the cumulative effects of other, deleted, non-imprinted genes.

The *Igf2r* gene codes for the type 2 receptor (IGF2R) of insulin-like growth factor II (IGF-II). Binding of IGF-II to the type 2 receptor results in internalization and degradation of the growth factor and is believed to regulate the fine tuning of its effects during development. The absence of the type 2 receptor in embryos with maternal T^{hp} or t^{lub2} deletions could thus result in increased concentrations of IGF-II in the blood. The assumption fits well with the increase in body mass, which was consistently observed in rescued newborn mice with T^{hp} and t^{lub2} maternal deletions (Forejt & Gregorová, 1992; J. Forejt & S. Gregorová, unpublished data).

Modification of the maternal T^{hp} *lethality in mice with paternal null* Igf2 *mutation*

Filson and co-workers (Filson *et al.*, 1993) proposed that the absence of IGF2R could result in a lethal overdose of IGF-II during development, thus explaining the lethality of the maternal *Tme* deletion. To test the hypothesis a genetic cross, C3H-T^{hp}/+ × 129/Sv-*Igf2*−/−, was set up, with the male parent homozygous for an engineered null mutation of the *Igf2* gene (Filson *et al.*, 1993). The idea was that if the overdose of IGF-II causes the lethality of the maternal T^{hp} deletion, then embryos with such a deletion and without a functional *Igf2* gene will have no reason to die. The mice with T^{hp} deletion were indeed born from this cross, but practically all of them died soon after birth and only one out of 114 scored progeny survived to adult age. However, this shift of the death window was significant, thus proving that the *Igf2* gene influences the *Tme* phenotype. The conclusions were, however, further extended to explain the rescue of T^{hp} lethality in the interspecies crosses with *Mus m. musculus* inbred strains, suggesting that in *Mus m. musculus* the IGF-II protein could be present at lower concentrations or have lower mitogenic activity (Filson *et al.*, 1993). Consequently, lowering the overdose of the growth factor would enable the embryo to survive. The main objection against this speculation is that if the lowering of the growth factor overdose were the cause of the T^{hp} rescue then a complete rescue should have been seen in $T^{hp\ maternal}$ mice without the functional *Igf2* gene and only partial rescue should have been observed in PWD hybrids. However, just the opposite was found to be the case (Table 3.1). The argument that the total absence of IGF-II could itself be lethal does not stand either, because homozygotes for the null allele are viable dwarf mice (DeChiara *et al.*, 1991). So it seems obvious that whatever is the mechanism of the rescue of maternal T^{hp} and t^{lub2} deletions, it does not operate by lowering the concentration of IGF-II.

Table 3.1. *Phenotypic features of maternal Tme rescue*

Genotype or cross[a]	Rescue efficacy[b]	Body mass	Tail phenotype	Development anomalies	Reference
t^{tub2}/T^{rprt}	63%	NR[c]	Kinky and/or short	Some animals displayed imperforate vaginas, vaginocolic fistulas, ambiguous external genitalia, testicular teratocarcinomas, extra toe	Tsai & Silver (1991)
(C3H-$T^{hp}/+$ × PWD) $T^{hp}/+$	70%	On average 18% heavier than their wild type littermates	Short (T^{null} effect)	In 65% of females vaginal atresia, enlarged uterus and ambiguous external genitalia. Sporadic omphalocele	Forejt & Gregorová (1992)
(C3H-$T^{hp}/+$ × 129Sv-Igf2−/−) $T^{hp}/+$	1.8%[d]	NR	Short (T^{null} effect)	One surviving male was fertile	Filson et al. (1993)
(129Sv-$t^{tub2}/+$ × PWD) $t^{tub2}/+$	100%	On average 14% heavier than their wild type littermates	Kinky and/or short	As in the cross: (C3H-$T^{hp}/+$ × PWD)$T^{hp}/+$	This chapter

[a] In the crosses, the first parent is always female.
[b] Observed/expected ratio of viable heterozygotes for maternal *Tme* deletion.
[c] NR, not reported.
[d] 49% of expected T^{hp} heterozygotes were born alive but most of them died within 48 h.

Genetic analysis from our laboratory indicates that, indeed, *Igf2* or a closely linked gene could play a major role in the lethal effect of the maternal *T^(hp)* deletion, but not in the rescue effect seen in the (C3H-*T^(hp)* × PWD) hybrids (see below). Admittedly, direct measurements of the concentrations of IGF-II in dying, rescued and wild type embryos still remain to be done; without these results, any conclusions are still tentative.

The phenotypes of rescued mice with deleted maternal Tme

The characteristic phenotypic anomalies observed in rescued viable animals with a deleted maternal *Tme* locus are summarized in Table 3.1. The accelerated growth and sporadic omphalocele seen in these newborn mice could resemble the symptoms of Beckwith–Wiedemann syndrome in humans, which is associated with increased concentrations of IGF-II and even biallelic expression of the *Igf2* gene (Weksberg *et al.*, 1993). This gene is normally expressed only from the paternal allele in humans as well as in mice (DeChiara *et al.*, 1991; Ohlsson *et al.*, 1993; Giannoukakis *et al.*, 1993). The cause of developmental abnormalities of the urogenital tract and tail is unclear. The fertility of the rescued males and of the females without genital malformations is normal.

Genetic analysis of the Tme rescue

Assuming that the *Tme* rescue in (C3H-*T^(hp)*/+ × PWD) is ensured by the PWD allele of a single gene, then in ♀ C3H-*T^(hp)*/+ × ♂ (C3H × PWD) cross the frequency of rescued *T^(hp)*/+ offspring should be half of that found in the former cross, which should represent 17.5% of the total progeny of the cross. This expected frequency did not differ significantly from the observed frequency (13.7%; $N = 328$), so the single gene hypothesis did not need to be rejected (Forejt & Gregorová, 1992). Moreover, if the *Tme* itself was responsible, for example by being insensitive to the imprinting machinery of the other subspecies, then all surviving *T^(hp)*/+ mice should receive from the (C3H × PWD)F₁ male the PWD allele of the *Tme* locus. However, the surviving *T^(hp)*/+ mice displayed randomly both alleles of the closely linked *D17Leh66D* locus (Table 3.2). Thus, control over the *Tme* rescue must be sought in a *trans*-acting gene, which was tentatively named *Imprintor1* (Forejt & Gregorová, 1992). Two possible candidates for a *trans*-acting gene, *M6pr*, a gene for a cation-dependent mannose 6-phosphate receptor on Chr 6, and the *Igf2* gene on Chr 7, were excluded by the analysis of the same cross (Table 3.2).

    In the genetic cross described above, only the viable part of the progeny were available for mapping; therefore, as the next experiment, the *Tme*-rescue

Table 3.2. *Genetic analysis of* Tme *imprinting in the backcross:* ♀ *C3H*-T^{hp}/+ ×
♂ *(C3H × PWD)*

		Number of viable T^{hp}/+ offspring with genotype[b]			
Chr.	Locus[a]	C3H/C3H	C3H/PWD	p	Reference
17	*D17Leh66*	11	6	0.5>*p*>0.2	Forejt & Gregorová (1992)
6	*M6pr*	10	6	0.5>*p*>0.2	Forejt & Gregorová (1992)
7	*Fgf3*	4	10	0.2>*p*>0.05	This chapter

[a] *D17Leh66* was used as a marker for *Igf2r*, located 0.5 cM distally. *M6pr* codes
for cation-dependent mannose 6-phosphate receptor. *Fgf3* (former name *Int2*)
was a marker for the *Igf2–H19* region, located 3 cM proximally.
[b] Only the results of typing of the short-tailed (*T^{hp}*/+) progeny are given here.
Each locus can be either homozygous for the allele of C3H origin, or
heterozygous for alleles from C3H and PWD strains. None of the three tested loci
revealed a non-random segregation of C3H and PWD alleles in surviving T^{hp}/+
offspring.

progeny test of BC1 males [(C3H × PWD) × C3H] was performed with the aim
to scan systematically for the genes involved in *Tme* rescue. Each BC1 male was
mated with several *T^{hp}*/+ females until 30 or more offspring were obtained and
the frequency of viable *T^{hp}*/+ short-tailed mice could be determined. Altogether
98 BC1 males gave enough progeny to be included in the analysis. According to
the single gene model two classes of BC1 males were expected to occur with
equal frequency: the homozygotes for the C3H allele, *Imp1^d/Imp1^d* (*d* stems
from *domesticus*), which should not rescue maternal *Tme* at all, and PWD/C3H
heterozygotes, *Imp1^m/Imp1^d* (*m* refers to *musculus*), which should rescue the
T^{hp}/+ genotype at the frequency observed in crosses of (C3H × PWD)F$_1$ hybrid
males. The results of the tests (Fig. 3.2) do not support the single gene
hypothesis; their analysis, albeit still incomplete, permits the following conclusions. (1) Unlike in previous crosses, where a *T$^{hp\ maternal}$*/+ genotype gave in most
cases either a fully viable phenotype or an embryonic lethal phenotype, the *Tme*-
rescue progeny-test cross frequently displayed a new phenotype, the apparently
normal *T^{hp}*/+ newborns dying within 48 h after birth. Their frequencies are
shown as light columns in Fig. 3.2. No relationship is obvious between frequencies of viable and dying short-tailed offspring. (2) Only 14 out of 98 BC1 males
analyzed did not produce any viable *T^{hp}*/+ offspring, whereas frequencies of

viable $T^{hp}/+$ mice in progenies of the remaining 84 BC1 males varied almost continuously from 2% to 20%. Thus it seems that more than two independently segregating genes control the viability of maternal *Tme* deletion. (3) The available data do not permit an unequivocal explanation of the difference between the results of C3H-$T^{hp}/+$ × PWD cross, indicating a single-gene control, and the *Tme*-rescue progeny test, indicating more than two loci. Nevertheless, the overall frequency of viable $T^{hp}/+$ offspring in the *Tme*-rescue progeny test, 264/4148 or 6.3%, is almost exactly what would be predicted according to the single-gene hypothesis interpretation of the CH3-$T^{hp}/+$ × PWD cross, namely $0.5 \times 13.7\% = 6.8\%$. (4) As a pilot experiment to the systematic mapping of the genes involved, we analyzed the possible role of several 'candidate' genes on Chr 7 by using the polymorphic microsatellite loci *D7MIT80*, *D7MIT83*, *D7MIT17* and *D7Nds4* (Dietrich *et al.*, 1992; W. Dietrich, personal communication). Because the variation in *Tme* rescue was almost continuous, we decided to genotype the BC1 males that reproduced the parental phenotypes, namely no *Tme* rescue as in the C3H parent and the maximum rescue as in the PWD parent. Thus 14 BC1 males that never rescued any maternal T^{hp} deletion (at the left extreme of the sorted graph in Fig. 3.2) were genotyped, together with 18 BC1 males that sired 13% or more of the surviving $T^{hp}/+$ offspring (from the extreme right of the same graph). Any gene that contributes to the lethality should be homozygous for the C3H allele in a statistically significant excess of individuals from the former set of 14 BC1 males, while a gene contributing to the survival of the $T^{hp}/+$ offspring should be heterozygous for the PWD allele in a non-random excess of individuals from the set of the 18 BC1 males. The preliminary results of this type of analysis (Table 3.3) indicate that a gene closely linked to the *D7Nds4* locus, which is approximately 3 cM distal to the *Igf2–H19* region on Chr 7, is associated with lethality of the $T^{hp\ maternal}/+$ genotype. However, the same gene shows a random segregation in the set of BC1 males with high efficiency of the *Tme* rescue, thus indicating that the lethality and a rescue from the lethality of the $T^{hp\ maternal}/+$ mice are controlled by different genetic mechanisms.

Imprintor or imprinted?

Admittedly, until now the genetic analysis of the *Tme* rescue has generated more questions than answers. The answer to the key question concerning the identity of the *Tme* with *Igf2r* will be known soon from the *Igf2r* knockout experiments. Provided that the *Igf2r* null mutation acts as a dominant lethal when transmitted from a female, thus confirming the identity with *Tme*, then what could be the mechanism of the *Tme* rescue in the ($T^{hp}/+$ × PWD) interspecies hybrids? Could

Table 3.3. *Tme rescue progeny test of BC1 males (C3H×PWD)×C3H; analysis of the selected microsatellite markers on chromosome 7*

Locus	BC1 males with no viable $T^{hp}/+$ progeny				BC1 males with most viable $T^{hp}/+$ progeny			
	C3H/C3H	C3H/PWD	χ^2	p	C3H/C3H	C3H/PWD	χ^2	p
D7MIT80	10	4	1.8	$0.2>p>0.05$	8	6	0.2	$0.8>p>0.5$
D7MIT83	10	4	1.8	$0.2>p>0.05$	8	9	0.07	$0.8>p>0.5$
D7MIT17	11	2	4.9	$0.05>p>0.01$	7	11	0.5	$0.5>p>0.2$
D7Nds4	12	2	5.8	$0.05>p>0.01$	7	10	0.5	$0.8>p>0.5$

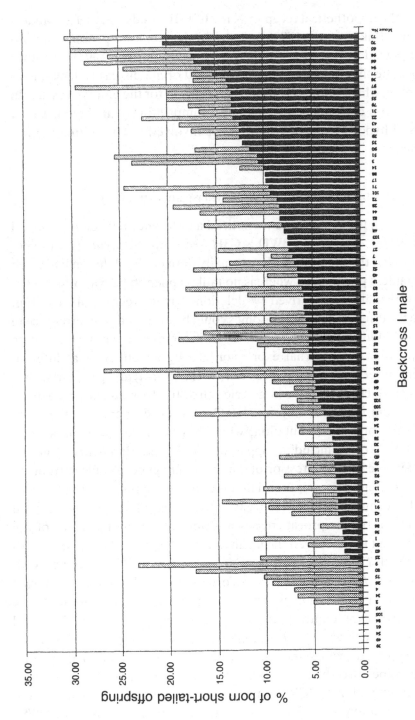

Backcross I male

Fig. 3.2. Genetic analysis of the rescue from maternal *Tme* lethality in the offspring of the crosses: ♀ C3H-*T*^{hp}/+ × ♂ [(C3H × PWD) × C3H]. Each column represents the percentage of viable (dark hatching) and perinatally dying (light hatching) *T*^{hp}/+ offspring of one BC1 male. Altogether 98 BC1 males were analyzed by this progeny test. They are sorted in this graph according to their ability to produce viable *T*^{hp}/+ progeny.

it be a gene for the hypothetical receptor X for IGF-II, predicted by Efstratiadis and co-workers (Baker *et al.*, 1993) and would this gene be genomically imprinted, as suggested by our genetic data (Forejt & Gregorová, 1992)? Another possibility could be that the paternal *Igf2r* of PWD origin displays a leaky, low-level transcription which, however, would be sufficient for the embryo rescue. In this case the gene(s) controlling the leakiness of imprinting could belong to the anticipated, still hypothetical, *Imprintor* genes involved in controlling the imprinting machinery.

Parental modification of *Brachyury* gene expression

In experiments with the *Tme* rescue we noticed a difference between reciprocal crosses, C3H-T^{hp}/+ × PWD and PWD × C3H-T^{hp}/+, in *Brachyury* phenotype. In the former cross, the offspring with paternally derived T^{hp} deletion had often no tail at all (tailless phenotype) whereas no tailless phenotype was observed in the offspring with maternally derived T^{hp} deletion from the reciprocal cross (Fig. 3.3). Because the effect of sex chromosomes could be excluded, the difference in the phenotypes could be explained either by an incomplete genomic imprinting (paternal expression > maternal expression) or by an effect of a different imprinted gene interfering with expression of the *Brachyury* gene or with a function of its product. The T^{hp} is a large deletion of 10 Mb or so, including many genes, one of them being the imprinted *Igf2r*; the experiment was therefore repeated with the original *T* mutation, which has been shown to be a small deletion of 160–200 kb, including apparently only the *Brachyury* gene. A significant difference in the expression of the *Brachyury* gene, as judged from the effect on the tail phenotype, was found in this cross, again pointing to the lower expression of the maternally derived PWD wild type allele (Fig. 3.3). The difference between the reciprocal crosses was not only in the incidence of the tailless progeny, but also between the mean tail length in the *T*/+ offspring with paternally derived *T* mutation (significantly shorter) and *T*/+ offspring with maternally derived *T* (data not shown). To determine whether this paternal effect on *Brachyury* expression is limited to interspecies *Mus musculus* × *M. domesticus* crosses, the intraspecies reciprocal crosses AKR/J × 129-*T* and 129-*T* × AKR/J were analyzed. The difference between these crosses was also significant and pointed again to the lower expression of the maternal allele (Fig. 3.3). To determine directly the steady-state content of *Brachyury* mRNA, RNase protection and RT PCR assays are being prepared to analyze the *Brachyury* transcription in e8.5 to e10.5 embryos from the PWD × 129/Sv reciprocal crosses. Our interest in this model is not only to find what is possibly another imprinted gene: provided that *Brachyury* does indeed show parental

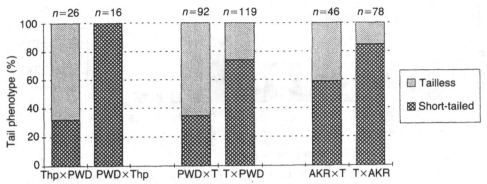

Fig. 3.3. The effect of the parental origin of the *T* or *T^{hp}* deletion on the tail phenotype of the offspring. In all three crosses the paternally derived deletion of the *Brachyury* locus resulted in significantly higher frequencies of tailless offspring than when the same deletion on the same genetic background was transmitted through the female parent.

differences in allelic transcription, then it could represent a model of a new type of parental imprinting with biallelic expression and quantitative, parent-of-origin-dependent regulation of allelic transcription.

Parental modification of spermatogenic arrest caused by a chromosomal translocation

Chromosomal reciprocal translocation T(16;17)43H displays one translocation break tightly linked to the *H-2* complex on Chr 17 and the other break inside the centromeric heterochromatin of Chr 16 (Searle *et al.*, 1974; Forejt *et al.*, 1980). T43H translocation causes male sterility (when heterozygous) by spermatogenic arrest at the pachytene stage of primary spermatocytes; the translocated autosomes are often heteropycnotic and attached to the X chromosome inside a specific compartment termed a sex vesicle. The female heterozygotes are fertile. The cause of spermatogenic arrest is unclear, but it was suggested that an interference with X chromosome inactivation in male pachytene cells could play a role (for review see Forejt, 1985). The T43H translocation was transferred onto the genetic background of C57BL/10SnPh (abbreviated B10) by repeated backcrossing, and made homozygous through fertile B10-T(16;17)43H/Rb(16;17)7Bnr double heterozygous males mated with B10-T43/+ females (Capková & Forejt, 1984). The Robertsonian translocation Rb7Bnr used in this cross was available on the B10 background. The resulting congenic strain B10-T43/T43 is fully viable and fertile in both sexes. It differs from the parental B10 strain only by the presence of chromosonal rearrangement and by closely linked flanks of DNA of undetermined size, not separated from the translocational

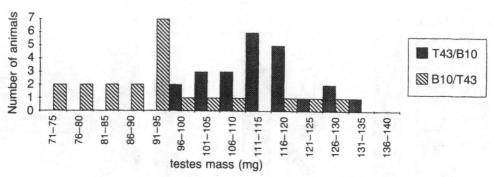

Fig. 3.4. The distribution of the fresh mass of paired testes of the sterile F_1 hybrid males from the following reciprocal crosses: (B10 × B10-T43/T43) and (B10-T43/T43 × B10). The chromosomal rearrangement coming from the male parent induces significantly lower testes mass ($p<0.0001$, Mann-Whitney U test) reflecting an earlier and/or more complete spermatogenic arrest. The effect of genetic background was effectively eliminated in this experiment by using the B10-T43/T43 congenic strain.

breaks by genetic recombination. However, when the B10-T43/T43 strain is outcrossed to any mice not carrying a T43H or Rb/7Bnr translocation, all male progeny are completely sterile. Thus, by definition, this male infertility is an extreme example of chromosomal hybrid sterility: the B10-T43/T43 mice are genetically identical to B10 inbred mice with the exception of the chromosomal rearrangement and the infertility is limited to the male T43/+ heterozygotes, whereas both homozygous forms (T43/T43 and +/+) are normally fertile (J. Capková, S. Gregorová & J. Forejt, unpublished data). For the purpose of this study, the reciprocal F_1 hybrids B10-T43/T43 × B10 and B10 × B10-T43/T43 were prepared and the mass of the testes, as an indicator of spermatogenic arrest, was determined. As shown in Fig. 3.4, the chromosomal translocation was associated with lower testes mass, causing more spermatogenic damage, when it came from the male parent. Because the effects of sex chromosomes or autosomal modifiers are practically excluded, it is most probable that the difference in spermatogenic damage is associated with an epigenetic modification of the rearranged chromosomes during gametogenesis in the homozygote parents. At present we are testing expression and methylation status of several genes linked to the translocation break in an attempt to find a differential mark possibly imposed by this rearrangement on DNA topology of this chromosome region.

The parental effect of a deletion in the region specific for Angelman and Prader–Willi syndromes on human chromosome 15 on DNA methylation of a distant *ZNF127* gene has been clearly demonstrated (Glenn *et al.*, 1993). Thus, the T43H translocation could become a mouse model for such long-ranging effects of chromosomal rearrangements dependent on parental legacy.

Acknowledgements

We thank Karl Pfeifer for critical reading of the manuscript. This work was supported in part by a grant from the NIH (GM 49097) to L. S. and J. F.

References

Baker, J., Liu, J.-P., Robertson, E. J. & Efstratiadis, A. (1993). Role of insulin-like growth factors in embryonic and postnatal growth. *Cell* **75**, 73–82.

Barlow, D. P. (1993). Methylation and imprinting: From host defence to gene regulation? *Science* **260**, 309–10.

Barlow, D. P., Stöger, R., Herrmann, B. G., Saito, K. & Schweifer, N. (1991). The mouse insulin-like growth factor type-2 receptor is imprinted and closely linked to the *Tme* locus. *Nature* **349**, 84–7.

Bartolomei, M. S. & Tilghman, S. M. (1992). Parental imprinting of mouse chromosome 7. *Semin. devel. Biol.* **3**, 107–17.

Bartolomei, M. S., Webber, A. L., Brunkow, M. E. & Tilghman, S. M. (1993). Epigenetic mechanisms underlying the imprinting of the mouse *H19* gene. *Genes Devel.* **7**, 1663–73.

Bartolomei, M. S., Zemel, S. & Tilghman, S. M. (1991). Parental imprinting of the mouse *H19* gene. *Nature* **351**, 153–5.

Brandeis, M., Kafri, T., Ariel, M., Chaillet, J. R., McCarrey, J., Razin, A. & Cedar, H. (1993). The ontogeny of allele-specific methylation associated with imprinted genes in the mouse. *EMBO J.* **12**, 3669–77.

Capková, J. & Forejt, J. (1984). Research news. *Mouse News Lett.* **71**, 43.

Cattanach, B. M. & Beechey, C. V. (1990). Autosomal and X-chromosome imprinting. *Development* (Suppl.), 63–72.

DeChiara, T. M., Robertson, E. J. & Efstratiadis, A. (1991). Parental imprinting of the mouse Insulin-like growth factor II gene. *Cell* **64**, 849–59.

Dietrich, W., Katz, H., Lincoln, S. E., Shin, H.-S., Friedman, J., Dracopoli, N. C. & Lander, E. S. (1992). A genetic map of the mouse suitable for typing intraspecific crosses. *Genetics* **131**, 423–47.

Efstratiadis, A. (1994). Parental imprinting of autosomal mammalian genes. *Curr. Opin. Genet. Devel.* **4**, 265–80.

Filson, A. J., Louvi, A., Efstratiadis, A. & Robertson, E. J. (1993). Rescue of the T-associated maternal effect in mice carrying null mutations in *Igf2* and *Igf2r*, two reciprocally imprinted genes. *Development* **118**, 731–6.

Forejt, J. (1985). Chromosomal and genic sterility of hybrid type in mice and man. *Exp. clin. Immunogenet.* **2**, 106–19.

Forejt, J., Capková, J. & Gregorová, S. (1980). T(16;17)43H translocation as a tool in analysis of the proximal part of chromosome 17 (including *T-t* complex) of the mouse. *Genet. Res., Camb.* **35**, 165–77.

Forejt, J. & Gregorová, S. (1992). Genetic analysis of genomic imprinting: An *Imprintor-1* gene controls inactivation of the paternal copy of the mouse *Tme* locus. *Cell* **70**, 443–50.

Giannoukakis, N., Deal, C., Paquette, J., Goodyer, C. G. & Polychronakos, C. (1993). Parental genomic imprinting of the human *Igf2* gene. *Nature Genet.* **4**, 98–101.

Giddings, S. J., King, C. D., Harman, K. W., Flood, J. F. & Carnaghi, L. R. (1994). Allele specific inactivation of insulin 1 and 2, in the mouse yolk sac, indicates imprinting. *Nature Genet.* **6**, 310–13.

Glenn, C. C., Nicholls, R. D., Robinson, W. P., Saitoh, S., Niikawa, N., Schinzel, A., Horsthemke, B. & Driscoll, D. J. (1993). Modification of 15q11–q13 DNA methylation imprints in unique Angelman and Prader–Willi patients. *Hum. molec. Genet.* **2**, 1377–82.

Hatada, I., Sugama, T. & Mukai, T. (1993). A new imprinted gene cloned by a methylation-sensitive genome scanning method. *Nucleic Acids Res.* **21**, 5577–82.

Hayashizaki, Y., Shibata, H., Hirotsune, S., Sugino, H., Okazaki, Y., Sasaki, N., Hirose, K., Imoto, H., Okuizumi, H., Muramatsu, H., Komatsubara, H., Shiroishi, T., Moriwaki, K., Katsuki, M., Hatano, N., Sasaki, H., Ueda, T., Mise, N., Takagi, N., Plass, C. & Chapman, V. M. (1994). Identification of an imprinted U2af binding protein related sequence on mouse chromosome 11 using the RLGS method. *Nature Genet.* **6**, 33–40.

Himmelbauer, H., Artzt, K., Barlow, D., Fisher-Lindahl, K., Lyon, M., Klein, J. & Silver, L. M. (1993). Mouse chromosome 17. *Mammalian Genome* **4**, S230–52.

Jinno, Y., Yun, K., Nishiwaki, K., Kubota, T., Ogawa, O., Reeve, A. E. & Niikawa, N. (1994). Mosaic and polymorphic imprinting of the *WT1* gene in humans. *Nature Genet.* **6**, 305–9.

Johnson, D. R. (1974). Hairpin-Tail: a case of postreductional gene action in the mouse egg? *Genetics* **76**, 795–805.

Kalscheuer, V. M., Mariman, E. C., Schepens, M. T., Rehder, H. & Ropers, H.-H. (1993). The insulin-like growth factor type-2 receptor gene is imprinted in the mouse but not in humans. *Nature Genet.* **5**, 74–8.

Kay, G. F., Penny, G. D., Patel, D., Ashworth, A., Brockdorff, N. & Rastan, S. (1993). Expression of *Xist* during mouse development suggests a role in the initiation of X chromosome inactivation. *Cell* **72**, 171–82.

Kitsberg, D., Selig, S., Brandeis, M., Simon, I., Keshet, I., Driscoll, D. J., Nicholls, R. D. & Cedar, H. (1993). Allele-specific replication of imprinted gene regions. *Nature* **364**, 459–63.

Leff, S. E., Brannan, C. I., Reed, M. L., Özcelik, T., Francke, U., Copeland, N. G. & Jenkins, N. A. (1992). Maternal imprinting of the mouse *Snrpn* gene and conserved linkage homology with the human Prader–Willi syndrome region. *Nature Genet.* **2**, 259–64.

Li, E., Beard, C. & Jaenisch, R. (1993). Role for DNA methylation in genomic imprinting. *Nature* **366**, 362–5.

Ogawa, O., Eccles, M. R., Szeto, J., McNoe, L. A., Yun, K., Maw, M. A., Smith, P. J. & Reeve, A. E. (1993). Constitutional relaxation of insulin-like growth factor II gene imprinting associated with Wilms' tumor and gigantism. *Nature* **362**, 749–51.

Ohlsson, R., Nystrom, A., Pfeifer-Ohlsson, S., Tohonen, V., Hedborg, F., Schofield, P., Flam, F. & Ekstrom, T. J. (1993). *IGF2* is parentally imprinted during human embryogenesis and in the Beckwith–Wiedemann syndrome. *Nature Genet.* **4**, 94–7.

Reik, W. & Allen, N. D. (1994). Imprinting with and without methylation. *Curr. Biol.* **4**, 145–7.

Ruvinsky, A. O. & Agulnik, A. I. (1990). Gametic imprinting and the manifestation of the *fused* gene in the house mouse. *Devel. Genet.* **11**, 263–9.

Sapienza, C. (1989). Genome imprinting and dominance modification. *Ann. N.Y. Acad. Sci.* **564**, 24–38.

Searle, A. G., Ford, C. E., Evans, E. P., Beechey, C. V., Burtenshaw, M. D. & Clegg, H. M. (1974). The induction of translocations in mouse spermatozoa. I. Kinetics of dose response with acute X-irradiation. *Mutation Res.* **22**, 157–74.

Solter, D. (1988). Differential imprinting and expression of maternal and paternal genomes. *A. Rev. Genet.* **22**, 127–46.

Stöger, R., Kubicka, P., Liu, C.-G., Kafri, T., Razin, A., Cedar, H. & Barlow, D. P. (1993). Maternal-specific methylation of the imprinted mouse *Igf2r* locus identifies the expressed locus as carrying the imprinted signal. *Cell* **73**, 61–71.

Tsai, J.-Y. & Silver, L. M. (1991). Escape from genomic imprinting at the mouse *T-associated maternal effect (Tme)* locus. *Genetics* **129**, 1159–66.

Varmusa, S. & Mann, M. (1994). Genomic imprinting – defusing the ovarian time bomb. *Trends Genet.* **10**, 118–23.

Weksberg, R., Shen, D. R., Fei, Y. L., Song, Q. L. & Squire, J. (1993). Disruption of insulin-like growth factor 2 imprinting in Beckwith–Wiedemann syndrome. *Nature Genet.* **5**, 143–50.

Winking, H. & Silver, L. M. (1984). Characterization of a recombinant mouset haplotype that expresses a dominant maternal effect. *Genetics* **108**, 1013–20.

Xu, Y., Goodyer, C. G., Deal, C. & Polychronakos, C. (1993). Functional polymorphism in the parental imprinting of the human *Igf2r* gene. *Biochem. biophys. Res. Commun.* **197**, 747–54.

II

Chromatin structure and DNA modifications

4

Epigenetic inheritance: the chromatin connection

ALAN P. WOLFFE

Abstract

This review describes the implications of chromatin structure for the regulation of differential gene expression in eukaryotes. I discuss hypotheses and experimental evidence concerning the molecular mechanisms that propagate stable states of gene activity or repression and how these may function to maintain an epigenetic imprint on gene expression.

Introduction

Within the eukaryotic nucleus homologous genes normally behave identically; however, this is not always the case. The rare exceptions in which copies of the same gene behave differently in the same nucleus are attributed to epigenetic mechanisms. The molecular basis for epigenetic effects is increasingly seen as involving the way in which a gene is packaged into chromatin and the chromosome. Because many epigenetic phenomena are stably inherited, it is important to understand not only how the packaging of a gene within the nucleus might influence the transcription process, but also how this packaging might be maintained through chromosomal replication. This review considers the events occurring at the eukaryotic replication fork, their consequences for preexisting chromosomal structures, and how chromosomal structures influencing gene expression might be duplicated.

The active state of a eukaryotic gene

The transcription of a eukaryotic gene can be influenced at several levels. The primary requirement for transcription is the association of the basal transcription machinery (including the TATA binding protein, TBP) with regulatory elements immediately upstream from the start site of transcription. This machinery directs the recruitment of RNA polymerase (I, II or III) dependent on the exact TBP associated factors (TAFs). Other sequence-specific transcription factors can influence either the initial recruitment of TBP, TAFs, the general transcription factors (GTFs, e.g. TFIIB) or RNA polymerase to the promoter or the subsequent activity of the proteins after they have been recruited (Fig. 4.1A). These sequence-specific transcription factors can be found many thousands of base pairs of DNA away from the promoter. However, they generally occur at clusters of binding sites, spread over several hundred base pairs, known as enhancers or locus control regions. I discuss later how the compaction of DNA mediated by various aspects of chromatin structure may facilitate communication between these dispersed regulatory elements (Fig. 4.1B).

Local position effect

Although transcription factors recognize DNA specifically, other nuclear proteins recognize DNA selectively, especially around the promoters of genes. These nuclear proteins include the histones, which have a major structural role in compacting DNA into nucleosomes. Each nucleosome contains over 160 bp of DNA wrapped in two superhelical turns around an octamer of the four core histones $(H2A, H2B, H3, H4)_2$. A fifth histone, H1, binds to the outside of this structure and interacts with the linker DNA between nucleosomes. The association of histone H1 stabilizes the folding of the nucleosomal array into the chromatin fiber. This structure is a loosely packed solenoid with approximately six to seven nucleosomes per turn. Each turn will include *ca.* 1000–1300 bp of DNA.

Transcription factors and the DNA sequence itself can direct the exact positioning of nucleosomes around promoter or enhancer regions (Simpson, 1991; Schild *et al.*, 1993; McPherson *et al.*, 1993). If a nucleosome includes the binding site for the basal transcriptional machinery, the gene is repressed; this is because the basal transcriptional machinery itself cannot disrupt a nucleosome (Clark & Wolffe, 1991; Workman & Roeder, 1987). Nevertheless, certain sequence-specific transcription factors can associate with nucleosomal templates. These proteins initiate a chain of events that leads to nucleosomal disruption over the promoter elements recognized by the basal transcriptional machinery (Workman *et al.*, 1991). Under physiological conditions, the association of transcription factors with repressed chromatin templates appears to depend on prior nucleosomal positioning, which maintains the necessary *cis*-acting elements in an accessible configuration (Richard-Foy & Hager, 1987; Straka & Horz, 1991). Nucleosome positioning may also have a role in maintaining *cis*-acting elements accessible during the chromatin assembly process in a way that allows transcription-factor entry into chromatin before nucleosomal structure is complete (see later). This is a 'local position effect' in which gene

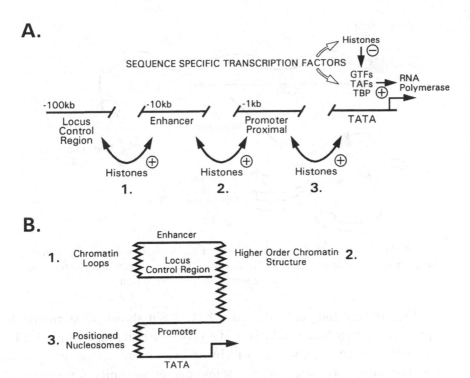

Fig. 4.1. Regulation of eukaryotic gene expression. Three types of *cis*-acting elements exist arbitrarily defined by their distance from the site of TBP binding at the TATA box. These are locus control regions, enhancers and promoter proximal elements, at which sequence-specific transcription factors (SSTFs) bind. Communication between transcription factors bound at these elements may be facilitated by packaging of the intervening DNA by the histone proteins. SSTFs influence the binding of general transcription factors (GTFs, e.g. TFIIB), TBP-associated factors (TAFs), TBP and potentially RNA polymerase itself. They may also direct the displacement of histones from the TATA box. The TAFs, GTFs, and TBP recruit RNA polymerase to the promoter and facilitate transcription.

expression depends upon the exact association of the histones with particular DNA sequences, and upon the three-dimensional folding of DNA directed by the histones.

The folding of DNA directed by the histones can actually facilitate the transcription process by mediating communication between dispersed regulatory elements. Each nucleosome brings regulatory elements separated by 80 bp into juxtaposition between adjacent superhelical turns of DNA on the surface of the histone octamer. Adjacent linker DNA segments separated linearly by 160–180 bp are also brought together by nucleosome formation (Fig. 4.2). Several examples exist of this type of structure being formed *in vivo* (Wallrath *et al.*,

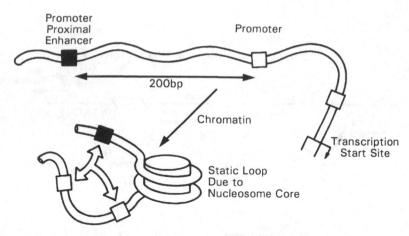

Fig. 4.2. Transcriptional potentiation through the formation of a nucleosome. The open arrows indicate facilitated transcription factor interactions. The hooked arrow represents the start site of transcription.

1994; Wolffe, 1994a) and such structures have been shown to stimulate the transcription process (Schild *et al.*, 1993). It is probable that longer-range folding of DNA within the chromatin fiber will bring even more distantly separated elements into proximity, thereby providing the opportunity for synergistic effects on transcription (Fig. 4.1B; see Cullen *et al.*, 1993).

Other proteins recognize DNA selectively. HMG1 and 2 preferentially interact with DNA that is distorted or bent (see Paull *et al.*, 1993; Giese *et al.*, 1992); others, such as MeCP1, recognize DNA that is modified through methylation of C in a CpG base pair (Boyes & Bird, 1991, 1992). The presence of this type of protein–DNA interaction could potentially modify both transcription factor (Ben-Hattar *et al.*, 1989) and histone interactions with DNA (Englander *et al.*, 1993). Methylation of DNA could also influence the binding of *trans*-acting factors directly. Thus transcriptional initiation can be influenced at several distinct stages through modification of the organization of promoter DNA, the displacement of histones and the recruitment of the basal transcriptional machinery and RNA polymerase (Fig. 4.1).

Once RNA polymerase has initiated transcription, other transcription factors concerned with the elongation process influence the processivity of the enzyme, as does chromatin structure itself (Izban & Luse, 1991; Hansen & Wolffe, 1992). Nucleosomes, either singly or in arrays, generally impede movement of RNA polymerase along the DNA molecule. These impediments depend in part on the folding of nucleosomal arrays into higher-order structures. This longer-range organization over several thousands of base pairs also has consequences for the transcription initiation process (Wolffe, 1994b).

In summary, active transcription requires the basal transcriptional machinery and RNA polymerase to associate with a promoter and also requires the polymerase to progress through the gene. The efficiency with which these events occur depends not only on sequence-specific transcription factors, but also on other parameters such as DNA modification and DNA binding proteins that alter the three-dimensional organization of the template. A major role in this organization lies with the histones, which are essential for the regulation of both local and long-range DNA packaging. These variables might, singly or in combination, contribute to epigenetic effects.

Long-range position effect

The functional organization of the chromosome into discrete domains has been increasingly recognized through experiments in *Drosophila* that make use of the phenomenon of position effect variegation (Schaffer *et al.*, 1993). These experiments employ a powerful combination of techniques including genetic analysis and cytological observation of the large polytene chromosomes. The introduction of a normally active gene into a chromosome at a position adjacent to a transcriptionally inactive, condensed heterochromatin domain will lead to a significant repression of the transcription process. This is believed to occur through a spreading of heterochromatin structure into the normally active gene. Thus, the expression of a gene depends on its chromosomal position, hence the term 'position effect'. This phenomenon provides a useful screen for genes and their products that will suppress or enhance the repression of transcription due to position effects on a suitable reporter gene, often one influencing *Drosophila* eye coloration. Many of the genes influencing position effect have been characterized and have been found to encode structural components of chromatin itself or to be capable of modifying the organization of chromatin through enzymatic mechanisms.

For example, position effect variegation depends upon the presence of normal levels of the histone proteins and post-translational modifications of the N-terminal tails of the core histones such as acetylation (Mottus *et al.*, 1980; Moore *et al.*, 1979). As we have discussed earlier, the histones are needed both for the formation of nucleosomes and for the subsequent formation of higher-order structures. Acetylation of the N-terminal tails alters the interaction of the histones with DNA and potentially alters the folding of nucleosomal arrays (Wolffe, 1992). Position effect variegation also depends on proteins that appear to recognize nucleosomal arrays, but not naked DNA, such as the chromodomain (*chromatin mo*dification organizer) proteins: HP1 and Polycomb (see Schaffer *et al.*, 1993). HP1 is associated only with inactive chromosomal regions, but Polycomb interacts with at least 50 different sites within *Drosophila* chromosomes, including developmentally important loci encoding homeodomain proteins (Orlando & Paro, 1993). However, mutations in a second gene family that interacts with the histone proteins will allow genes associated with Polycomb to remain active (Tamkun *et al.*, 1992). Thus, Polycomb is likely to exert its effects on gene expression via chromatin structures dependent on the histone proteins.

Position effect variegation is now recognized as a universal phenomenon in eukaryotic chromosomes. Genes integrated into yeast chromosomes near the silent mating loci or close to the telomeres are repressed in a way that reflects their proximity to these sites in the chromosome. This silencing effect can spread over at least 5–10 kb of contiguous DNA, but not as much as 20–30 kb in yeast. Thus, the level of chromatin organization exerting a position effect in yeast would appear to be the chromatin fiber, each turn of which will contain approximately 1 kb of DNA. As in *Drosophila*, the genes influencing position effect in yeast encode structural components of chromatin or enzymes associated with the modification of chromatin (Laurensen & Rine, 1992).

Position effects in mammalian chromosomes have been a recurrent problem for transgenic research, because highly variable levels of transcriptional activity follow from the random introduction of reporter genes into the genome (Grosveld *et al.*, 1987; Steif *et al.*, 1989). These effects can be relieved by the introduction of locus control regions (LCRs) that exert a dominant transcriptional activation function over a chromatin domain (10–100 kb). The mechanism of this activation function remains to be determined; however, communication of the LCRs with enhancers and promoters, either directly or through modification of chromatin structural components, are favored hypotheses to explain transcriptional activation (Wolffe & Dimitrov, 1993; Felsenfeld, 1992). Thus, the presence of heterochromatin domains that can transmit repressive effects and the definition of the extensive long-range activation function of LCRs over chromatin domains emphasizes the necessary compartmentalization of the chromosome into discrete functional units (see Fig. 4.3). Remarkably, these discrete functional units are prevented from influencing each other in the natural chromosomal context through the presence of special chromosomal regions that prevent the transmission of chromatin structural features associated with repressive or active domains. These special regions are known as insulators (Chung *et al.*, 1993; Wolffe, 1994c).

Several models for the action of LCRs and enhancers exist (Fig. 4.3). They may function as entry points for transcription factors, RNA polymerase or general activators such as the SWI1, 2, 3, snf5, 6 complex that might track along DNA to the promoter (Fig. 4.3A, Entry). The LCR or enhancer complex might associate with the promoter complex by stable looping of intervening DNA or

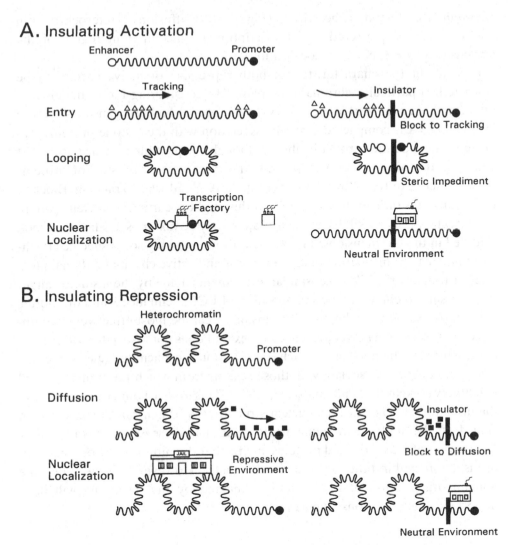

Fig. 4.3. Model for the action of LCRs, heterochromatin and insulators (see text for details).

chromatin to assemble a complex that can more effectively recruit and utilize RNA polymerase (Fig. 4.3A, Looping). Alternatively, the LCR or enhancer complex may lead the gene to assemble into chromatin structures that are capacitated for transcription through association with nuclear organelles that function as transcription factories or that associate with proteins that modify repressive chromatin structure by disrupting nucleosomes, for example the SWI1, 2, 3, snf5, 6 complex or histone acetyltransferase (Fig. 4.3A, Nuclear Localization). Several models for the repressive chromatin proteins also exist. There may be local diffusion of repressive chromatin proteins, such as HP1 in

Drosophila or histone-deacetylases (Fig. 4.3B, Diffusion). Heterochromatin might also be sequestered in a transcriptionally incompetent region of the nucleus (Fig. 4.3B, Nuclear Localization).

How might the characteristics of both repressive or active chromatin be restricted to particular chromatin domains? In considering these models it is important to recognize that the eukaryotic nucleus is a highly organized structure in which DNA is compacted through association with the histone proteins into nucleosomes and the chromatin fiber. Although it is possible that insulators that delineate domains function to prevent the tracking or diffusion of proteins between active or repressive domains (Fig. 4.3A, B, Block to Tracking, Block to Diffusion), it is difficult to envisage how this might occur in the nucleus (where DNA segments many kilobases linearly apart may be juxtaposed when the DNA is folded in three dimensions; Fig. 4.1B) without invoking some specific attachment of inactive chromatin domain, insulator and active chromatin domain to a nuclear framework. Likewise, similar attachments made by the insulator might be necessary to eliminate the juxtaposition of LCRs, enhancers and promoters (Fig. 4.3A, Steric Impediment). The insulator can be most effectively hypothesized to represent a nucleoprotein complex that does not associate with regions or structures of the nucleus in which transcription is capacitated (Jackson *et al.*, 1993) and does not associate with those regions from which the transcriptional machinery is excluded (Palladino *et al.*, 1993). This model would necessitate that the insulator associates with a nuclear structure that is neutral for transcription (Fig. 4.3A, B, Neutral Environment). Resolution of these issues will only follow purification of the associated proteins and further definition of the organization of insulators within functional eukaryotic nuclei. However, it is clear that the domain organization of the nucleus delineated by the insulators will have important functional consequences.

The fate of nucleoprotein complexes conferring active and repressed states during replication

It has long been thought that, once established, the nucleoprotein complexes determining gene activity or repression might be capable of reproducing these structures during replication (Tsanev & Sendov, 1971; Brown, 1984; Weintraub, 1985). The capacity of these complexes to duplicate will clearly depend upon the fate of a particular complex during the replication process.

Nucleosomes are disrupted by replication (Sogo *et al.*, 1986; Gruss *et al.*, 1993). Histones are at least transiently displaced from DNA, and nucleosomes appear to reassemble *de novo* with a sequential deposition of histones H3/H4 followed by histones H2A/H2B (Jackson, 1990; Gruss *et al.*, 1990; see later). In spite of this disruption, histones originally associated with a region of replicating DNA (1–2 kb) will prefer to remain associated with that same region of DNA (Randall & Kelly, 1992). This means that histones possessing a particular marked state of modification will remain in the vicinity of a particular gene (Perry *et al.*, 1993). Moreover, nucleosomes within arrays will segregate randomly to either of the two daughter DNA molecules, but will do so in small groups (3–4 nucleosomes) (Sogo *et al.*, 1986). Thus a regional state of histone modification, such as acetylation, extending over more than one thousand base pairs is likely to be discontinuously maintained after replication. This could provide a platform for the retention of proteins such as Polycomb, histone acetyltransferases or deacetylases within a particular chromatin domain. Nevertheless, preexisting chromatin proteins can only account for the assembly of 50% of the daughter DNA into chromatin. Thus preexisting chromatin must serve only to 'seed' the reassembly of similar structures within a domain. If enzymes that modify chromatin, such as histone acetyltransferase, are retained, their ensuing activity would lead to modification of the entire domain; alternatively, cooperative interaction between proteins such as Polycomb might occur to retain a hetero-chromatic state.

The basal transcriptional machinery also appears to be removed from promoter elements by the passage of a replication fork (Wolffe & Brown, 1986). Replication is found to be dominant to the transcription process, and a direct consequence of replication fork progression through an active 5S rRNA gene is the displacement of transcription factors. Several correlations from work *in vivo* support the generality of this observation. There is a clear antagonism between transcription and replication on efficiently replicating SV40 DNA molecules (Lebkowski *et al.*, 1985; Lewis & Manley, 1985). Replication forks invade the transcriptionally active ribosomal RNA genes in yeast (Saffer & Miller, 1986; Lucchini & Sogo, 1994). Thus replication will transiently erase both functional transcription complexes and repressive histone–DNA interactions from promoters. The component protein molecules that assemble activating or repressive structures may rapidly reassociate with DNA. However they will have to associate not with naked DNA but with a nascent chromatin template (Fig. 4.4).

It is possible that structures that establish functional domains within the nucleus, but that are not assembled directly upon DNA might also duplicate during S phase. For example, cytoplasmic structures such as the centriole duplicate with every cell division; likewise, nuclear machines necessary for the assembly of replication or transcription factories might also have to duplicate. The establishment or maintenance of contact between DNA and these hypothetical structures could also potentially influence gene expression and other nuclear functions.

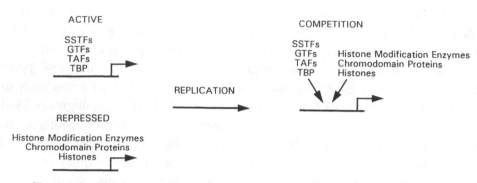

Fig. 4.4. Replication may facilitate a competition between regulatory molecules that maintain stable active or repressed states for the regulatory elements of genes.

Nucleosome and transcription complex assembly on replicating DNA

In vivo, the process of chromatin assembly is coupled to the replication of DNA. Thus newly synthesized DNA is immediately packaged by histone proteins derived both from preexisting nucleosomes and from those that are newly synthesized during S phase. Nascent DNA is assembled into a chromatin structure that is more sensitive to nucleases (and presumably to other DNA binding proteins) than mature chromatin. The maturation of this nascent chromatin from a nuclease-sensitive conformation takes approximately 10–20 min in a mammalian cell (Kempnauer *et al.*, 1980; Cusick *et al.*, 1983). Fractionation of nascent chromatin at various times following replication demonstrated that histones H3 and H4 are sequestered onto DNA before histones H2A and H2B. Histone H1 is the last histone to be stably incorporated into chromatin (Senshu *et al.*, 1978; Worcel *et al.*, 1978; Cremisi & Yaniv, 1980). This observation is related to the structure of the nucleosome, since histones H3 and H4 form the core of the structure, whereas histones H2A and H2B bind at the periphery of the nucleosome and histone H1 can only associate in its proper place once two superhelical turns of DNA are wrapped around the core histones.

The histone H4 incorporated into nascent chromatin is also post-translationally modified by acetylation before nucleosome assembly. Deacetylation of histone H4 correlates with the stable sequestration of histone H1 and the folding up of nucleosomal arrays into higher-order structures (Perry & Annunziato, 1989). Acetylation of the histones also influences transcription factor access to DNA (see below).

Nascent chromatin structures are more accessible to transcription factors than are mature chromatin structures (Wolffe, 1991). The complex of the 5S rRNA gene with the histone tetramer $(H3/H4)_2$ is not repressive to transcription (Tremethick *et al.*, 1990; Wolffe, 1989a,b; Almouzni *et al.*, 1991) whereas the complete octamer of core histones (H2A, H2B, H3, H4)$_2$ is repressive (Clark & Wolffe, 1991). Moreover, acetylation of the core histones facilitates transcription factor access to DNA even when the complete octamer is bound (Lee *et al.*, 1993). The histone tetramer $(H3/H4)_2$ recognizes the DNA sequences that position the nucleosome containing the 5S rRNA gene; hence it is probable that the formation of a specific chromatin structure also has a role in allowing transcription factors access to the template. Thus, following replication, it is probable that both sequence-specific DNA binding proteins and preexisting chromatin structural proteins will have opportunities to reassociate with the daughter DNA molecules (Fig. 4.4). The competition between these potentially activating and repressive influences will determine the association and utilization of the basal transcriptional machinery (GTFs, TAFs and TBP) at the promoter.

It is possible that proteins such as Polycomb might maintain states of transcriptional activity through the cell cycle by influencing the outcome of this competition in a particular direction (Epstein, 1992). Examples of this type of activity are proteins that organize nucleosomes into particular positions (Roth *et al.*, 1992; Chasman *et al.*, 1990). Other molecular chaperones facilitate nucleosome assembly (Smith & Stillman, 1991). The assembly of chromatin assists in the establishment of a transcriptionally repressed state (Almouzni & Wolffe, 1993). Proteins that bind after the core histones have associated with DNA, such as histone H1, can still influence gene expression towards more stable states of repression (Wolffe, 1989b; Chipev & Wolffe, 1992; Bouvet *et al.*, 1994). It is also possible that certain domains of chromatin might be sequestered in a region of the nucleus where transcription factors are more or less abundant (Fig. 4.3; Epstein, 1992).

Hypotheses to explain the inheritance of chromatin states

As we have discussed, the available evidence suggests that the transient disruption of preexisting active and repressive chromatin structures will occur during the replication process. Nevertheless, experimental work also demonstrates that proteins displaced by the elongating replication fork will also have a window of opportunity to reassociate with the daughter DNA molecule. The following hypotheses that attempt to explain how stable states of gene activity or repression might be maintained through replication build on this foundation.

The simplest situation that would lead to continued gene activity would be if a superabundance of transcription factors specific for a given gene were available within the nucleus throughout the cell cycle, including S phase. The factors would always be able to bind to their regulatory elements and to recruit the basal

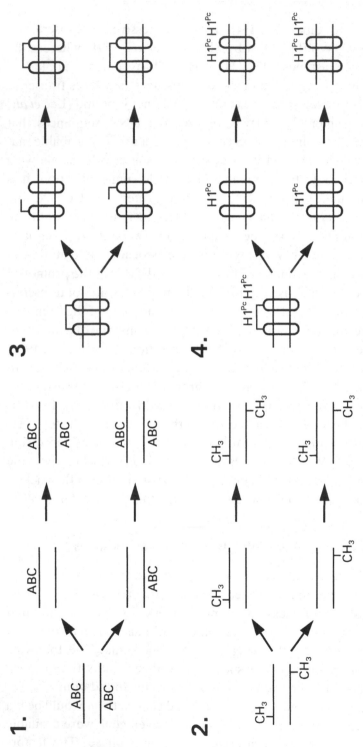

Fig. 4.5. Hypothetical mechanisms for imprinting. (1) Maintenance of specific *trans*-acting factor (ABC) interactions through replication (first arrows) followed by cooperative sequestration of additional transcription factors (second arrows). (2) Maintenance of methylation. Methylated cytosine in a CpG sequence is segregated to daughter DNA duplexes following replication (first arrows). Methyltransferase preferentially methylates CpG at a hemimethylated site (second arrows). (3) Maintenance of nucleosomal structure. Following replication (first arrows), positioned nucleosomes segregate to daughter DNA duplexes, but direct the phasing of adjacent nucleosomes (second arrows). (4) Maintenance of long-range chromatin structure. Following replication (first arrows), repressive proteins such as histone H1 or Polycomb (Pc) are reduced in abundance. Direct or indirect cooperativity between these proteins, or structure-dependent features, might direct the sequestration of additional H1 or Pc (second arrows).

transcriptional machinery to the nascent promoter DNA, and thereby to prevent histones or other proteins binding to the TATA homology. The factors might even be of the type that can displace histones from the promoter (Workman *et al.*, 1991). The promoter would in this situation be constitutively active. It is, however, possible that the transcription factors cannot themselves invade chromatin and displace repressive histones; consequently, any chromatin structures that form over their binding sites would be stably repressive. However, if the transcription factors are already bound to the regulatory elements of the gene in multiple copies, the preexisting multimeric protein complex might be split during replication, segregating copies of the transcription factors to both daughter DNA duplexes (Fig. 4.5, panel 1). These transcription factors bound to the gene could then either directly sequester other factors from the nucleoplasm, making use of protein–protein interactions, or maintain the gene accessible in the face of ongoing chromatin assembly, such that when other factors became available they could bind to DNA (Brown, 1984).

The maintenance of specific transcription factor–DNA interactions might be facilitated by considering the promoter, the enhancer and locus control regions not as separate entities, but as contributory components to a single structure (Fig. 4.1B; Wolffe, 1990). This could be achieved through protein–protein interactions between the distinct nucleoprotein complexes assembled at each regulatory element. One reason for the separation of these regulatory elements over extensive distances may be that any one structure might be independently disrupted by DNA replication, while the other would remain intact. If protein binding to one sequence element influences the binding of proteins to the other, then the intact nucleoprotein complex might facilitate the reformation of the disrupted one (Fig. 4.6).

Stable propagated covalent modifications of DNA such as cytosine methylation (Fig. 4.5, panel 2) might influence the association of transcription factors directly (Ben-Hattar *et al.*, 1989), maintain the association of repressive proteins such as MeCP1 and MeCP2 (Boyes & Bird, 1991, 1992) or influence nucleosome positioning (Englander *et al.*, 1993). If a positioned nucleosome includes a key DNA regulatory element such that a particular transcription factor cannot bind to it, the gene will be repressed. Histones themselves may bind to nucleosome positioning sequences or interact with transcription factors such that nucleosome positioning occurs (Simpson, 1991). The potential access of transcription factors and RNA polymerase to the template may consequently be restricted by nucleosomes, or alternatively the formation of a particular chromatin structure may allow a process to occur more effectively (Schild *et al.*, 1993).

We have discussed how the histones already on the template during replication will be segregated randomly to the daughter DNA duplexes, but within the

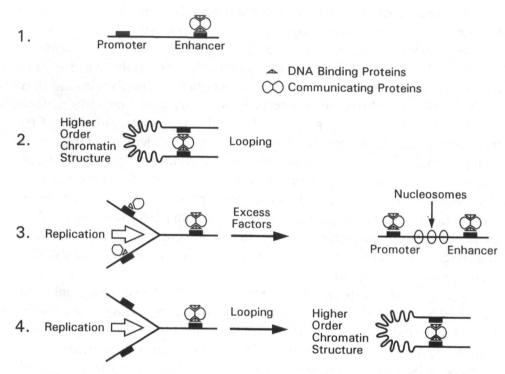

Fig. 4.6. Models for the maintenance of transcription complexes through replication. The regulatory regions of a gene are shown as a promoter and an enhancer (bars). Open boxes are DNA binding or non-DNA binding components of a transcription complex. (1) In this case similar factors are shared between enhancers and promoters. (2) The sequestration of transcription factors onto the promoter (and its activation) is facilitated by looping of the intervening DNA between enhancer and promoter. Common DNA binding proteins associate with both the enhancer and promoter. The bound proteins interact with a common non-DNA binding protein. (3) DNA replication disrupts the transcription complex on the promoter, splitting it in half. The remaining transcription factors can sequester free factors from solution, generating a complete transcription complex on each daughter chromatid. In this case the enhancer is required for establishment, but not maintenance of the transcription complex. (4) Alternatively DNA replication again disrupts the complex on the promoter, displacing transcription factors; however, because of the distance between enhancer and promoter, the enhancer complex remains intact. DNA looping can establish a new transcription complex on the promoter. Here, the enhancer is required for both establishment and maintenance of the transcription complex through cell division.

context of small groups of nucleosomes (Fig. 4.5, panel 3). If proteins that modify the subsequent folding of nucleosomal arrays or that modify histones themselves, for example by acetylation or deacetylation, are also partitioned in this way, the properties of a chromatin domain might be stably propagated (Fig.

4.5, panel 4). Chromodomain proteins that initiate the formation of hetereochromatin, such as Polycomb and HP1, are also good candidates for this type of maintenance mechanism. These models for the duplication of chromatin states are summarized in Figs. 4.5 and 4.6.

Replication and transcription activity are potentially linked in other ways. This is most clearly seen in yeast, where components of the origin recognition complex that regulates the initiation of replication within the chromosome are also involved in directing the repression of transcription within the same chromosomal domain (Bell *et al.*, 1993). The yeast origin recognition complex may be a greatly streamlined version of the replication factories of larger eukaryotes (Cook, 1991). The molecular mechanisms responsible for the repression of transcription directed by the origin recognition complex are unknown. However, one possible explanation for repression is that the origin recognition complex influences the type of chromatin assembled in that domain, or influences the organization of the domain within the nucleus (see Fig. 4.3). The final result could be that a gene adjacent to the origin is directed by the origin recognition complex to reside in a replication-competent but transcriptionally incompetent environment (Fig. 4.3). Components of the origin recognition complex remain associated with the origin throughout the cell cycle (J. Diffley, personal communication). Thus the origin recognition complex provides one biological example of the maintenance of sequence-specific protein–DNA interactions through the replication process. It provides a precedent for the potential maintenance of other structures such as insulators. However, because the origin recognition complex also serves to initiate the replication process, its maintenance may occur under circumstances distinct from the transcription complexes or chromatin structures that are exposed to the fully assembled elongation complex at the replication fork.

Chromatin organization outside of the origin recognition complex may also have significance for the initiation of replication and the timing of this initiation in S phase. If replication disrupts both active and repressed chromatin structures, then the entire nucleus has to be remodeled after each replication event. I have suggested a means of accomplishing this remodeling; however, the reformation of nuclear structures has other implications. If there are limiting transcription factors available in a cell, then a gene that is replicated early in S phase has more opportunity for the assembly of an active transcription complex than a gene that replicates late. This is simply because the gene that replicates early is available for transcription factors to bind before all of the early replicating portion of the genome has sequestered these factors. A late replicating gene will therefore experience a relative deficiency in factor availability (Gottesfeld & Bloomer, 1982; Wormington *et al.*, 1982). Conversely, it is also possible that the type of chromatin assembled early in S phase is more accessible to transcription factors than chromatin assembled late in S phase. For example, early-replicating chromatin may sequester histones that are more highly acetylated, and consequently favor continued transcription activity. Transcriptionally active genes replicate early in S phase (Goldman *et al.*, 1984; Gilbert, 1986; Guinta & Korn, 1986; Wolffe, 1993). The reason for this early replication is unknown, but possibilities include the local disruption of chromatin structure by transcription complexes, such that the DNA within those chromatin domains becomes more accessible to the replication machinery (Wolffe & Brown, 1988). Many transcription factors are also replication factors (De Pamphilis, 1988); consequently, local concentrations of transcription factors may favor the assembly of replication initiation complexes.

Testing the hypotheses with experiment: the examples of the X chromosome, *Igf-2*, *Igf-2r*, *H19* and *Snrpn*

Within each somatic cell nucleus of the female mammal lie two X chromosomes; one is transcriptionally active and the other is not. Active and inactive states are maintained through replication. These two different X chromosomes provide an excellent case of both epigenetic effects and the inheritance of chromatin states. Do any of the hypotheses we have discussed explain the selective transcriptional inactivity of one of the pair of identical X chromosomes, and the maintenance of this inactivation? In addition, imprinting within the paternal and maternal genomes in the mouse has been studied in detail for *Igf2*, *Igf2r*, *H19* and *Snrpn* genes. Substantial recent process has been made in examining the mechanism of this imprinting (Surani, 1993); useful similarities and distinctions emerge from comparison with the X chromosome.

Many genes in the inactive X chromosome are heavily methylated, in contrast to those of the active X chromosome (Grant & Chapman, 1988). However, the kinetics with which the X-linked genes became methylated during the differentiation of embryonic female somatic cells do not always correlate with the timing of transcriptional inactivation (Lock *et al.*, 1987). Thus other mechanisms must supplement any influence of DNA methylation on transcription within the inactive X chromosome. In contrast, if methylation is impaired in the developing mouse embryo by restricting the activity of DNA methyltransferase, major changes occur in the expression pattern of imprinted genes (Li *et al.*, 1993). Reduction in DNA methylation leads to activation of the normally silent paternal allele of *H19*, the repression of the normally active paternal allele of the *Igf2* gene, and the repression of the normally active maternal allele of the *Igf2r* gene. These results dramatically demonstrate a key role for DNA methylation in imprinting.

The active X chromosome normally replicates early in S phase, whereas the inactive X chromosome replicates late (Takagi, 1974). However, female lymphoma cell lines have been isolated in which the converse occurs (Yoshida *et al.*, 1993). Thus the inactive X chromosome does not have to replicate late in S phase in order to be transcriptionally quiescent. Likewise, although the replication timing patterns of maternal and paternal alleles of the imprinted genes *Igf2*, *Igf2r*, *H19* and *Snrpn* differ, with the paternal allele always being early-replicating, there is no simple correlation with gene activity (Kitsberg *et al.*, 1993). Nevertheless, the differential replication timing phenomenon is useful in demonstrating that the imprinted genes are embedded in large chromatin domains that have distinct replication patterns. Formation of such domains may provide a structural imprint on gene activity (Fig. 4.3; Kitsberg *et al.*, 1993).

Promoters in the inactive X chromosome appear to be incorporated into positioned nucleosomes, whereas promoters in the active X chromosome are free of such structures and have transcription factors bound to them (Riggs & Pfeifer, 1992). Thus specific chromatin structures clearly appear to have a role in regulating differential gene activity between the two X chromosomes. Moreover, nucleosomes on the active X chromosome contain predominantly acetylated histones whereas those on the inactive X chromosome are not acetylated (Jeppesen & Turner, 1993). Thus the establishment and maintenance of specific chromatin structures containing modified histones is an excellent candidate mechanism for establishing and maintaining differential expression of genes between the two X chromosomes. Differential methylation and replication timing may serve to stabilize these different states of gene activity.

Summary

The packaging of regulatory DNA within the eukaryotic chromosome has considerable potential not only for modulating the transcriptional activity of genes, but also for propagating states that are permissive or restrictive for transcription. Sequence-specific transcription factors, histones and their modifications, chromodomain proteins and enzymes that modify histones, DNA methylation and proteins that recognize methylated DNA could all play independent or interrelated roles in regulating gene activity. They all also have the potential of propagating their interactions with nascent DNA following replication. This is clearly seen for the imprinted *Igf2*, *Igf2r* and *H19* genes in the mouse. In contrast, observations on the phenomenon of X chromosome inactivation suggest that the formation and stability of specific histone–DNA interactions through replication may be central to the inheritance of chromatin states, and that other molecular mechanisms have supporting roles. The future offers the exciting prospect of reconstructing the propagation of stable active or repressed chromatin states *in vitro*, and consequently understanding the events occurring at the replication fork in molecular detail.

References

Almouzni, G., Méchali, M. & Wolffe, A. P. (1991). Transcription complex disruption caused by a transition in chromatin structure. *Molec. Cell Biol.* **11**, 655–65.

Almouzni, G. & Wolffe, A. P. (1993). Replication coupled chromatin assembly is required for the repression of basal transcription *in vivo*. *Genes Devel.* **7**, 2033–47.

Bell, S. P., Kobayashi, R. & Stillman, B. (1993). Yeast origin recognition complex functions in transcription silencing and DNA replication. *Science* **262**, 1844–9.

Ben-Hattar, J., Beard, P. & Jiricny, J. (1989). Cytosine methylation in CTF and SP1 recognition sites of an HSV tK promoter: effects on transcription *in vivo* and on factor binding *in vitro*. *Nucleic Acids Res.* **17**, 10179–90.

Bouvet, P., Dimitrov, S. & Wolffe, A. P. (1994). Specific regulation of *Xenopus* chromosomal 5S rRNA gene transcription by histone H1. *Genes Devel.* **8**, 1147–59.

Boyes, J. & Bird, A. (1991). DNA methylation inhibits transcription indirectly via a methyl-CpG binding protein. *Cell* **64**, 1123–34.

Boyes, J. & Bird, A. (1992). Repression of genes by DNA methylation depends on CpG density and promoter strength: evidence for involvement of a methyl-CpG binding protein. *EMBO J.* **11**, 327–33.

Brown, D. D. (1984). The role of stable complexes that repress and activate eukaryotic genes. *Cell* **37**, 359–65.

Chasman, D. I., Lue, N. F., Buchman, A. R., LaPointe, J. W., Lorch, Y. & Kornberg, R. D. (1990). A yeast protein that influences the chromatin structure of UAS_G and functions as a powerful auxiliary gene activator. *Genes Devel.* **4**, 503–14.

Chipev, C. C. & Wolffe, A. P. (1992). Chromosomal organization of *Xenopus laevis* oocyte and somatic 5S rRNA genes *in vivo*. *Molec. Cell Biol.* **12**, 45–55.

Chung, J. H., Whiteley, M. & Felsenfeld, G. (1993). A 5′ element of the chicken β-globin domain serves as an insulator in human erythroid cells and protects against position effect in *Drosophila*. *Cell* **74**, 505–14.

Clark, D. J. & Wolffe, A. P. (1991). Superhelical stress and nucleosome mediated repression of 5S RNA gene transcription *in vitro*. *EMBO J.* **10**, 3419–28.

Cook, P. R. (1991). The nucleoskeleton and the topology of replication. *Cell* **66**, 627–37.

Cremisi, C. & Yaniv, M. (1980). Sequential assembly of newly synthesized histones on replicating SV40 DNA. *Biochem. biophys. Res. Commun.* **92**, 1117–23.

Cullen, K. E., Kladde, M. P. & Seyfred, M. A. (1993). Interaction between transcription regulatory regions of prolactin chromatin. *Science* **261**, 203–6.

Cusick, M. E., Lee, K. S., DePamphilis, M. L. & Wasserman, P. M. (1983). Structure of chromatin at deoxyribonucleic acid replication forks: nuclease hypersensitivity results from both prenucleosomal deoxyribonucleic acid and an immature chromatin structure. *Biochemistry* **22**, 3873–84.

DePamphilis, M. L. (1988). Transcriptional elements as components of eukaryotic origins of DNA replication. *Cell* **52**, 635–8.

Englander, E. W., Wolffe, A. P. & Howard, B. H. (1993). Nucleosome interactions with a human Alu element: Transcriptional repression and effects of template methylation. *J. biol. Chem.* **268**, 19565–73.

Epstein, H. (1992). Polycomb and friends. *BioEssays* **14**, 411–13.

Felsenfeld, G. (1992). Chromatin: an essential part of the transcriptional apparatus. *Nature* **335**, 219–24.

Giese, K., Cox, J. & Grosschedl, R. (1992). The HMG domain of lymphoid enhancer factor 1 bends DNA and facilitates assembly of functional nucleoprotein structures. *Cell* **69**, 185–95.

Gilbert, D. M. (1986). Temporal order of replication of *Xenopus laevis* 5S ribosomal RNA genes in somatic cells. *Proc. Natl. Acad. Sci. USA* **83**, 2924–8.

Goldman, M. A., Holmquist, G. P., Gray, M. C., Caston, L. A. & Nag, A. (1984). Replication timing of genes and middle repetitive sequences. *Science* **224**, 686–92.

Gottesfeld, J. & Bloomer, L. S. (1982). Assembly of transcriptionally active 5S RNA gene chromatin *in vitro*. *Cell* **28**, 781–91.

Grant, S. G. & Chapman, V. M. (1988). Mechanisms of X-chromosome regulation. *A. Rev. Genet.* **22**, 199–233.

Grosveld, F., Van Assendelft, G. B., Greaves, D. & Kollias, G. (1987). Position-independent, high level expression of the human β-globin gene in transgenic mice. *Cell* **51**, 975–85.

Gruss, C., Gutierrez, C., Burhans, W. C., DePamphilis, M. L., Koller, T. & Sogo, J. M. (1990). Nucleosome assembly in mammalian cell extracts before and after DNA replication. *EMBO J.* **9**, 2911–22.

Gruss, C., Wu, J., Koller, T. & Sogo, J. M. (1993). Disruption of nucleosomes at replication forks. *EMBO J.* **12**, 4533–45.

Guinta, D. R. & Korn, L. J. (1986). Differential order of replication of *Xenopus laevis* 5S RNA genes. *Molec. Cell Biol.* **6**, 2536–42.

Hansen, J. & Wolffe, A. P. (1992). Influence of chromatin folding on transcription initiation and elongation by RNA polymerase III. *Biochemistry* **31**, 7977–88.

Izban, M. G. & Luse, D. S. (1991). Transcription on nucleosomal templates by RNA polymerase II *in vitro*: inhibition of elongation with enhancement of sequence-specific pausing. *Genes Devel.* **5**, 683–96.

Jackson, D. A., Hassan, A. B., Errington, R. J. & Cook, P. R. (1993). Visualization of focal sites of transcription within human nuclei. *EMBO J.* **12**, 1059–65.

Jackson, V. (1990). *In vivo* studies on the dynamics of histone-DNA interaction: evidence for nucleosome dissolution during replication and transcription and a low level of dissolution independent of both. *Biochemistry* **29**, 719–31.

Jeppesen, P. & Turner, B. M. (1993). The inactive X chromosome in female mammals is distinguished by a lack of histone H4 acetylation, a cytogenetic marker for gene expression. *Cell* **74**, 281–89.

Kempnauer, K. H., Fanning, E., Oho, B. & Knippers, R. (1980). Maturation of newly replicated chromatin of simian virus 40 and its host cell. *J. molec. Biol.* **136**, 359–74.

Kitsberg, D., Selig, S., Brandeis, M., Simon, I., Keshet, I., Driscoll, D. J., Nicholls, R. D. & Cedar, H. (1993). Allele-specific replication timing of imprinted gene regions. *Nature* **364**, 459–63.

Laurensen, P. & Rine, J. (1992). Silencers, silencing and heritable transcriptional states. *Microbiol. Rev.* **56**, 543–92.

Lebkowski, J. S., Clancy, S. & Calos, M. P. (1985). Simian virus 40 replication in adenovirus-transformed human cells antagonizes gene expression. *Nature* **317**, 169–71.

Lee, D. Y., Hayes, J. J., Pruss, D. & Wolffe, A. P. (1993). A positive role for histone acetylation in transcription factor binding to nucleosomal DNA. *Cell* **72**, 73–84.

Lewis, E. D. & Manley, J. L. (1985). Repression of simian virus 40 early transcription by viral DNA replication in human 293 cells. *Nature* **317**, 172–5.

Li, E., Beard, C. & Jaenisch, R. (1993). Role of DNA methylation in genomic imprinting. *Nature* **366**, 362–5.

Lock, L. F., Takagi, N. & Martin, G. R. (1987). Methylation of the hprt gene on the inactive X occurs after chromosome inactivation. *Cell* **48**, 36–46.

Lucchini, R. & Sogo, J. M. (1994). Chromatin structure and transcriptional activity around the replication forks arrested at the 3′ end of the yeast rRNA genes. *Molec. Cell Biol.* **14**, 318–26.

McPherson, C. E., Shim, E. Y., Friedman, D. S. & Zaret, K. S. (1993). An active tissue-specific enhancer and bound transcription factors existing in a precisely positioned nucleosomal array. *Cell* **75**, 387–98.

Moore, G. D., Procunier, J. D., Cross, D. P. & Grigliatti, T. A. (1979). Histone gene deficiencies and position-effect variegation in *Drosophila*. *Nature* **282**, 312–14.

Mottus, R., Reeves, R. & Grigliatti, T. A. (1980). Butyrate suppression of position effect variegation in *Drosophila melanogaster*. *Molec. gen. Genet.* **178**, 465–9.

Orlando, V. & Paro, R. (1993). Mapping Polycomb-repressed domains in the bithorax complex using in vivo formaldehyde cross-linked chromatin. *Cell* **75**, 1187–98.

Palladino, F., Laroche, T., Gilson, E., Axelrod, A., Pillus, L. & Gasser, S. M. (1993). SIR3 and SIR4 proteins are required for the positioning and integrity of yeast telomeres. *Cell* **75**, 543–55.

Paull, T. T., Haykinson, M. J. & Johnson, R. C. (1993). The non specific DNA-binding and -bending proteins HMG1 and HMG2 promote the assembly of complex nucleoprotein structures. *Genes Devel.* **7**, 1521–34.

Perry, C. A., Allis, C. D. & Annunziato, A. T. (1993). Parental nucleosomes segregated to newly replicated chromatin are underacetylated relative to those assembled *de novo*. *Biochemistry* **32**, 13615–23.

Perry, C. A. & Annunziato, A. T. (1989). Influence of histone acetylation on the solubility, H1 content and DNase I sensitivity of newly assembled chromatin. *Nucl. Acids Res.* **17**, 4275–91.

Randall, S. K. & Kelly, T. J. (1992). The fate of parental nucleosomes during SV40 DNA replication. *J. biol. Chem.* **267**, 14259–65.

Richard-Foy, H. & Hager, G. L. (1987). Sequence-specific positioning of nucleosomes over the steroid-inducible MMTV promoter. *EMBO J.* **6**, 2321–8.

Riggs, A. P. & Pfeifer, G. P. (1992). X-chromosome inactivation and cell memory. *Trends Genet.* **8**, 169–74.

Roth, S. Y., Shimizu, M., Johnson, L., Grunstein, M. & Simpson, R. T. (1992). Stable nucleosome positioning and complete repression by the yeast α2 repressor are disrupted by amino-terminal mutation in histone H4. *Genes Devel.* **6**, 411–25.

Saffer, D. L. & Miller, O. L. Jr. (1986). Electron microscopic study of Saccharomyces cerevisiae rDNA chromatin replication. *Molec. Cell Biol.* **6**, 1147–57.

Schaffer, C. D., Wallrath, L. L. & Elgin, S. C. R. (1993). Regulating genes by packaging domains: bits of heterochromatin in euchromatin. *Trends Genet.* **9**, 35–7.

Schild, C., Claret, F.-X., Wahli, W. & Wolffe, A. P. (1993). A nucleosome-dependent static loop potentiates estrogen-regulated transcription from the *Xenopus* vitellogenin B1 promoter *in vitro*. *EMBO J.* **12**, 423–33.

Senshu, T., Fukada, M. & Ohashi, M. (1978). Preferential association of newly synthesized H3 and H4 histones with newly synthesized replicated DNA. *J. Biochem.* **84**, 985–8.

Simpson, R. T. (1991). Nucleosome positioning: occurrence, mechanisms and functional consequences. *Prog. Nucl. Acids Res. molec. Biol.* **40**, 143–84.

Smith, S. & Stillman, B. (1991). Stepwise assembly of chromatin during DNA replication *in vitro*. *EMBO J.* **10**, 971–80.

Sogo, J. M., Stahl, H., Koller, T. & Knippers, R. (1986). Structure of the replicating SV40 minichromosomes: The replication fork, core histone segregation and terminal structures. *J. molec. Biol.* **189**, 189–204.

Steif, A., Winter, D. M., Stratling, W. H. & Sippel, A. E. (1989). A nuclear DNA attachment element mediates elevated and position-independent gene activity. *Nature* **341**, 343–5.

Straka, C. & Horz, W. (1991). A functional role for nucleosomes in the represssion of a yeast promoter. *EMBO J.* **10**, 361–8.

Surani, M. A. (1993). Genomic imprinting: silence of the genes. *Nature* **366**, 302–3.

Takagi, N. (1974). Differentiation of X chromosomes in early female mouse embryos. *Exp. Cell Res.* **86**, 127–35.

Tamkun, J. W., Deuring, R., Scott, M. P., Kissinger, M., Patlatucci, A. M., Kaufman, T. C. & Kennison, J. A. (1992). Brahma: a regulator of *Drosophila* homeotic genes structurally related to the yeast transcriptional activator SNF2/SWI2. *Cell* **68**, 561–73.

Tremethick, D., Zucker, D. & Worcel, A. (1990). The transcription complex of the 5S RNA gene, but not transcription factor TFIIIA alone, prevents nucleosomal repression of transcription. *J. biol. Chem.* **265**, 5014–23.

Tsanev, R. & Sendov, B. (1971). Possible molecular mechanism for cell differentiation in multicellular organisms. *J. theor. Biol.* **30**, 337–93.

Wallrath, L. L., Lu, Q., Granock, H. & Elgin, S. C. R. (1994). Architectural variations of inducible eukaryotic promoters: preset and remodeling chromatin structures. *BioEssays* **16**, 165–70.

Weintraub, H. (1985). Assembly and propagation of repressed and derepressed chromosomal states. *Cell* **42**, 705–11.

Wolffe, A. P. (1989a). Transcriptional activation of *Xenopus* class III genes in chromatin isolated from sperm and somatic nuclei. *Nucleic Acids Res.* **17**, 767–80.

Wolffe, A. P. (1989b). Dominant and specific repression of *Xenopus* oocyte 5S RNA genes and satellite I DNA by histone H1. *EMBO J.* **8**, 527–37.

Wolffe, A. P. (1990). Transcription complexes. *Prog. clin. biol. Res.* **322**, 171–86.

Wolffe, A. P. (1991). Implications of DNA replication for eukaryotic gene expression. *J. Cell Sci.* **99**, 201–6.

Wolffe, A. P. (1992). *Chromatin: Structure and Function*. London: Academic Press.

Wolffe, A. P. (1993). Replication timing and *Xenopus* 5S RNA gene transcription *in vitro*. *Devel. Biol.* **157**, 224–31.

Wolffe, A. P. (1994a). Transcription: in tune with the histones. *Cell* **77**, 1–20.

Wolffe, A. P. (1994b). A general and dominant role for chromatin compaction in the regulation of transcription. In *Structural Biology: the State of the Art*, ed. R. H. Sarma, pp. 109–24. New York: Adenine Press.

Wolffe, A. P. (1994c). Insulating chromatin. *Curr. Biol.* **4**, 85–7.

Wolffe, A. P. & Brown, D. D. (1986). DNA replication *in vitro* erases a *Xenopus* 5S RNA gene transcription complex. *Cell* **47**, 217–27.

Wolffe, A. P. & Brown, D. D. (1988). Developmental regulation of two 5S ribosomal RNA genes. *Science* **241**, 1626–32.

Wolffe, A. P. & Dimitrov, S. (1993). Histone modulated gene activity: developmental implications. *CRC Crit. Rev. Euk. Gene Exp.* **3**, 167–91.

Worcel, A., Han, S. & Wong, M. L. (1978). Assembly of newly replicated chromatin. *Cell* **15**, 969–77.

Workman, J. L. & Roeder, R. G. (1987). Binding of transcription factor TFIID to the major late promoter during *in vitro* nucleosome assembly potentiates subsequent initiation by RNA polymerase II. *Cell* **51**, 613–22.

Workman, J. L., Taylor, I. C. A. & Kingston, R. E. (1991). Activation domains of stably bound Gal4 derivatives alleviate repression of promoters by nucleosomes. *Cell* **64**, 533–44.

Wormington, W. M., Schlissel, M. & Brown, D. D. (1982). Developmental regulation of *Xenopus* 5S RNA genes. *Cold Spring Harbor Symp. quant. Biol.* **47**, 879–84.

Yoshida, I., Kashio, N. & Takagi, N. (1993). Cell fusion-induced quick change in replication time of the inactive mouse X chromosome: an implication for the maintenance mechanism of late replication. *EMBO J.* **12**, 4397–405.

5

Chromobox genes and the molecular mechanisms of cellular determination

PRIM B. SINGH AND THARAPPEL C. JAMES

The attraction that the heterochromatic regions of the chromosomes holds for investigators resides in the fact that they are differentiated chromosome regions. This fact provides the possibility that by their study, one might gain insight into some quality which could itself serve as a guide to generalities of the nature and function of all genes.

Jack Schultz, 1956

Introduction

During regulative development, embryonic cells undergo a restriction in developmental potential (reviewed by Slack, 1983). Early on, cells retain a degree of pluripotency (Illmensee, 1972; Kelly, 1977) that enables them to follow any one of several different developmental pathways; their commitment to one particular fate is poor. The fate of cells is malleable during this time and is largely under the instruction of extracellular factors. However, as development proceeds cells undergo a transition – often unaccompanied by overt changes in cellular phenotype – whereupon their fates become determined (Kieny *et al.*, 1972; Simcox & Sang, 1983; De Robertis *et al.*, 1991) and essentially irreversible. This transition from a situation where developmental fate is governed by cell-extrinsic factors to one where it becomes cell-intrinsic, and is maintained independent of environment, represents the problem we wish to address here. Our approach is essentially to look at the problem in reverse: to describe the detailed information we have about the mechanisms that can change the expressibility of genes (and therefore of cellular fate) in a way that is heritable from one cellular generation to the next, and then to examine how these states of expressibility are established. We also discuss how the molecular mechanisms involved in establishing determined states provide an excellent framework for understanding parental imprinting phenomena.

71

We begin with heterochromatin, which is a well-known example of a heritable state of gene inactivity (Brown, 1966; Cattanach, 1975). The notion that hetero-chromatin is a repressive chromosomal environment stems from the observation that the effect of heterochromatin on gene repression is pervasive. If, for example, a euchromatic segment is artificially relocated next to hetero-chromatin, its genes are repressed in their activity, resulting in an *epigenetic* silencing that is faithfully inherited through many cellular generations. Such chromosomal rearrangements often lead to phenotypic variegation in tissues where the translocated gene is normally expressed, a feature most clearly exemplified by a long-known genetic phenomenon, first described in *Drosophila*, called position effect variegation (PEV). PEV is almost invariably associated with chromosomal rearrangements, where one or both of the breakpoints lie within heterochromatin (Baker, 1958; Spofford, 1976). It is a reliable phenomenon. Indeed, in *Drosophila*, PEV obeys certain rules (Schultz, 1941; Morgan & Schultz, 1942; Baker, 1953) which can predict the effects of rearrangements involving heterochromatin, and which have enabled the biology of PEV to be described in some detail (Table 5.1). The clear genetical basis to PEV, the consistency and ease with which the effects can be observed, especially when using *white* mottling, has made PEV a useful system for the study of development in *Drosophila* (Schultz, 1941).

The notions of determination and differentiation as they relate to PEV

The phenomenon of *white* mottling provides an excellent assay for the repression of gene activity that results from position effect (Fig. 5.1). This property has not gone unnoticed, and has been used effectively to determine the precise time during *Drosophila* development when the decision is made to inactivate the *white* gene (Baker, 1963). Careful study of the pigmentation patterns from several hundred eyes has shown that they are, in general, continuous and not a random salt-and-pepper distribution and, when compared, that many of the geographical zones of the patterns are shared. Finally, both positive and negative images of the same pattern can be obtained (Figs. 5.2b–g).

Information about these patterns has been usefully integrated with lineage analysis (Fig. 5.2a) (Becker, 1957), which has shown that at the end of the first larval instar there are eight cells in the eye disk whose descendants will form the ommatidia and part of the hypodermis of the ventral half of the head. The relatively regular cell lineage in the ventral half makes it possible to delineate the size and location of the eight sectors that are derived from the eight cells (Fig. 5.2a). Comparison of the patterns in Figs. 5.2b–g with the sectors of common cell lineage in Fig. 5.2a shows that the patterns cover entire sectors or more than one

Table 5.1. *Characteristics of PEV*

The features of PEV given here apply only to variegating euchromatic genes. It should be noted that genes that lie within heterochromatin variegate when placed in distal euchromatic locations by rearrangement (see Wakimoto & Hearn, 1990). Many of the features typically associated with the euchromatic genes, and given below, are reversed when considering variegating heterochromatic genes.

Characteristic feature	Reference
I. Variegation usually acts in *cis* (although see VIII) and is the result of inactivation of gene expression at the level of transcription.	Baker, 1958; Nix, 1973; Henikoff, 1981
II. Practically any gene can be affected in *Drosophila*.	Baker, 1958
III. Inactivation spreads along the chromosome in a polarized fashion, with the genes closer to the breakpoint exhibiting the more extreme variegation. The distances involved can be enormous. In one case in *Drosophila virilis*, genes that lie almost a third of a chromosome away (several Mb) can be affected.	Schultz, 1941; Demerec, 1941; Baker, 1958
IV. Inactivation occurs early during development and is, like heterochromatin, clonally inherited.	Becker, 1957; Baker, 1958
V. For variegating euchromatic loci the addition of heterochromatin (e.g. the Y chromosome) suppresses variegation, whereas removal of heterochromatin enhances variegation.	Gowan & Gay, 1933b
VI. Inactivation is likely to be the result of a change in chromatin structure, since the variegating gene assumes the condensed morphology of the adjacent heterochromatin in cells where the gene is inactivated.	Prokofyeva-Belgovskaya, 1941; Henikoff, 1981
VII. Study of modifiers of PEV support the notion that repression is the result of a change in chromatin structure, since they include the histones and proteins that localize to heterochromatin (see Table 5.2).	Tartof *et al.*, 1989; Grigliatti, 1991; Reuter & Spierer, 1992
VIII. Although PEV is usually recessive, in certain cases it can be dominant. When a variegating *brown* locus is localized close to the normal copy on the unrearranged chromosome, there is often a inter-homolog effect whereby the normal copy is repressed. This 'trans-heterochromatinization' is the one important exception in the *cis*-dominant rule.	Slatis, 1955; Henikoff, 1990

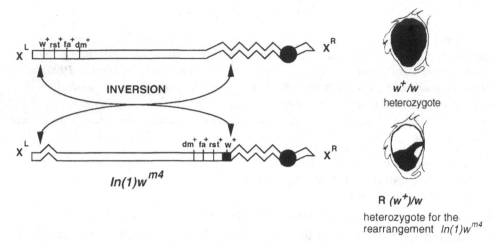

Fig. 5.1. A schematic illustration of *white* variegation in the X chromosome inversion *In(1)w^{m4}*. The distal region of the X chromosome contains a cluster of genes, including *white (w+)*, *roughest (rst+)*, *facet (fa+)* and *diminutive (dm+)* that have been useful in the study of variegating eye phenotypes. In strains that possess the *In(1)w^{m4}* chromosome these genes are brought close to hetero-chromatin by chromosomal rearrangement (zig-zag line), such that the *white* gene is now only 25 kb away from constitutive heterochromatin (Tartof *et al.*, 1984). In heterozygotes for the rearrangement, where the rearranged chromosome bears the dominant allele of *white*, *w+*, the eye has a distinctive mottled appearance. This is because in some cells *w+* has been repressed by its proximity to heterochromatin, and the recessive allele carried on the normal unrearranged chromosome has gained phenotypic expression. In all figures, the black parts of the eye represent pigmented wild-type coloration, while the colourless parts represent non-pigmented, mutant areas.

sector, a result which means that in most cases the determinative event of whether or not to inactivate the *white* locus occurs in one or more of the eight cells during the first larval instar. For example, in pair b and c the entire sector I is affected; in pair d and e sectors IV, V, VI and VII are the same; and in pair f and g sectors I, VI, VII and VIII are affected. The presence of both positive and negative images of the same pattern also suggests that the decision is arrived at by a stochastic process and there is no predisposition of the cells to inactivate the *white* gene or not. However, once the decision is made it is final and is stored for many cellular generations while the cells divide, forming the eight sectors that differ with regard to the activity of the rearranged genes. The decision only becomes phenotypically manifest during the final stages of differentiation of the eye, during the mid-pupal stage of development, when the genes responsible for pigment formation are transcribed and pigment first appears within the eye. This is some seven days after the determinative event. On the basis of these and other

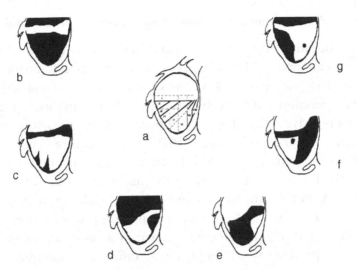

Fig. 5.2. Patterns of eye variegation in the eyes of *Drosophila melanogaster* with the duplication $Dp(1;3)N^{264-58a}$. Eyes b and c, d and e, and f and g are pairs of positive and negative images. Eye a indicates diagrammatically the areas filled by descendants of the eight cells present at the end of the first larval instar, which will form the ventral half of the eye. After Becker (1957), but redrawn from Baker (1963), with permission.

findings (Hadorn, 1965) it has become well known that the acquisition of the potential to express a pattern of genes (determination) precedes the overt expression of this potential (differentiation) and that these two processes are separable in developmental time.

   The nature of the inactivation of the variegating *white* gene is clearly central to the mechanism of determination. Some clues have come from the inspection of variegating euchromatic loci in polytene nuclei, where it has been shown that the frequency with which a locus is packaged into heterochromatin correlates well with the frequency with which the genes residing within the locus are inactivated in a tissue (Schultz & Caspersson, 1939; Prokofyeva-Belgovskaya, 1941). This latter observation has suggested that the inactivation seen in PEV and put into place at the first larval instar stage of development is not due to somatic gene loss, since revertants to wild-type can be recovered (Dubinin & Sidorov, 1935; Panshin, 1935), but rather that inactivation is mediated by a change in chromatin packaging, a change that can be followed for a variegating euchromatic gene as a cytological transition from a euchromatic conformation to one that is decidedly heterochromatic (Henikoff, 1981).

Modifiers of PEV and the mass-action model of heterochromatin formation

Over several decades many environmental and genetical factors have been described that can modify PEV. Changes in environmental temperature have a dramatic effect on variegation: lowering of the temperature at specific times during embryogenesis normally enhances variegation, and raising the temperature has a suppressive effect (Fig. 5.3) (Gowan & Gay, 1933a). There are two sensitive periods for the modulation of PEV by temperature. The first is before the time of determination, at around the time of cellularization of the embryo (Spofford, 1976); the second is during the mid-pupal stage of development (Chen, 1948). Although little was known of the molecular mechanisms underlying PEV at the time, these effects were interpreted, prophetically, as being an indication that PEV might be a consequence of a self-assembly process that involved many proteins which form a macromolecular complex (Spofford, 1976). Like all macromolecular complexes, its stability would be temperature-dependent, being more stable at lower temperatures. At higher temperatures enough thermal energy could be provided for dissolution of an ordered structure into its constituent parts. In the light of this prescient explanation, the time at which the sensitive periods occur during development might be understandable. The first is around the time that heterochromatin becomes recognizable within the nuclei (Cooper, 1959): a temperature shift at this time could have an effect on the *initial steps* involved in heterochromatin assembly. The second is at the time that the genes responsible for pigment formation are transcribed, and heat shock at this time might allow transcription factors to have access to the otherwise heterochromatized *white* gene. A key feature is that both these sensitive periods represent windows within which the determined state can be changed.

As for genetic modifiers of PEV, they can have two types of effect on variegation. *Suppressors of PEV (Suvar)* convert the mottled phenotype to one that is essentially indistinguishable from the wild type, whereas *Enhancers of PEV (Evar)* have the opposite effect and alter the phenotype to a more mutant form (Fig. 5.3). The function(s) of *Suvars* and *Evars* are clearly pertinent to the mechanism by which heterochromatin domains are established. The observation that the degree of enhancement or suppression of variegation caused by two modifiers of PEV can be directly correlated with the extent of heterochromatization at a variegating breakpoint (Reuter *et al.*, 1982) suggests that they might encode structural components of heterochromatin. Moreover, the reciprocal effects of the *Suvars* and *Evars* suggest that they have opposite effects on heterochromatin formation: *Suvars* are thought to be involved in the formation of heterochromatin, through encoding either components of the compact state or enzymes that modify these components, whereas the *Evars* promote the

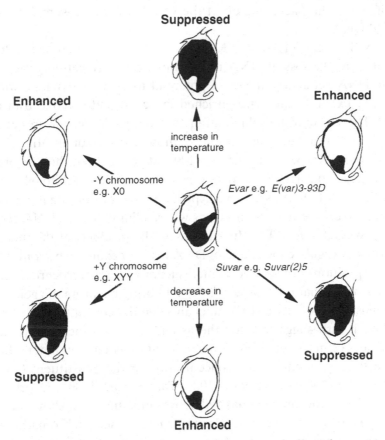

Fig. 5.3. Both genetic and environmental factors can affect the process of determination and therefore the degree of variegation within a tissue. The central eye illustrates an idealized variegation of the *white* gene in an XY male. In general, an increase in temperature or addition of heterochromatin to the genome via an extra Y chromosome leads to a reduction in variegation. The reverse, that is cooling or the removal of heterochromatin, has the opposite effect of enhancing variegation. Euchromatic modifiers of position-effect variegation have two types of effect. Suppressor mutations such as *Suvar(2)5* convert the mottled phenotype to one that is almost wild type, whereas Enhancer mutations such as *E(var)3–93D* have the opposite effect and convert the mottled phenotype to one that is more mutant. Not given here is the modifying effect of butyrate (Reuter & Spierer, 1992), which has a suppressing effect on variegation; this effect has been explained by an increase in histone acetylation.

euchromatic state, perhaps by binding hypothetical boundary elements (Tartof *et al.*, 1984) that stop the spreading of heterochromatin. Analysis of the *Suvar*s also provided firm evidence for a connection between PEV and chromatin, since one of the first *Suvar*s to be described was the group of genes encoding the core histones (Moore *et al.*, 1979), a result which hinted strongly that repression seen in PEV involves the packaging of, at the very least, nucleosomal if not chromatosomal DNA.

Karpen & Spradling (1990) and Karpen (1994) have proposed that PEV may also result from the loss of DNA representing the variegating gene. Heterochromatic DNA sequences have the potential to be very dynamic within the genome. For example, they are enriched in active and inactive transposable elements. The chromosome diminution that occurs in certain insects is also proceeded by heterochromatinization of those chromosomes. In a carefully controlled study, Karpen & Spradling (1990) demonstrated the loss of specific DNA sequences from a heterochromatic ring chromosome. Although there is no proof for the loss of DNA as the sole explanation of PEV in somatic tissues, it is conceivable that there may be instances where elimination of DNA sequences might be responsible for PEV. In such cases, the products of the modifiers of variegation may regulate the extent of DNA loss, for example by controlling the rate of transpositions of movable elements from within heterochromatin, or by other mechanisms that might affect the neighboring euchromatic genes.

The exquisite sensitivity of PEV to changes in the concentration of modifier protein has in turn suggested that the assembly of heterochromatic domains obeys the laws of mass-action, with the amount of assembled heterochromatin being directly dependent on the concentration of the constituent (structural) components (Fig. 5.4) (Locke *et al.*, 1988; Tartof *et al.*, 1989). As predicted by the mass-action model and emphasized above, modifiers that show such dosage effects are likely to encode structural components of heterochromatin, whereas modifiers that do not are more likely to encode enzymes that post-translationally modify the components. The mass-action model also provides an explanation for the observation that extra Y chromosomes present in the genome suppresses variegation of the euchromatic *white* gene (Fig. 5.3) (Gowan & Gay, 1933b). This effect can be explained as a titration of components necessary for heterochromatin assembly by the Y chromosome (Zuckerkandl, 1974), which in the somatic tissues of *Drosophila* is entirely heterochromatic. Thus the Y chromosome acts as a sink for components that would otherwise be used to repress genes by the formation of heterochromatin at the variegating breakpoint.

Some of the structural components of heterochromatin, apart from the histones, have now been characterized at the molecular level (Table 5.2). The first to be identified, and consequently the best studied, is heterochromatin protein 1 (James & Elgin, 1986).

Heterochromatin protein 1: the archetypal modifier of PEV

As part of a study to identify monoclonal antibodies that bind to specific regions on polytene chromosomes one of them, C1A9, was found to possess a reproducible pattern of staining on polytene chromosomes that included the whole length of chromosome 4, a few discrete sites in the arms, of which the most noticeable was the cytological interval 31–32 on the second chromosome, and, most strikingly, the entire β-heterochromatin of the chromocenter (Fig. 5.5A,B; James & Elgin, 1986; James *et al.*, 1989). In some preparations the telomeres were also labeled (James *et al.*, 1989). The gene encoding the C1A9 antigen, now called heterochromatin protein 1 (HP1), has been cloned (James & Elgin, 1986) and more recently shown, through the isolation and sequencing of two mutant alleles, to be the wild type allele of the position effect suppressor *Suvar(2)5* (Eissenberg *et al.*, 1990, 1992). Studies on the overexpression of the HP1 gene have shown that an increase in concentration of HP1 protein leads to an enhancement of variegation (Eissenberg *et al.*, 1992) and can rescue to some extent the recessive lethality of the homozygous mutant (Eissenberg & Hartnett, 1993). In a clinching experiment, HP1 protein was also found to localize to many of the euchromatic regions that become cytologically hetero-chromatinized by their translocation next to constitutive heterochromatin (Belyaeva *et al.*, 1993), a result which suggests that the dosage-dependent effects of the HP1 gene on PEV can be directly related to the compaction of euchromatin into heterochromatin that occurs at variegating breakpoints and, more importantly, that HP1 is usually a component of this repressive, hetero-chromatic, environment. That HP1 did not localize to all variegating break-points confirms the previous observation that heterochromatin itself is made up of different domains, some of which share many structural components and some of which contain components that are unique to a domain (Belyaeva & Zhimulev, 1991; Bishop, 1992).

Despite its crucial role in PEV, the true function of HP1 must lie elsewhere. Some clues as to the true physiology of HP1 have come from the isolation of HP1-like genes from mammals (Singh *et al.*, 1991). The protein product of one of these genes, M31, localizes to centromeric heterochromatin in both murine and human metaphase chromosomes (Fig. 5.5C) (Wreggett *et al.*, 1994). This conserved localization, which crosses the divide between methylation (mam-mals) and non-methylation (*Drosophila*), is suggestive in that HP1-like proteins might be required as part of highly condensed constitutive heterochromatin for proper centromere function. Some support for this contention has come from a detailed analysis of the null HP1 mutant phenotype in *Drosophila* embryos (Kellum & Alberts, 1995). In mutant embryos the principal effect of the

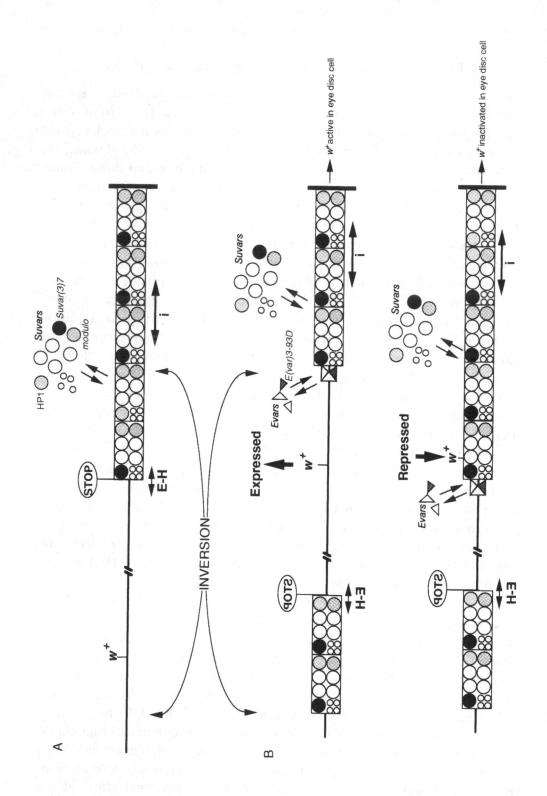

A

w⁺

STOP   E-H   i

HP1   Suvars   Suvar(3)7   modulo

INVERSION

B   Expressed

Evars   E(var)3-93D

w⁺

H-3   STOP

Suvars

i   w⁺ active in eye disc cell

Repressed

Evars

w⁺

H-3   STOP

Suvars

i   w⁺ inactivated in eye disc cell

Suvar(2)5 mutation is seen during anaphase where chromosomes are seen lagging between the segregating sister chromatids, leading to a lack of separation of the chromosomes during anaphase B of the cell cycle. Thus the null mutant appears to compromise centromere function. However, detailed examination of the staining pattern for HP1 on polytene chromosomes suggest that this is not likely to be the whole story.

The association of HP1 with bands 31–32 on the second chromosome is intriguing in that it highlights a small cluster of euchromatic genes, including the locus *abnormal oocyte (abo)*, that are known to interact with heterochromatin (Sandler, 1977; Pimpinelli *et al.*, 1985). *Drosophila* eggs that do not possess any product of the *abo* locus fail to develop, although they can be rescued by

Fig. 5.4. A highly schematic diagram illustrating the *cis*- and *trans*-acting factors that are likely to be involved in heterochromatic position effects. Based on the mass-action model of Tartof and his school (Locke *et al.*, 1988; Tartof *et al.*, 1989). (A) The normal chromosome where heterochromatin components (circles) encoded by *Suvars* (Table 5.2) such as HP1, *Suvar(3)7* and *modulo* assemble into a core complex (boxes with circles in them) that reiterates along the chromosome, forming a condensed heterochromatin domain. Genetic analysis shows that the core complex may include nucleosomal DNA (Moore *et al.*, 1979) which is represented by the line passing through the middle of the boxes. According to the model, the core complex can contain components that are required in more than one copy. A case is shown where four copies of the smallest circles are required per core complex. The domain is propagated in *cis* from an initiation site (i) that may consist of arrays of middle repetitive sequences such as Dr. D (Miklos & Costell, 1990). Termination of the complex occurs at a natural boundary or stop signal and forms the euchromatin–heterochromatin (E–H) junction. (B) A chromosomal inversion which has one breakpoint between i and the stop signal and permits the spreading of heterochromatin into a normally euchromatic region of the chromosome. According to the mass-action model, the final degree of spreading is dependent on a variety of factors, which include both the concentration of the *Suvar* components that form the heterochromatin itself and the *Envars* (triangles in the figure), such as *En(var)3–93D* (Table 5.2). The *Envars* have an antagonistic effect to the *Suvars*, in stopping the spreading of heterochromatin, and promoting euchromatin. The sensitivity to concentration changes is heightened if any of the components are required in more than one copy (e.g. the small circles). It is the outcome of the equilibrium brought about by these interactions that regulates the degree of spreading; as the concentration of any one of the many components in this equilibrium is likely to vary from cell to cell, the spreading also varies from cell to cell. For example, if, in one of the eight cells of the eye disk the spreading terminates before the *white* gene, the gene remains transcriptionally competent (expressible) and is transcribed in the progeny of the cell – at around the mid-pupal stage of development – giving rise to a sector that has the normal wild type coloration. On the other hand, if the spreading encapsulates the *white* gene, the gene is heterochromatinized (nonexpressible), and remains inactive, eventually giving rise to a colorless, mutant sector.

Table 5.2. *Molecular characterization of modifiers of PEV*

Over 150 modifiers of PEV have been described in the literature; they can either suppress or enhance variegation (Spofford, 1976; Henikoff, 1979; Tartof et al., 1989; Grigliatti 1991; Reuter & Spierer, 1992; Dorn et al., 1993a,b). This table contains only those that have been characterized at the molecular level. The placement of mus209/Pcna and Suvar(2)16 as enzymatic components is tentative, and is only on the basis of their suggested role in the remodeling of chromatin during DNA replication.

		References
Suppressors of PEV: structural components		
Histone genes	Deletion of part of the histone gene cluster suppresses variegation. This result formalized the relationship of chromatin to gene repression brought about by position effects.	Moore et al., 1979
Heterochromatin protein 1 (HP1)	The 26 kDa HP1 protein is diagnostic for β-heterochromatin and its gene is allelic to the *Suvar(2)5* mutation that is located at 29A on the second chromosome. Homozygous mutants do not survive, as is the case with all strong suppressors of PEV. Its binding to polytene chromosomes is co-extensive with the middle repetitive sequence Dr.D. The gene is transcribed during oogenesis, but the protein can only be detected in the nuclei of late blastoderm embryos.	James & Elgin, 1986; James et al., 1989; Eissenberg et al., 1990
Suvar(3)7	Duplications of the *Suvar(3)7* gene, which lies at 87E on the third chromosome, enhance variegation, and deficiencies suppress variegation. The gene is transcribed in the egg, and the mutation has a strong maternal effect. The gene product consists of a zinc-finger protein with five widely spaced fingers. This spacing is thought to be important in its suggested role in the packaging of heterochromatin. It has many phosphorylation sites that are used for regulation of its activity. The *Suvar(3)7* gene product has not been located with antibodies to heterochromatin in polytene chromosomes, and its role in heterochromatin formation is inferred from the dosage effects on variegation. Its absence in polytene chromosomes might reflect a restricted role for *Suvar(3)7* in the initial steps of heterochromatin formation.	Reuter et al., 1990; Reuter & Spierer, 1992
modulo	*modulo* lies at 100F on the third chromosome and deficiencies in this gene suppress variegation; *modulo*, like *Suvar(3)7*, has many phosphorylation sites that might be involved in its regulation. *modulo* binds the chromocenter and about 100 euchromatic sites in the arms. *modulo* mRNA is produced during embryogenesis up until the preblastoderm stage of development, when it is translated. During embryogenesis its zygotic expression is lineage-specific, being restricted to primordia that develop into endomesodermal and cephalopharyngeal structures. These observations suggest that *modulo* may be involved in regulation of euchromatic genes through regional compaction of chromatin.	Krejci et al., 1989; Grazino et al., 1992

Suppressors of PEV: enzymatic components

Suvar(2)16

Suvar(2)16 lies at position 31E on chromosome two, which is within a cluster of suppressors that had been described previously. The antimorphic nature of the original allele (216A) originally suggested that the gene encoded by *Suvar(2)16* might be a structural component of heterochromatin. However, P-element tagging of the gene has led to its isolation and it shares 70% homology with the yeast protein kinase *cdc2*, which plays a crucial role in determining the timing of entrance into M-phase. The known H1-kinase activity of *cdc2* indicates a possible role in phosphorylation of chromatin components during chromatin assembly at around the time of cell division.

Grigliatti, 1991

mus209/Pcna

mus209/Pcna maps within the 56F5-15 region of the second chromosome. PCNA is the well-known proliferating cell nuclear antigen and is an essential component of the replication machinery. Mutations in PCNA are pleiotrophic and are thought to have a common basis in problems with DNA replication. A requirement for replication in the assembly of heterochromatin or repressed chromosomal domains at the silent mating-type loci has been known for some time, and suggests that replication may also be important for the assembly of heterochromatin domains in PEV; the site for assembly of heterochromatin and heterochromatin-like complexes may be origins of replication. The suggested role of PCNA in PEV is thought to be as a factor required for chromatin assembly at the time of DNA replication, perhaps in concert with a molecule like CAF-1. Thus PCNA has more in common with an enzymatic component than a structural component, hence its tentative placement in this section.

Henderson *et al.*, 1994

Suvar(3)6

Suvar(3)6 is at position 87B on the third chromosome and encodes a protein phosphatase (PP1). PP1 is thought to be involved in the phosphorylation-dependent regulation of *Suvar(3)7*. Like many suppressors of PEV that are enzymes it does not show any dosage effects, even when in three copies in the genome. The large number of phosphorylatable sites in *Suvar(3)7* and *modulo* make them ideal targets for regulation by secondary messenger systems. PP1 might be a component of such a system that regulates heterochromatin formation.

Dombardi & Cohen, 1992

Enhancer of PEV: structural component

E(var)3–93D

E(var)3–93D is located in region 93D of the third chromosome. It had previously been transposon-tagged in a screen for modifier loci, and is the first enhancer of PEV to be characterized molecularly. *E(var)3–93D* appears to interact with suppressors of PEV directly, as mutations in *E(var)3–93D* suppress the dominant suppressor effect of the mutations *Suvar(2)1, Suvar(2)5* (HP1), *Suvar(3)3* and *Suvar(3)9*. This observation has suggested that *E(var)3–93D* is a chromatin component required for the maintenance of an 'open' expressible chromatin configuration. *E(var)3–93D* is also a positive regulator of the bithorax complex, an observation that again suggests a mechanistic link between PEV and maintenance of the homeogene expression patterns. The *E(var)3–93D* mutation also leaves an epigenetic mark on the Y chromosome, which can be paternally transmitted for several generations.

Dorn *et al.*, 1993a,b

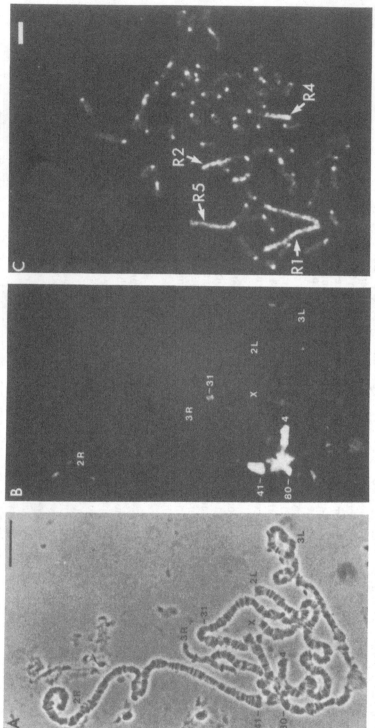

Fig. 5.5. Distribution pattern of HP1 and a murine HP1-like protein, M31, on polytene and metaphase chromosomes, respectively. (A) A phase contrast micrograph of a polytene chromosome spread. (B) A fluorescence micrograph of the same spread stained with the anti-HP1 antibody C1A9. HP1 protein localizes to the chromocenter, the fourth chromosome and regions 41, 80 and 31. The bar in A is 50 µm. Reproduced, with permission, from James *et al.* (1989). (C) Fluorescence micrograph of a metaphase spread from the murine methotrexate-resistant cell line PG19T3::MTX$_R^{10-4M}$ after staining with the anti-M31 monoclonal antibody AFRC MAC353. M31 localizes to the centromeric heterochromatin of the normal metaphase chromosomes and to the large blocks of constitutive heterochromatin in the four giant chromosomes, R2, R3, R4 and R5, which are found in this cell line. The bar is 5 µm. Reproduced, with permission, from Wreggett *et al.* (1994).

paternally derived *abo* gene product contributed by the sperm. The degree to which the embryo may be rescued depends on whether the *abo* gene derived from the father is located within heterochromatin or euchromatin. There are three heterochromatic copies of *abo*, designated *ABO*: one lies in the basal heterochromatin of the X chromosome and there is one copy in each of the arms of the Y. When a single heterochromatic *ABO* gene is introduced into the zygote via the sperm, rescue is effected only during the first stages of development, well before the activation of the zygotic genome. This early rescue is short-lived, for when the zygotic genome switches on and heterochromatin (and HP1) (James *et al.*, 1989) becomes cytologically visible within the nucleus, development is again halted and the embryos die. In stark contrast, a wild-type euchromatic *abo* gene contributed by the sperm completely rescues the egg, as expected. These results suggest that *Drosophila* HP1 may, as part of a repressor complex, be involved in epigenetically silencing genes that act very early during development, when the zygotic genome is largely silent. In addition, the localization of HP1 to the cytologically euchromatic (banded) fourth chromosome, and the observation that translocations involving this chromosome can sometimes give rise to variegation (Griffen & Stone, 1940), provides strong support for the notion that repression through higher-order chromatin packaging, involving HP1-like proteins, might also determine the transcriptional fate of genes within euchromatin.

Thus, careful study of the binding pattern of HP1 has led to the suggestion that mechanisms similar to those proposed for the formation of heterochromatin domains might also exist for domains within euchromatin (Singh *et al.*, 1991). It almost follows that if such packaging is widespread within the genome that we might, perhaps, expect a large class of proteins to be involved in this regional compaction of euchromatin into *heterochromatin-like* complexes. It is the finding that HP1 does indeed share a region of homology with another *Drosophila* protein, namely Polycomb (Pc) (Paro & Hogness, 1991), a protein also involved in the heritable inactivation of genes, which has added support to the suggestion that chromatin compaction, similar to that found in heterochromatin, is likely to exist elsewhere in the genome.

Role of the *Polycomb* gene in cellular determination

The early determination and clonal inheritance of gene expression patterns which characterize PEV are also an intrinsic feature of normal development in *Drosophila* and are clearly recognizable in the many studies that have been made on the homeogenes (Akam, 1987; Duncan, 1987). Homeogenes are determinants of cellular fate in flies, mice and, by extrapolation, humans (for review, see McGinnis & Krumlauf, 1992). It is through their spatially restricted patterns of expression that they set up the identities of the structures and appendages along the anterior–posterior (A–P) axis of the body. When the expression of the homeogenes is aberrant or missing, through mutation, and they are expressed inappropriately, dramatic shifts in cellular fate can take place. For example, rearrangements that place the *Antennapedia (Antp)* gene under the control of head-specific regulatory elements lead to the inappropriate expression of *Antp* in cells which will form the eye-antennal disk, and result in the classical transformation of the antennae into legs (Boulet & Scott, 1988). Moreover, mis-expression of the homeogenes can change cellular fate at any time during development (Struhl, 1981). Thus, for completion of normal development the spatially restricted homeogene expression patterns must be maintained, i.e. homeogenes must be active within their normal realms of expression and be repressed outside of them. These two states must also be maintained through many mitotic divisions until development is complete.

In *Drosophila*, the *trithorax*-Group (*trx*-G) (Kennison, 1993) and the *Polycomb*-Group (*Pc*-G) (Jurgens, 1985) of genes play a crucial role in maintaining, respectively, the active and repressed state of the homeotic genes. Some clues to the means whereby the *Pc*-G might heritably repress homeogene activity has come from the isolation and sequencing of the group's namesake, *Pc*. *Pc* shares a 37 amino acid domain, called the chromodomain, with HP1 (see Fig. 5.7) (Paro & Hogness, 1991). Identification of this motif brought together two different classes of genes that are involved in the repression of gene activity and, most importantly, suggested that the *Pc*-G of genes might exert their effect through heritable changes in chromatin structure. By analogy with the mass-action model for heterochromatin assembly (Locke *et al.*, 1988; Tartof *et al.*, 1989) the *Pc*-G genes are also thought to encode proteins that form a multimeric complex (Gaunt & Singh, 1990; Paro, 1990) (Fig. 5.6D), a contention that has recently been borne out by elegant immunoprecipitation experiments (Franke *et al.*, 1992).

Immunostaining of polytene chromosomes with anti-*Pc* antibodies has shown that the Pc protein binds to over 100 specific sites on polytene chromosomes (Zink & Paro, 1989), many of which are shared by other members of the *Pc*-G (Rastelli *et al.*, 1993); the latter finding is a prediction of previous models (Gaunt & Singh, 1990; Paro, 1990). From this initial observation a considerable amount of data has accumulated on both the *cis*-acting sequences and *trans*-acting factors required to direct the assembly of the *Pc*-G complex at specific sites within the fly genome. Indirect evidence that sequences surrounding the homeogenes are likely to contain sites required for *Pc*-G assembly came from transgenic experiments. For example, three *cis*-acting elements known to regulate genes within the *bithorax* complex, namely *bxd, iab-2* and *iab-3*, have been coupled to *LacZ* and shown to be able to faithfully reproduce the anterior boundaries of the corresponding homeogene (Muller & Bienz, 1991; Simon *et al.*, 1993). These expression patterns are dependent upon members of the *Pc*-G, as mutation in any one of eight members of the *Pc*-G results in the aberrant expression of *LacZ* in parasegments anterior to the normal expression domain. An interesting feature of these experiments is that the sequences required to specify the assembly of the *Pc*-G complex – which may represent binding sites for segmentation genes – are separable for the sequences required for the assembly of the *Pc*-G complex itself (Simon *et al.*, 1993). The latter sequences may, in fact, be generic: when they are coupled to any one of a variety of different regulatory elements they can direct the silencing of the element in anterior parasegments where the element does not normally act (Muller & Bienz, 1991; Simon *et al.*, 1993).

More direct evidence for Pc-binding sites has come from co-immuno-precipitation experiments where antibodies have localized Pc protein to specific sites within the abdominal region of the *bithorax* complex, such as *Mcp* and *Fab-7* (Orlando & Paro, 1993). These sites had previously been designated as boundaries (Eissenberg & Elgin, 1991) that insulate homeogenes from the possible promiscuous activities of parasegment-specific enhancers (Peifer *et al.*, 1987; Galloni *et al.*, 1993). Pc protein was also found in chromatin immuno-precipitated from the *Antp-P1* and *Abd-B* promoters (Orlando & Paro, 1993), a result which suggests that the sequences required for *Pc*-G silencing of these genes may be closely associated with the sequences normally required for their activation. Transgenic experiments have also shown that as little as 2.9 kb of flanking sequence linked to a *white* marker gene is sufficient to assemble the *Pc*-G complex, when assayed by antibody binding to the product of *Polyhomeotic (Ph)* (Fauvarque & Dura, 1993). Interestingly, the *white* gene exhibited noticeable variegation, indicating that the realm of action of the *Pc*-G complex did not always extend the full 2.9 kb required for repression.

Taken together, these experiments provide formal proof that *cis*-acting sequences are necessary for the binding of *Pc*-G proteins and the assembly of a repressed chromosomal domain. They also suggest that the assembly of a *heterochromatin-like* complex can regulate gene expression *locally*, on a gene-by-gene basis, and may only need to complex sequences required for activation (promoters or enhancers) in order to effectively silence a gene. The assembly of the *Pc*-G complex also appears to be able to act as a boundary that can insulate a gene from neighboring *cis*-acting enhancer elements (Galloni *et al.*, 1993). This feature may be particularly relevant to models, to be discussed, of the reciprocal imprinting of the *Igf2* and *H19* genes (Bartolomei *et al.*, 1993; Efstratiadis, 1994).

Whereas the *cis*-acting DNA fragments required for proper assembly of the

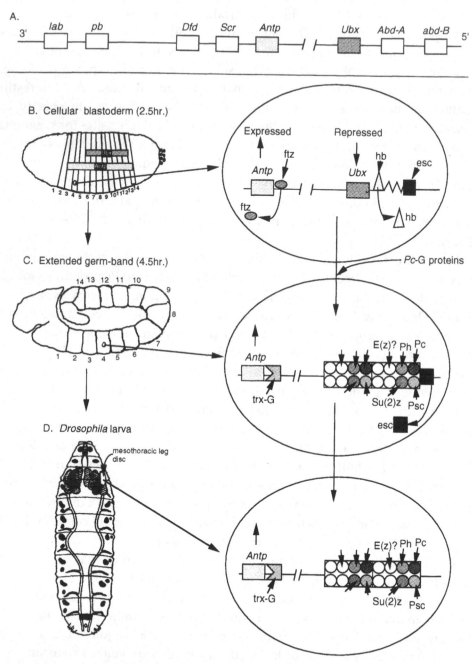

Fig. 5.6. A schematic diagram illustrating the stepwise progression towards cell fate determination. (A) The homeobox genes in *Drosophila* are divided into two clusters known as the *Bithorax* and *Antennapedia* complexes. The homeobox genes are ordered (5'–3') as follows: *Abdominal-B* (*Abd-B*), *abdominal-A* (*abd-A*), *Ultrabithorax* (*Ubx*), *Antennapedia* (*Antp*), *Sex combs reduced* (*Scr*), *Deformed* (*Dfd*), *proboscipedia* (*pb*), *labial* (*lab*). (B) At the cellular blastoderm

Caption for Fig. 5.6 (*cont.*)

stage of development the parasegmentally restricted pattern of homeogene expression determines the fate of cells along the A–P axis. Here I focus only on the *Antp* and *Ubx* homeotic genes, whose realms of expression encompass parasegments 3–14 and 5–13, respectively. In a cell taken from parasegment 4 of the cellular blastoderm the *Antp* gene is active, and it is through the exclusive expression of the *Antp* gene in parasegment 4 that the cell is fated to become part of the mesothoracic leg. Also, because this domain is anterior to the normal realm of expression of the *Ubx* gene, the *Ubx* gene is inactive, and must remain so if the fate of the cell is to be sealed. The initial repression of the *Ubx* gene is through the binding of a transcriptional repressor, *hunchback* (*hb*). The hb protein acts as an 'imprintor' that imprints a site on the DNA that will direct the assembly of the *Pc*-G complex. The binding of the hunchback protein is only transient and because of this we suggest that its binding is recognized by another protein, perhaps by the product of the *extra sex combs* (*esc*) gene, which is an early-acting member of the *Pc*-G. The recognition of hb binding by esc is not direct; instead esc is envisaged to recognize local, transient, changes in chromatin structure (zig-zag line), which result from binding of hb to its recognition sequence. The *Pc*-G may assemble at, or around, the same time as esc binds. (C) In a cell (progeny of the cell above) taken from parasegment 4 of the extended germ-band embryo, the *Pc*-G complex has already assembled on the site marked by *esc*. Note the similarity of the *Pc*-G complex and the heterochromatin complex described in Fig. 5.4. Of the *Pc*-G members, the protein products of *Polycomb* (*Pc*), *Polyhomeotic* (*Ph*), *Posterior sex combs* (*Psc*) and *Suppressor* (*2*) *of zeste* (*Su(2)z*) have been immunolocalized to the homeotic genes of polytene chromosomes. The mutant phenotype of *Enhancer of zeste* (*E(z)*) suggests that it may be part of the *Pc*-G complex (Rastelli *et al.*, 1993), although it has yet to be shown to localize to the homeotic genes. Immunochemical studies have also shown that the *Pc*-G complex does not contain H1 histone (Franke *et al.*, 1992) and may only therefore contain nucleosomal DNA. The activation of *Antp* in parasegment 4 by the fushi tarazu (ftz) protein (Ingham & Martinez-Arias, 1986) is also translated into a more permanent form of activation by the *trithorax*-group of genes (*trx*-G). The *trx*-G keeps the chromatin surrounding the *Antp* in an open 'expressible' state that maintains expression of *Antp* throughout embryogenesis. Two of the major, but no means only, players in the *trx*-G are the group's namesake *trithorax* (Mazo *et al.*, 1990) and the *brahma* gene (Tamkun *et al.*, 1992). *En(var)3–93D* also appears to be involved in maintaining the activity of the homeogenes and may therefore be a member of both the *trx*-G and the *Evar*s. Beyond the extended germ-band stage of development the need for *esc* is removed. (D) Cells that expressed the *Antp* gene in parasegment 4 of the early embryo have greatly expanded and now form part of the mesothoracic leg disk within the *Drosophila* larva. The disk will differentiate into the mesothoracic leg during metamorphosis. A cell taken from this disk possesses the final, heritable, state of chromatin that determines the transcriptional fate of the *Antp* and *Ubx* genes: the *Antp* gene is maintained in an expressible state by the *trx*-G of genes, while the *Ubx* gene is rendered inexpressible by the *Pc*-G of genes.

Pc-G can be broadly defined by the experiments above, the *trans*-acting factors required for specific assembly have been less well characterized. However, some clues to the means whereby the *Pc*-G complex binds to specific sites within the cluster have come from mutational analysis of a segmentation gene, *hunchback* (*hb*), a gene known to be involved in setting up the homeogene expression patterns (White & Lehmann, 1986). Particular emphasis in these experiments has been given to the repression of the *Ubx* gene, whose normal realm of activity encompasses parasegments 5–13 (Akam, 1987) (Fig. 5.6B). Anterior to these parasegments it has been proposed that initial *Ubx* repression is by the hb protein (Zhang & Bienz, 1992) and it is this initial binding of hb that may direct the specific assembly of the *Pc*-G complex (Fig. 5.6B). The imprint provided by the hb protein is developmentally labile and is stable for just a few cell divisions, because the maternal and segmentation genes in *Drosophila* are only expressed maximally for a brief period during embryogenesis, for the 2 h before the cellular blastoderm stage of development, whereupon their concentrations fall rapidly (Akam, 1987). At the time the concentration of hb is falling, cells along the A–P axis have begun to express homeogenes or set of homeogenes that will determine their fates (Simcox & Sang, 1983). It is this pattern of homeogene expression that must be maintained, and so the transient repression of *Ubx* mediated by hb protein has to be translated into a more permanent form of repression.

Transduction of the initial binding of hb into the more stable repression conferred by the *Pc*-G complex may be via an intermediary molecule, of which the most likely candidate is extra sex combs (esc) (Struhl, 1981). This is the earliest-acting member of the *Pc*-G and is, like hb, developmentally labile, being required for repression of the homeogenes only up until the extended germ-band stage (Fig. 5.6C) (Struhl, 1981, 1983). The *esc* gene is also specific for the selector genes within the clusters, as it is not required for determination of the transcriptional fate of another selector gene, *engrailed (en)* (Moazed & O'Farrell, 1992). Interestingly, the final state of determination of *en* requires the repression conferred by the rest of the *Pc*-G of genes (Heemskerk *et al.*, 1991). No direct interaction of hb with esc is envisaged, since the sites for initiation and maintenance of the homeogene expression patterns are separable (Simon *et al.*, 1993); instead esc may recognize the local, transient, changes in chromatin structure that accompany the temporary repression of *Ubx* by hb. According to this scheme, binding of esc enables the assembly of the rest of the *Pc*-G repressor complex (Fig. 5.6C). Four products of the *Pc*-G have so far been immunolocalized to the homeogenes: *Pc* (Zink & Paro, 1989), *Ph* (DeCamillis *et al.*, 1992), *Posterior sex combs* (*Psc*) (Brunk *et al.*, 1991) and *Suppressor (2) of zeste* (*Su(2)z*) (Rastelli *et al.*, 1993). Once assembled, the requirement for esc protein after the extended germ-band stage is removed and the complex renucleates on the site(s) identified by *hb* and *esc*, during further rounds of DNA replication (Fig. 5.6D).

The final assembly of the *Pc*-G complex (Fig. 5.6D) represents half of the requirement for the maintenance of the homeogene expression patterns, since another group of genes are required for maintaining the activity of homeogenes, namely the *trx-G* (reviewed by Kennison, 1993). It is beyond the scope of the present discussion to describe this important group in detail; however, it is noteworthy that the *Evar(3)93D* enhancer mutation (Table 5.2) does have an effect on the homeogene expression patterns, suggesting that the *Evar*s have much in common with the *trx*-G. In addition, mutation in the *Psc* results in the suppression of PEV (D. A. R. Sinclair *et al.*, unpublished; cited in Wu, 1993), suggesting that the *Pc*-G of genes are analogous to the *Suvar*s.

Once the activities of the *trx*-G and *Pc*-G genes are brought into place the fate of cells is sealed and, as in PEV, remains so through many mitotic divisions to the end of development. Indeed, the ability of imaginal disks (Fig. 5.6D) to differentiate appropriately even after the time between determination and differentiation has been greatly expanded (Hadorn, 1965), in some cases from days to years, implies that the state of determination, as regulated by the *trx*-G and *Pc*-G of genes, is very stable. We have suggested previously (Gaunt & Singh, 1990) that the occasional lapses from stability (transdetermination) are due to changes in the epigenetic regulation of homeogene expression by the *trx*-G and *Pc*-G genes, leading to inappropriate expression, or repression, of homeogenes within imaginal disk cells.

The mechanisms of repression that involve HP1 and *Pc* are likely to be conserved. Sequences that hybridize with the chromobox are found in a wide variety of animal and plant species (Singh *et al.*, 1991); moreover, the motif can be used to clone genes from other organisms that are either HP1-like or *Pc*-like (Fig. 5.7A).

The chromobox gene family

The original members of the chromobox gene family were HP1 and *Pc*; and the 37 amino acid region of homology between these two proteins defines the minimal chromodomain (Fig. 5.7A) (Paro & Hogness, 1991). Of these 37 amino acids, which lie towards the N-termini of both proteins, 24 are identical. The chromobox gene family is expanding all the time. New members have been cloned from a variety of organisms including humans (Singh *et al.*, 1991; Saunders *et al.*, 1993), mouse (Singh *et al.*, 1991; Pearce *et al.*, 1992; Saunders *et al.*, 1993), mealy bug (Epstein *et al.*, 1992) and yeast (Lorentz *et al.*, 1994). They can be placed into either the HP1 or the *Pc* subfamily, not only on the basis of

A

The HP1 and *Polycomb* Chromodomain protein subfamilies

Pc-like chromodomain proteins

```
Pc consensus  - - - - - V - A Q E - I - - K R - - K G - - E Y - - V K M - G M - - - N - N E P E - N - L D - - R L - -
M33           S V G E Q V F A A E C I L S K R L R K G K L E Y - L V K W R G W S S - K H N S W E P E E N I L D - P R L L A P Q K K E H E

Pc            D P V D L V - A A E I I Q K R V K K G V V E Y - R Y N K G W N Q - R Y N T W E P E V N - I L D - - R R L I D I Y E Q T N K S
                        1 -                 10 -              20 -            30 -                40 -               50 -
HP1           E E E E E - A V R K I I D R R V R R G K V E Y - Y L K W K G Y P E - T E N T W E P E N N - L D C Q D L I Q Q Y E A S R K D

DV HP1        E E E E E E Y A V E K I L D R R V R K G K V E Y - Y L K W K G Y A E - T E N T W E P E G N - L D C Q D L I Q Q Y E L S R K D
HSM1          E E E E E E Y V V E K V L D R R V V K G K V E Y - L L K W K G F S D - E D N T W E P E E N - L D C P D L I A E P L L S Q K T
M31           E E E E E E Y V V E K V L D R R V V K G K V E Y - L L K W K G F S D - E D N T W E P E E N - L D C P D L I A E P L L S Q K T
M32           E A E E E F V V E K V L D R R V V N G K V E Y - P L K W K G F T D - A D N T W E P E E N - L D C P D L I E D F L N S Q K K A
HP1(hsu)      S E D E E E Y V V E K V L D R R V V K G Q V E Y - L L K W K G F S E - E H N T W E P E K N - L D C P E L I S E F M K K Y K K
Pchet 1       G S E E E E Y V V E K I I D K R T V N G K V Q Y - P L K W K G Y D E - S E N T W E P E E N - L E C P E L I A E P E K K W E K
Pchet 2       P A V E E E P I V E K I L D K R T E P D G S V R Y L L K W K G Y G D - E D N T W E P E E N - K D C E D L L E E P E K K L S K
Swi-6         E E E D E D Y V V E K I L H R M A R K G G G Y E L L K W E G Y D D P S D N T W S S E A D C S G C K Q L I E A Y W N E H G G
HP1 consensus e e e e e - Q y v v E k v l d r r v r k g k v e y - l Q K M k G y p e - - d N T W e p E e n - l d C p d - l i - - f - - s - - k -
```

HP1-like chromodomain proteins

B

Chromodomain helicase DNA binding (ChD) protein subfamily

```
Pc            D P V D L V - A A E I I Q K R V K K G V V E Y - R V K K - G W N Q R Y N T W E P E V N - I L D - - R R L I D I Y E Q T N K S
                        1 -                 10 -              20 -            30 -                40 -               50 -
HP1           E E E E E - A V R K I I D R R V R R G K V E Y - Y L K W K - G Y P E B N T W E P E N N - L - D C Q D L I Q Q Y E A S R K D

ChD-1         G A T T I Y A V E - 15 RESIDUES - G D I Q Y - L I K W K - G W S H I H N T W E T E E T L - - K Q - - -
Yeast ChD-1   - - - - - - - - - - - - - - N Y E F - L I K W T - D E S H L H N T W E T Y E S I - - G Q - - -
ChD consensus - - - - - - - - - - - - - - - - - - L I K M - - S H - N T W E T - E - - Q - - -
```

sequence homology to the canonical member of each subfamily (HP1 or Pc) but also on size: the Pc-like proteins are much bigger than the HP1-like proteins (Pearce *et al.*, 1992; Messemer *et al.*, 1992; Clarke & Elgin, 1992). The *Pc*-like genes also share a C-terminal homology (Pearce *et al.*, 1992). Comparison of the HP1-like and Pc-like proteins within the chromodomain has revealed only a few residues that remain invariant across both subfamilies, such as those present at positions 4, 20, 21, 23, 29, 31, 33 and 34. Moreover, sequences around the chromodomain can also be identified as being peculiar to either the HP1 or Pc subfamilies, thus extending the chromodomain for each subfamily to around 48 amino acids (Fig. 5.7A) (Pearce *et al.*, 1992; Messemer *et al.*, 1992; Clarke & Elgin, 1992). For example, immediately adjacent to the chromodomain of HP1-like proteins is a stretch of negatively charged amino acids (usually glutamic acid) that is a striking feature and diagnostic of this subfamily. The negatively charged group of residues is also found in the newest member of the HP1 class, Swi-6 (Lorentz *et al.*, 1994), a protein that is crucial for silencing of the donor mating type loci in *Schizosaccharomyces pombe* (Klar & Bonaduce, 1991; Lorentz *et al.*, 1992). In this context it is pertinent to draw attention to the growing similarity – which stems from the central role played by chromodomain proteins – between

Fig. 5.7. Compilation of chromodomain amino acid sequences. (A) The HP1 and *Pc* chromodomain subfamilies. The shaded box represents the minimal chromodomain with the sequence of *Pc* given above the HP1 sequence. All sequences are aligned with respect to this sequence; gaps in the sequences, required for alignment, are represented by dashes. The *Pc* consensus sequence is derived from the comparison of M33 (Pearce *et al.*, 1992), the murine homolog of *Pc*, and *Pc* (Paro & Hogness, 1991). The upper-case letters represent residues that remain invariant in the *Pc* subfamily but can sometimes be found in members of the HP1 subfamily. Boxes around the upper-case letters represent residues that are invariant across both subfamilies; circles around the residues denote subfamily-specific residues. Enough HP1 subfamily members have now been cloned from *Drosophila melanogaster* (James & Elgin, 1986), *D. virilis* (Clarke & Elgin, 1992), the mouse (Singh *et al.*, 1991), humans (Singh *et al.*, 1991; Saunders *et al.*, 1993) and the mealy bug (Epstein *et al.*, 1992) that a more complete consensus sequence of the HP1 chromodomain can be given. Lower-case letters in the consensus sequence denote conservation in at least five out of nine sequences. A dash in the consensus indicates that fewer than five out of nine residues at this location are conserved. The designation for the upper-case letters is as for the *Pc* consensus. (B) ChD-1 chromodomain subfamily. The consensus sequence shows that the region of homology between the ChD-1 protein and the minimal chromodomain is limited to the left half. Both these proteins do, however, share an extensive region of homology towards their C-termini that has high homology with DNA helicases. The ChD-1 proteins may therefore have more in common with chromatin activation than with repression. The ChD-1 sequence is from Delmas *et al.* (1993). The yeast ChD-1 sequence is, as yet, unpublished but is in the EMBL data base under the accession number L10718.

the suggested mechanisms of repression involved in PEV (Fig. 5.4) and the maintenance of the homeogene expression patterns (Fig. 5.6). With the discovery of the swi-6 protein, the original mass-action model (Fig. 5.4) can be extended to repression of the silent mating type loci.

The structure of the chromodomain is, as yet, unknown. It does not appear to be involved in protein–DNA interactions, as determined by South Western analysis (T. C. James, unpublished), and is therefore more likely to be involved in protein–protein interactions. Its role in Pc and HP1 function has been tested by deletion analysis, but no firm conclusion can yet be drawn. Selective deletions or non-conservative substitutions within the chromodomain of the Pc protein has shown that an intact chromodomain is required for proper localization of the Pc protein to polytene chromosomes: mutant Pc protein appears to aggregate into large disorganized masses within the nucleus (Messemer *et al.*, 1992). Conversely, a similar study using β-gal fusions of mutated forms of HP1 (Powers & Eissenberg, 1993) has shown that the chromodomain is not required for proper localization of the rest of the protein to heterochromatin.

However, any function ascribed to the chromodomain must now incorporate the finding of a chromodomain motif, albeit distantly related, in the ChD-1 (Chromodomain-*h*elicase-*D*NA binding) proteins (Fig. 5.4B) (Delmas *et al.*, 1993; Mulligen *et al.*, 1993), which also possesses a DNA helicase motif reminiscent of those found in the SW12/SNF2 protein in yeast (Peterson & Herskowitz, 1992) and the brahma protein in *Drosophila* (Tamkun *et al.*, 1992). The latter proteins are known to be involved in relieving the repressive effect of chromatin, suggesting that ChD-1 proteins may have more in common with the *Envars* (Table 5.2) and thus may be important in maintaining the *active* state of genes. The presence of chromodomains in proteins that are known to be involved in repression (HP1, Pc, swi-6) and in a protein likely – but not yet proven – to be involved in maintaining gene activity (ChD-1) suggests that the chromodomain might be involved in a variety of different protein–protein interactions. On the other hand, it may be that the protein (or proteins) that interacts with the chromodomain may be similar for all chromodomain-containing proteins (a histone, perhaps?) and the effect of this interaction on gene expression, that is repression or activation, is determined by the rest of the molecule.

In the next section we discuss the relevance, if any, of the epigenetic mechanisms we have described above to the parental imprinting phenomena that form the central theme of this volume.

Parental imprinting and PEV: insights into the nature of the imprint

A remarkable result that has received little attention is the observation that the degree of PEV is dependent upon whether the rearranged chromosome is derived through the sperm or the egg (Morgan *et al.*, 1937; Noujdin, 1944; especially Spofford, 1959, 1961; Hessler, 1961). The most convincing demonstration of the non-equivalence of reciprocal crosses is with the autosomally inherited rearrangement $Dp(1;3)N^{264-58a}$, which involves an insertion of around 20 bands from the X chromosome into the proximal heterochromatin of 3L (Fig. 5.8A). The insertion includes the *white* gene in an inverted orientation such that the *white-diminutive* (w^+-dm^+) segment is reversed in its polarity in relation to the centromere. This rearrangement brings about marked variegation within the eyes for *white*. Moreover, in all tissues examined the mutant areas are much less extensive when $Dp(1;3)N^{264-58a}$ is transmitted through the sperm than through the egg.

This parental-origin effect is not due to any differences that might arise from conditioning of egg cytoplasm by the premeiotic presence or absence of the rearrangement in the mother. In crosses where *both* parents harbor $Dp(1;3)N^{264-58a}$, and in fathers the non-rearranged homolog is marked, the parental origin of the duplication can be determined in sons with certainty. This is because homozygosity for the duplication in males is lethal. Thus in the cross $Dp(1;3)N^{264-58a}/+$ (mothers) × $Dp(1;3)N^{264-58a}/W$ (fathers) where the dominant marker for the normal third chromosome is *Wrinkled* (*W*; wrinkled wings), the *W* sons have the maternal duplication whereas the duplication in non-*W* sons is paternally derived (Fig. 5.8B). Comparison of the degree of variegation showed that non-*W* sons have 4–5 times as much pigment as *W* sons (Baker, 1963). To rule out the possibility of the difference being attributed to *W*-bearing (normal) and unmarked (rearranged) third chromosomes, the reciprocal cross was also examined, with the paternal derivation of the duplication again giving rise to more pigment in sons.

These results represent one of the early examples of parental imprinting, where the rearrangement, derived from the father, has on it a mark or 'imprint' (see Appendix, p. 100), which leads to a reduction of the mutant phenotype (and therefore of repression) in his progeny. This imprint is epigenetic: in grand-children that inherit the duplication from daughters of the cross it is reversed, and the variegation (and therefore the repression) is enhanced (Spofford, 1959). Reversibility is an essential component of the original definition of chromosomal imprinting (Crouse, 1960) and makes this example distinct from Y chromosome imprinting (Reuter *et al.*, 1982; Dorn *et al.*, 1993a) where the imprint on the Y chromosome appears to be permanent, since the direction of its effect on

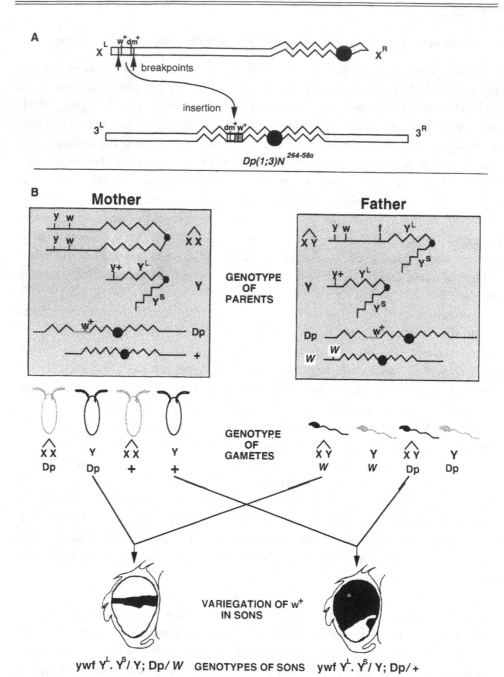

Fig. 5.8. The degree of variegation in PEV is affected by parental origin of the rearrangement. (A) The $Dp(1;3)N^{264-58a}$ chromosome is an inverted insertion of 20 chromosome bands from the X chromosome into the proximal hetero-chromatin of the left arm of chromosome 3. (B) Cytological and genetical constitution of the flies used to show that variegation caused by position effect of $Dp(1;3)N^{264-58a}$ can be affected by parental origin. Both parents contain

variegation in sons is the same whether the 'imprinted' Y chromosome is inherited from an XY father or indirectly through a XX/Y mother.

Because the parental origin of the rearrangement changes the number of pigmented sectors within the mottled eye (Fig. 5.8B) it can be concluded that the imprint acts via the normal mechanism of determination (Baker, 1963; cf. Fig. 5.2). By analogy with the explanation suggested for the known effect of heat shock during the first temperature-sensitive period (Fig. 5.3) (Spofford, 1976), the imprint might modulate – perhaps by being part of – the *initial steps* involved in the assembly of heterochromatin at the variegating breakpoint.

That the imprint might affect the initial assembly of heterochromatin puts us in mind of the role of the hb and esc proteins in directing the assembly of the *Pc*-G complex (Singh, 1994). Some parental imprints may, in fact, have much in common with proteins like hb; they may be developmentally labile and change during gametogenesis or embryogeny through intermediary molecules like *esc*, before becoming permanent later in development through heritable changes in chromatin structure, including those brought about by DNA methylation in mammals. Because there is a demand for specificity in parental imprinting effects (specific genes are imprinted), the initial 'imprintor' (see Appendix, p. 100) is unlikely to be methyltransferase: a single enzyme cannot be responsible, alone, for all the observed, specific effects.

The original studies on parental imprinting provide firm evidence that a parental imprint can be stored for several cellular generations before becoming permanent through later changes in chromatin structure. In male coccids of the species *Plannococcus citri*, both chromosomal sets are euchromatic and indistinguishable during the early divisions, and it is only at the time that the nuclei migrate to the periphery of the egg, just before cellularization, that the paternal chromosome set is heterochromatinized and rendered genetically inert (Brown & Nur, 1975). A similar observation has been made in *Sciara coprophila*, where the first few divisions are normal and, again, as the nuclei begin to migrate to the

Caption for Fig. 5.8 (*cont.*)

Dp(1;3)N²⁶⁴⁻⁵⁸ᵃ; however, in fathers the normal unrearranged chromosome bears a dominant marker, *W* (Wrinkled wings), which can be used to identify the parental origin of the normal, unrearranged third chromosome. The *W* marker does not affect variegation itself. Both parents also possess a Y chromosome, which suppresses variegation and makes it easier to score differences between the offspring. The attached-Y and attached-X chromosomes reduce the number of segregating elements in the crosses. The gametes that give rise to the informative progeny are drawn in solid line. The effect of parental origin can be unequivocally shown in sons, since males homozygous for the duplication die. In sons that inherit *Dp(1;3)N²⁶⁴⁻⁵⁸ᵃ* from the father, the mutant areas within the eye are much less extensive than when *Dp(1;3)N²⁶⁴⁻⁵⁸ᵃ* is inherited from the mother.

periphery the paternal X chromosomes are eliminated (Du Bois, 1933). Study of nine reciprocal X:autosome translocations has shown that the element that controls this selective elimination lies within heterochromomere II, adjacent to the centromere of the X chromosome (Crouse, 1979). The heterochromatic nature of the controlling element, and the fact that the eliminations occur at around the time heterochromatin is first observed, has suggested that the controlling element acts by affecting X centromere function via a spreading effect, similar to that seen in PEV (John, 1988).

The most recent studies on the nature of the imprint in mammals have also revealed many striking similarities with PEV and the other insect systems. For example, both mammalian X chromosomes remain active in undifferentiated female ES cells through several cellular generations, but upon differentiation the paternal X chromosome is preferentially inactivated in yolk-sac derivatives containing visceral mesoderm and endoderm (Tada *et al.*, 1993). This observation recapitulates *in vitro* the situation in embryos (Takagi & Sasaki, 1975) and suggests that the imprint responsible for the preferential inactivation can be stored in undifferentiated cells – whether in embryos or in tissue culture – and seems unlikely to be methylation, because the preferential inactivation takes place even in the presence of demethylating agents.

As always, the studies on the X chromosome have been closely shadowed by studies on autosomally imprinted genes. Both *Igf2r* and *Igf2* are codominantly expressed within the preimplantation mouse embryo (Latham *et al.*, 1994), yet are reciprocally imprinted and expressed only from the paternal and maternal genomes, respectively, in the fetal and adult mouse (Barlow *et al.*, 1991; DeChiara *et al.*, 1991). Here again, the imprint is stored during early embryogeny and only becomes liminal later on. The nature of the imprint found on the *Igf2* and *H19* genes during early embryogeny appears not to involve methylation, as no differences in allelic methylation can be observed up until the blastocyst stage and, moreover, no differences can be observed in the respective parental germlines (Brandeis *et al.*, 1993). The *Igf2r* gene is, however, different from the other two imprinted genes. *Igf2r* has an unconventional CpG-rich intron, which is highly methylated on the expressed maternal allele in adults (Stöger *et al.*, 1993). Some of this intronic methylation is also present in oocytes, suggesting that it might be the maternal imprint. A possible role for the methylation within the second intron of *Igf2r* has been posited; methylation on the maternal chromosome may inhibit the binding of proteins to a silencer within the intron and thus enable the gene to be expressed (Stöger *et al.*, 1993). Conversely, a lack of methylation on the paternal chromosome is thought to allow the assembly of a repressed chromosomal domain, which silences the *Igf2r* gene. Interestingly, a precedent for the silencing may come from *Drosophila*, where the *iab-2* regulatory sequence, found within the fourth intron of the *abd-A* gene of the *bithorax* complex, can nucleate the assembly of the *Pc*-G complex and thus result in repression of the *abd-A* gene (Simon *et al.*, 1993).

Findings from the study of boundary elements within the *bithorax* complex may also be applicable to a model of the reciprocal imprinting of the *Igf2* and *H19* genes by competition of enhancers (Bartolomei *et al.*, 1993; Efstradiatis, 1994). In the most recent model (Efstradiatis, 1994) the suggestion is that sharing of the *H19* enhancers by both *H19* and *Igf2* is regulated by a postulated boundary element that lies between the genes. The boundary is assembled on the maternal chromosome as a consequence of a maternal imprint (that appears not to be methylation; Brandeis *et al.*, 1993) and its role is to direct the activities of the enhancers to the *H19* gene alone. The *Igf2* gene is therefore effectively silenced by proxy, by being insulated away from the *H19* enhancers. Inhibiting the assembly of the boundary element on the paternal chromosome – perhaps by analogy with the *Igf2r* intron, through methylation – allows the enhancers to act on the *Igf2* gene (Efstradiatis, 1994). A feature of this model is that the *Igf2* gene remains in an expressible conformation throughout, and in this way explains the low, but detectable, levels of transcription of *Igf2* on the maternal chromosome (Sasaki *et al.*, 1992). Again, a precedent for such a scenario has been found in the study of the *Fab-7* boundary element, which lies between the *iab-6* and *iab-7 cis*-regulatory sequences of the abdominal region of the *bithorax* complex (Galioni *et al.*, 1993). The *iab-7* gene is normally active in parasegment 12 and regulates the *Abd-B* gene in this parasegment. However, deletion of *Fab-7* results in the ectopic activation of *iab-7* in parasegment 11, where the *iab-6* regulatory element normally functions (Galloni *et al.*, 1993). Thus, the *Fab-7* element acts as a boundary (Eissenberg & Elgin, 1991) and directs the activities of enhancer elements to their cognate targets within the appropriate parasegment. *Fab-7* also binds Pc protein (Orlando & Paro, 1993), suggesting that the boundary is the *Pc*-G repressor complex (see Fig. 5.6). Interestingly, in both the *Igf2r* and *H19–Igf2* imprinting models the role of methylation is to inhibit the formation of a repressed chromosomal domain, and is therefore distinct from the more typical role of methylation in repression of gene activity (Bird, 1992).

In summary, the final epigenetic states of both the inactive X chromosome and the autosomally imprinted genes discussed above are likely to involve methylation (Kaslow & Midgeon 1987; Li *et al.*, 1993). However, it seems unlikely in these examples that methylation is the sole imprint – except, perhaps, for the *Igf2r* gene – retained during early (especially preimplantation) embryogenesis. Instead the molecular mechanisms that lead to the final epigenetic, yet heritable, state of an imprinted gene or chromosome may have much in common with the mechanisms described for the stepwise determination of cell fate (Fig. 5.6). In this way, imprinted genes are seen as sharing much of the regulatory machinery used by many other developmentally regulated genes. For parentally imprinted genes the difference is that the initial 'imprintor' must act very early, when the parental genomes are separate. Only thus can the maternal and paternal alleles (or chromosome) be imprinted differently and therefore function in opposite ways, at some time after the formation of the zygote. This first step may take place in the respective germlines (Crouse, 1960) or be completely under maternal control: the 'imprintor' acting during female meiosis and/or during the period that the sperm is being assembled into the paternal pronucleus by the ooplasm (Brown & Nur, 1975).

We also note that many of the nuclear–cytoplasmic effects that cause epigenetic modifications with phenotypic consequences later in development (Babinet *et al.*, 1990) could be explained by perturbations in the process of cellular determination, and be similar, in many ways, to the environmental effects of temperature on PEV (Gowan & Gay, 1933a) (Fig. 5.3).

Appendix: definition of terms used in the text

Imprintor: A molecule (could be a protein or a nucleic acid) that marks out a region of the genome that will be changed in its expressibility at some later stage of development. An example would be the hb protein, which targets the assembly of the *Pc*-G complex (Fig. 5.6). The imprintee is the DNA sequence to which the imprintor binds.

Imprint: A combination of imprintor and imprintee. However, in the example discussed the imprintor may change during development (hb to esc) (Fig. 5.6). Nevertheless, it remains true that the same region marked out by the initial imprintor will be heritably changed in its expressibility, sometime during development; the imprint must be at least partially stable for a few rounds of DNA replication before it directs more permanent changes. It may constitute a methylation imprint in mammals.

Up until the time there are permanent changes in the expressibility of an imprinted gene, it may be regulated in any way and independently of the final change in expressibility that is a consequence of the imprint (for example, preferential inactivation of the paternal X chromosome occurs despite both both X chromosomes being active initially). Beyond this point the transcriptional fate of a gene is determined. Only in special cases (e.g. de-heterochromatinization of the paternal chromosome set in the gut of male coccids (Nur, 1967) and biallelic expression of *Igf2* in choroid plexus (DeChiara *et al.*, 1991)) can determination be reversed. In mammals, this stage involves methylation (Li *et al.*, 1993).

Acknowledgements

Work in the laboratory of T.C.J. was supported by a grant from the National Institutes of General Medical Sciences (RO1GM42813).

References

Akam, M. (1987). The molecular basis of the metameric pattern in *Drosophila* embryos. *Development* **101**, 1–22.

Babinet, C., Richoux, V., Guenet, J.-L. & Renard, J.-P. (1990). The DDK inbred strain as a model for the study of interactions between parental genomes and egg cytoplasm in mouse preimplantation development. In *Genomic Imprinting*, ed. M. Monk & M. A. H. Surani, pp. 81–7. Cambridge: Company of Biologists Ltd.

Baker, W. K. (1953). V-type position effects of a gene normally located in heterochromatin. *Genetics* **38**, 328–44.

Baker, W. K. (1958). Position-effect variegation. *Adv. Genet.* **14**, 133–69.

Baker, W. K. (1963). Genetic control of pigment differentiation in somatic cells. *Am. Zool.* **3**, 57–69.

Barlow, D. P., Stöger, R., Herrmann, B. G., Saito, K. & Schweifer, N. (1991). The mouse insulin-like growth factor type-2 receptor is imprinted and closely linked to the *Tme* locus. *Nature* **349**, 84–7.

Bartolomei, M. S., Webber, A. L., Brunkow, M. E. & Tilghman, S. M. (1993). Epigenetic mechanisms underlying the imprinting of the mouse *H19* gene. *Genes Devel.* **7**, 1633–73.

Becker, H. J. (1957). Uber Rotgenmosaikflecken und Defektmutationen am Auge von *Drosophila* und die Entwicklungsphysiologie des Auges. *Z. indukt. Abstammungs-Verebungsl.* **88**, 333–73.

Becker, H. J. (1961). Untersuchungen zur Wirkung des Heterochromatins auf die Genmanifestierung bei *Drosophila melanogaster*. *Verh. Dt. zool. Ges.* Suppl. **24**, 283–91.

Belyaeva, E. S., Demakova, O. V., Umbetova, G. H. & Zhimulev, I. F. (1993). Cytogenetic and molecular aspects of position-effect variegation in *Drosophila melanogaster*. V. Heterochromatin-associated protein HP1 appears in euchromatic chromosomal regions that are inactivated as a result of position-effect variegation. *Chromosoma* **102**, 583–90.

Belyaeva, E. S. & Zhimulev, I. F. (1991). Cytogenetic and molecular aspects of position effect variegation in *Drosophila*. III. Continuous and discontinuous compaction of chromosomal material as a result of position-effect variegation. *Chromosoma* **100**, 453–66.

Bird, A. P. (1992). The essentials of DNA methylation. *Cell* **70**, 5–8.

Bishop, C. E. (1992). Evidence for intrinsic differences in the formation of chromatin domains in *Drosophila melanogaster*. *Genetics* **132**, 1063–9.

Boulet, A. M. & Scott, M. P. (1988). Control elements of the P2 promoter of the *Antennapedia* gene. *Genes Dev.* **2**, 1600–14.

Brandeis, M., Kafri, T., Ariel, M., Challiet, J. R., Razin, A. & Cedar, H. (1993). The ontogeny of allele-specific methylation associated with imprinted genes in the mouse. *EMBO J.* **12**, 3669–77.

Brown, S. W. (1966). Heterochromatin. *Science* **151**, 417–25.

Brown, S. W. & Nur, U. (1975). Heterochromatic chromosomes in the Coccids. *Science* **145**, 130–6.

Brunk, B. P., Martin, E. C. & Adler, P. N. (1991). *Drosophila* genes *Posterior Sex Combs* and *Suppressor two of Zeste* encode proteins with homology to the murine *bmi-1* oncogene. *Nature* **353**, 351–3.

Cattanach, B. M. (1974). Position-effect variegation in the mouse. *Genet. Res., Camb.* **23**, 291–306.

Cattanach, B. M. (1975). Control of chromosome inactivation. *A. Rev. Genet.* **9**, 1–18.

Chandra, H. S. & Brown, S. W. (1975). Chromosome imprinting and the mammalian X chromosome. *Nature* **253**, 165–8.

Chen, S.-Y. (1948). Action de la temperature sur trois mutants a panachure de *Drosophila melanogaster*:w^{258-18},w^{m5} et z. *Bull. Biol. France Belg.* **82**, 114–29.

Clarke, R. F. & Elgin, S. C. R. (1992). Heterochromatin protein 1, a known suppressor of position-effect variegation. *Nucl. Acids Res.* **20**, 6067–74.

Cooper, K. W. (1959). Cytogenic analysis of major heterochromatic elements (especially Xh and Y) in *Drosophila melanogaster*, and the theory of heterochromatin. *Chromosoma* **10**, 535–88.

Crouse, H. V. (1960). The controlling element in sex chromosome behaviour in *Sciara*. *Genetics* **45**, 1425–43.

Crouse, H. V. (1979). X heterochromatin subdivision and cytogenetic analysis in *Sciara coprophila* (Diptera, Sciaridae). II. The controlling element. *Chromosoma* **74**, 219–39.

DeCamillis, M., Cheng, N. S., Pierre, D. & Brock, H. W. (1992). The *polyhomeotic* gene of Drosophila encodes a chromatin protein that shares polytene chromosome-binding sites with *Polycomb*. *Genes Dev.* **6**, 223–32.

DeChiara, T., Robertson, E. & Efstratiadis, A. (1991). Parental imprinting of the mouse *insulin-like growth factor II* gene. *Cell* **64**, 849–59.

Delmas, V., Stokes, D. G. & Perry, R. P. (1993). A mammalian DNA binding protein that contains a chromodomain and an SNF2/SW12-like helicase domain. *Proc. Natl. Acad. Sci. USA* **90**, 2414–18.

Demerec, M. (1941). The nature of changes in the white-Notch region of the X-chromosome of *Drosophila melanogaster*. *Proc. 7th Internatl. Congr. Genet. Edinburgh, 1939*, pp. 99–103.

DeRobertis, E. M., Morita, A. & Cho, K. W. Y. (1991). Gradient fields and homeobox genes. *Development* **112**, 669–78.

Dombardi, V. & Cohen, P. T. (1992). Protein phosphorylation is involved in the regulation of chromatin condensation during interphase. *FEBS Lett.* **312**, 21–6.

Dorn, R., Krauss, V., Reuter, G. & Saumweber, H. (1993a). The enhancer of position-effect variegation, *E(var)3-39D*, codes for a chromatin protein containing a conserved domain common to several transcriptional regulators. *Proc. Natl. Acad. Sci. USA.* **90**, 11376–80.

Dorn, R., Szidonya, J., Korge, G., Sehnert, M., Taubert, H., Archoukieh, E., Tschiersch, B., Moraweitz, H., Wustman, G., Hoffmann, G. & Reuter, G. (1993b). P transposon-induced dominant mutations of position effect variegation in *Drosophila melanogaster*. *Genetics* **133**, 279–90.

Dubinin, N. P. & Sidorov, B. N. (1935). The postion-effect of the hairy gene. *Biol. Zh. Mosk.* **4**, 555–68.

Du Bois, A. M. (1933). Chromosome behaviour during the cleavage in the eggs of *Sciara coprophila* (Diptera) in relation to the problem of sex determination. *Z. Zellforsch.* **19**, 595–614.

Duncan, I. M. (1987). The bithorax complex. *A. Rev. Genet.* **21**, 285–319.

Efstratiadis, A. (1994). Parental imprinting of autosomal mammalian genes. *Curr. Opin. Genet. Dev.* **4**, 265–80.

Eissenberg, J. C. & Elgin, S. C. R. (1991). Boundary functions in the control of gene expression. *Trends Genet.* **7**, 335–40.

Eissenberg, J. C. & Hartnett, T. (1993). A heat shock-activated cDNA rescues the recessive lethality of mutations in the heterochromatin-associated protein HP1 of Drosophila melanogaster. *Molec. gen. Genet.* **240**, 333–8.

Eissenberg, J. C., James, T. C., Foster-Hartnett, D. M., Hartnett, T., Ngan, V. & Elgin, S. C. R. (1990). Mutation in a heterochromatin-specific chromosomal protein is associated with the suppression of position-effect variegation in *Drosophila melanogaster*. *Proc. Natl. Acad. Sci. USA* **87**, 9923–7.

Eissenberg, J. C., Morris, G. D., Reuter, G. & Hartnett, T. (1992). The heterochromatin association protein HP1 is an essential protein in *Drosophila* with dosage-dependent effects on position-effect variegation. *Genetics* **131**, 345–52.

Epstein, H. (1992). Polycomb and friends. *Bioessays* **14**, 411–13.

Epstein, H., James, T. C. & Singh, P. B. (1992). Cloning and expression of *Drosophila* HP1 homologues from a mealybug, *Planococcus citri*. *J. Cell Sci.* **10**, 463–74.

Fauvarque, M. & Dura, J. (1993). Polyhomeotic regulatory sequences induce developmental regulator-dependent variegation and targeted P-element insertion in *Drosophila*. *Genes Dev.* **7**, 1508–20.

Franke, A., DeCamillis, M., Zink, D., Cheng, N., Brock, H. W. & Paro, R. (1992). Polycomb and Polyhomeotic are constituents of a multi-meric protein complex in chromatin of Drosophila melanogaster. *EMBO J.* **11**, 2941–50.

Galloni, M., Gyrurkovics, H., Schedl, P. & Karch, F. (1993). The bluetail transposon: evidence for independent cis-regulatory domains and domain boundaries in the bithorax complex. *EMBO J.* **12**, 1087–97.

Gaunt, S. J. & Singh, P. B. (1990). Homeogene expression patterns and chromosomal imprinting. *Trends Genet.* **6**, 208–12.

Gowan, J. H. & Gay, E. H. (1933a). Effect of temperature on eversporting eye colour in *Drosophila melanogaster*. *Science* **77**, 312.

Gowan, J. H. & Gay, E. H. (1933b). Eversporting as a function of the Y chromosome in *Drosophila melanogaster*. *Proc. Natl. Acad. Sci. USA* **19**, 122–6.

Grazino, V., Pereira, A., Laurenti, P., Graba, Y., Levis, R. W., Parco Le, Y. & Pradel, J. (1992). Cell lineage-specific expression of *modulo*, a dose-dependent modifier of variegation in *Drosophila*. *EMBO J.* **11**, 4471–9.

Griffen, A. B. & Stone, W. S. (1940). The w^{m5} and its derivatives. *Univ. Texas Publ.* No. 4032, 190–200.

Grigliatti, T. (1991). Position-effect variegation: an essay for non-histone chromosomal proteins and chromatin modifying factors. In *Functional Organisation of the Nucleus*, ed. B. A. Hamkalo & S. C. R. Elgin, pp. 588–628. San Diego: Academic Press.

Hadorn, E. (1965). Problems of determination and transdetermination. In *Genetic Control of Differentiation*, vol. 18, pp. 148–61. New York: Upton.

Heemskerk, J., DiNardo, S., Kostriken, R. & O'Farrell, P. H. (1991). Multiple modes of engrailed expression in the progression towards cell fate determination. *Nature* **352**, 404–10.

Henderson, D. S., Banga, S. S., Grigliatti, T. A. & Boyd, J. B. (1994). Mutagen sensitivity and suppression of position-effect variegation result from mutation in *mus209*, the *Drosophila* gene encoding PCNA. *EMBO J.* **13**, 1450–9.

Henikoff, S. (1979). Position-effect and variegation enhancers in an autosomal region of *Drosophila melanogaster*. *Genetics* **81**, 705–21.

Henikoff, S. (1981). Position-effect variegation and the chromosome structure of a heat shock puff in *Drosophila*. *Chromosoma* **83**, 381–93.

Henikoff, S. (1990). Position-effect variegation after 60 years. *Trends Genet.* **6**, 422–6.

Hessler, A. Y. (1961). A study of parental modifications of variegated position effects. *Genetics* **46**, 463–84.

Illmensee, K. (1972). Developmental potencies of nuclei from cleavage, preblastoderm and syncytial blastoderm transplanted into unfertilised eggs of *Drosophila melanogaster*. *Wilhelm Roux's Arch. Entwicklungsmech. Org.* **170**, 267–78.

Ingham, P. W. & Martinez-Arias, A. (1986). The correct activation of *Antennapedia* and bithorax complex requires the *fushi tarazu* gene. *Nature* **324**, 592–7.

James, T. C., Eissenberg, J. C., Craig, C., Dietrich, V., Hobson, A. & Elgin, S. C. R. (1989). Distribution patterns of HP1, a heterochromatin-associated nonhistone chromosomal protein of *Drosophila*. *Eur. J. Cell Biol.* **50**, 170–80.

James, T. C. & Elgin, S. C. R. (1986). Identification of a nonhistone chromosomal protein associated with heterochromatin in *Drosophila melanogaster* and its gene. *Molec. Cell Biol.* **6**, 3862–72.

John, B. (1988). The biology of heterochromatin. In *Heterochromatin: Molecular and Structural Aspects*, ed. R. S. Verma, pp. 1–147. Cambridge University Press.

Jurgens, G. (1985). A group of genes controlling spatial expression of the *bithorax* complex in *Drosophila*. *Nature* **316**, 153–5.

Karpen, G. H. (1994). Position-effect variegation and the new biology of heterochromatin. *Curr. Opin. Genet. Dev.* **4**, 281–91.

Karpen, G. H. & Spradling, A. C. (1990). Reduced DNA polytenisation of a minichromosome region undergoing position-effect variegation in *Drosophila*. *Cell* **63**, 97–107.

Kaslow, D. C. & Midgeon, B. R. (1987). DNA methylation stabilises X chromosome inactivation in eutherians but not in marsupials: evidence for multistep maintenance of mammalian X dosage compensation. *Proc. Natl. Acad. Sci. USA* **84**, 6210–14.

Kellum, R. & Alberts, B. M. (1995). The heterochromatin-associated protein, heterochromatin protein-1 is required for correct segregation in *Drosophila* embryos. *J. Cell Sci.* (in press).

Kelly, S. J. (1977). Studies on the development potential of 4- and 8-cell stage mouse embryos. *J. exp. Zool.* **200**, 365–76.

Kennison, J. A. (1993). Transcriptional activation of *Drosophila* homeotic genes from distant regulatory elements. *Trends Genet.* **9**, 75–9.

Kieny, M., Mauger, A. & Sengel, P. (1972). Early regionalization of the somitic mesoderm as studied by development of the axial skeleton of the chick embryo. *Dev. Biol.* **28**, 142–61.

Kitsberg, D., Selig, S., Brandeis, M., Simon, I., Keshet, I., Driscoll, D. J., Nicholls, R. D. & Cedar, H. (1993). Allele-specific replication timing of imprinted gene regions. *Nature* **366**, 362–5.

Klar, A. J. S. & Bonaduce, M. J. (1991). *swi6*, a gene required for mating-type switching, prohibits meiotic recombination in the *mat2-mat3* 'cold-spot' of fission yeast. *Genetics* **129**, 1033–42.

Krejci, E., Grazino, V., Mary, C., Bennani, N. & Pradel, J. (1989). Modulo, a new maternally expressed *Drosophila* gene encodes a DNA-binding protein with distinct acidic and basic regions. *Nucl. Acids Res.* **17**, 8101–15.

Latham, K. E., Doherty, A. S., Scott, C. D. & Schultz, R. M. (1994). *Igf2r* and *Igf2* gene expression in androgenetic, gynogenetic, and parthenogenetic preimplantation mouse embryos: absence of regulation by genomic imprinting. *Genes Dev.* **8**, 290–9.

Lewis, E. B. (1950). The phenomenon of position effect. *Adv Genet.* **3**, 73–115.

Lewis, E. B. (1978). A gene complex controlling segmentation in *Drosophila*. *Nature* **276**, 565–70.

Li, E., Beard, C. & Jaenisch, R. (1993). Role of DNA methylation in genomic imprinting. *Nature* **366**, 362–5.

Locke, J., Kotarski, M. A. & Tartof, K. D. (1988). Dosage-dependent modifiers of position-effect variegation in *Drosophila* and a mass-action model to explain their effect. *Genetics* **120**, 181–98.

Lorentz, A., Heim, L. & Schmidt, H. (1992). The switching gene *swi6* affects recombination and gene expression in the mating-type region of *Schizosaccharomyces pombe. Molec. gen. Genet.* **233**, 436–42.

Lorentz, A., Ostermann, K., Fleck, O. & Schmidt, H. (1994). The switching gene *swi6*, involved in the repression of the silent mating-type loci in fission yeast, encodes a homologue of chromatin-associated proteins from *Drosophila* and mammals. *Gene* **143**, 139–43.

Mazo, A., Huang, D., Mozer, B. & Dawid, I. (1990). The *trithorax* gene, a regulator of the bithorax complex in *Drosophila*, encodes a protein with zinc-binding domains. *Proc. Natl. Acad. Sci. USA* **87**, 2112–16.

McGinnis, W. & Krumlauf, R. (1992). Homeobox genes and axial patterning. *Cell* **120**, 181–98.

Messemer, S., Franke, A. & Paro, R. (1992). Analysis of the functional role of the Polycomb chromo domain in *Drosophila melanogaster. Genes Dev.* **6**, 1241–54.

Miklos, G. L. G. & Costell, J. N. (1990). Chromosome structure at interfaces between major chromatin types: *alpha-* and *beta*-heterochromatin. *Bioessays* **12**, 1–6.

Moazed, D. & O'Farrell, P. H. (1992). Maintenance of the engrailed pattern by polycomb group genes in *Drosophila. Development* **16**, 805–10.

Moore, G. D., Procunier, J. D., Cross, D. P. & Grigliatti, T. A. (1979). Histone deficiencies and position-effect variegation in *Drosophila. Nature* **282**, 312–14.

Morgan, T. H., Bridges, C. B. & Schultz, J. (1937). Investigations on the constitution of the germinal material in relation to heredity. *Yearbk. Carnegie Inst.* **36**, 298–305.

Morgan, T. H. & Schultz, J. (1942). Investigations on the constitution of the germinal material in relation to heredity. *Yearbk. Carnegie Inst.* **41**, 242–5.

Muller, J. & Bienz, M. (1991). Long range repression conferring boundaries of *Ultrabithorax* expression in the *Drosophila* embryo. *EMBO J.* **10**, 1241–54.

Mulligen, J. T., Dietrich, F. S., Hennessey, K. M., Sehl, P., Komp, C., Wei, Y., Taylor, P., Nakahara, K., Roberts, D. & Davis, R. W. (1993). Hypothetical yeast ChD-1-like protein. *EMBL*: L10718.

Nix, C. (1973). Suppression of transcription of the ribosomal RNA cistrons of *Drosophila melanogaster* in a structurally rearranged chromosome. *Biochem. Genet.* **10**, 1–12.

Noujdin, N. I. (1944). The regularities of heterochromatin influence on mosaicism. *J. gen. Biol. (USSR)* **5**, 357–88.

Nur, U. (1967). Reversal of heterochromatinisation and the activity of the paternal chromosome set in the male mealybug. *Genetics* **56**, 375–89.

Orlando, V. & Paro, R. (1993). Mapping polycomb-repressed domains in the bithorax complex using in vivo formaldehyde cross-linked chromatin. *Cell* **75**, 1187–98.

Panshin, I. B. (1935). New evidence for the position-effect hypothesis. *C.R. (Doklady) Acad. Sci. U.R.S.S.* **9**(4), 85–8.

Paro, R. (1990). Imprinting the determined state into the chromatin of *Drosophila melanogaster*. *Trends Genet.* **6**, 416–21.

Paro, R. & Hogness, D. S. (1991). The Polycomb protein shares a homologous region with a heterochromatin-associated protein of *Drosophila*. *Proc. Natl. Acad. Sci. USA* **88**, 263–7.

Pearce, J. J. H., Singh, P. B. & Gaunt, S. J. (1992). The mouse has a *Polycomb*-like chromobox gene. *Development* **114**, 921–30.

Peifer, M., Karch, F. & Bender, W. (1987). The bithorax complex: Control of segment identity. *Genes. Dev.* **1**, 891–8.

Peterson, C. & Herskowitz, I. (1992). Characterisation of the yeast *SWI1*, *SWI2*, and *SWI3* genes, which encode a global activator of transcription. *Cell* **68**, 573–83.

Pimpinelli, S., Sullivan, W., Prout, M. & Sandler, L. (1985). On biological functions that map to the heterochromatin of *Drosophila melanogaster*. *Genetics* **109**, 701–24.

Powers, J. A. & Eissenberg, J. C. (1993). Domains of the heterochromatin-associated protein HP1 mediate nuclear localisation and heterochromatin binding. *J. Cell Biol.* **120**, 291–9.

Prokofyeva-Belgovskaya, A. A. (1941). Cytological properties of inert chromosome regions and their bearing on the mechanics of mosaicism and chromosome rearrangement. *Dros. Inf. Serv.* **15**, 34–5.

Rastelli, L., Chan, C. S. & Pirrotta, V. (1993). Related chromosome binding sites for zeste, suppressors of zeste and the polycomb group of proteins in *Drosophila* and their dependence on the Enhancer of zeste function. *EMBO J.* **12**, 1513–22.

Reuter, G., Giarre, M., Farah, J., Gausz, J., Spierer, A. & Spierer, P. (1990). Dependence of position-effect variegation in *Drosophila* on dose of a gene encoding an unusual zinc-finger protein. *Nature* **344**, 219–23.

Reuter, G. & Spierer, P. (1992). Position-effect variegation and chromatin proteins. *Bioessays* **14**, 605–12.

Reuter, G., Werner, W. & Hoffman, H. J. (1982). Mutants affecting position-effect heterochromatinisation in *Drosophila melanogaster*. *Chromosoma* **85**, 539–51.

Sandler, L. (1977). Evidence for a set of closely linked autosomal genes that interact with sex-chromosome heterochromatin in *Drosophila melanogaster*. *Genetics* **86**, 567–82.

Sasaki, H., Jones, P. A., Challiet, R. J., Ferguson-Smith, A. C., Barton, S. C., Reik, W. & Surani, M. A. (1992). Parental imprinting: Potentially active chromatin of the repressed maternal allele of the mouse Insulin-like growth factor II (*IGF2*) gene. *Genes Dev.* **6**, 1843–56.

Saunders, W. S., Chue, C., Goebl, M., Craig, C., Clarke, R. F., Powers, J. A., Eissenberg, J. C., Elgin, S. C. R., Rothfield, N. F. & Earnshaw, W. C. (1993). Molecular cloning of a human homologue of *Drosophila* heterochromatin protein HP1 using anti-centromere autoantibodies with *anti-chromo* specificity. *J. Cell Sci.* **104**, 573–82.

Schultz, J. (1941). The function of heterochromatin. *Proc. 7th Internatl. Congr. Genet. Edinburgh, 1939*, pp. 257–62.

Schultz, J. (1956). The relation of the heterochromatin chromosome regions to the nucleic acids of the cell. *Cold Spring Harbor Symp. quant. Biol.* **21**, 307–28.

Schultz, J. & Caspersson, T. (1939). Heterochromatic regions and the nucleic acid metabolism of the chromosomes. *Arch. exp. Zellforsch*, **22**, 650–4.

Simcox, A. & Sang, J. H. (1983). When does determination occur in *Drosophila* embryos? *Dev. Biol.* **97**, 212–21.

Simon, J., Chiang, A., Bender, W., Shimell, M. J. & O'Conner, M. (1993). Elements of the *Drosophila* bithorax complex that mediate repression by *Polycomb* group products. *Dev. Biol.* **158**, 131–44.

Singh, P. B. (1994). Molecular mechanisms of cellular determination; their relation to chromatin structure and parental imprinting. *J. Cell Sci.* **107**, 2653–68.

Singh, P. B., Miller, J. R., Pearce, J. J., Burton, R. D., Paro, R., James, T. C. & Gaunt, S. J. (1991). A sequence motif found in a *Drosophila* heterochromatin protein is conserved in animals and plants. *Nucl. Acids Res.* **19**, 789–93.

Slack, J. W. M. (1983). *From Egg to Embryo: Determinative Events in Early Development.* In *Developmental and Cell Biology* Series, ed. P. W. Barlow, P. B. Green & C. C. Wylie. Cambridge University Press.

Slatis, H. M. (1955). Position-effects at the brown locus in *Drosophila melanogaster.* *Genetics* **40**, 5–23.

Spofford, J. (1959). Parental control of position-effect variegation. I. Parental heterochromatin and expression of the *white* locus in compound X *Drosophila melanogaster. Proc. Natl. Acad. Sci. USA* **45**, 1003–7.

Spofford, J. (1961). Parental control of position-effect variegation. II. Effect of sex of parent contributing white-mottled rearrangement in *Drosophila melanogaster. Genetics* **46**, 1151–67.

Spofford, J. (1976). Position-effect variegation in *Drosophila*. In *The Genetics and Biology of* Drosophila, vol. 1c, ed. M. Ashburner & E. Novitski, pp. 955–1018. New York: Academic Press.

Stocum, D. L. & Fallon, J. F. (1982). Control of pattern formation in urodele limb ontogeny: a review and a hypothesis. *J. Embryol. exp. Morphol.* **69**, 7–36.

Stöger, R., Kubicka, P., Liu, C.-G., Kafri, T., Razin, A., Cedar, H. & Barlow, D. P. (1993). Maternal-specific methylation of the imprinted mouse *Igf2r* locus identifies the expressed locus as carrying the imprinting signal. *Cell* **73**, 61–71.

Struhl, G. (1981). A gene product required for correct initiation of segmental determination in Drosophila. *Nature* **293**, 36–41.

Struhl, G. (1983). Role of the *esc*[+] gene product in ensuring the selective expression of segment-specific homeotic genes in *Drosophila. J. Embryol. exp. Morphol.* **76**, 297–331.

Tada, T., Tada, M. & Takagki, N. (1993). X chromosome retains the memory of its parental origin in murine embryonic stem cells. *Development* **119**, 813–21.

Takagi, N. & Sasaki, M. (1975). Preferential inactivation of the paternally-derived X chromosome in the extraembryonic membranes of the mouse. *Nature* **256**, 640–42.

Tamkun, J. W., Deuring, R., Scott, M. P., Kissenger, M., Pattatucci, A. M., Kaufman, T. C. & Kennison, J. A. (1992). *brahma*, A regulator of *Drosophila* homeotic genes structurally related to the yeast transcriptional activator SNF2/SWI2. *Cell* **68**, 561–72.

Tartof, K. D., Bishop, C., Jones, M., Hobbs, C. A. & Locke, J. (1989). Towards an
    understanding of position-effect variegation. *Dev. Genet.* **10**, 162–76.
Tartof, K. D., Hobbs, C. & Jones, M. (1984). A structural basis for variegating position
    effects. *Cell* **37**, 869–78.
Turner, B. M. (1991). Histone acetylation and control of gene expression. *J. Cell Sci.* **99**,
    13–20.
van Holde, K. E. (1988). *Chromatin.* New York: Springer-Verlag.
Wakimoto, B. T. & Hearn, M. G. (1990). The effects of chromosome rearrangements on
    the expression of heterochromatic genes in chromosome 2L of *Drosophila
    melanogaster. Genetics* **125**, 141–54.
White, R. A. H. & Lehmann, R. (1986). A gap gene, *hunchback*, regulates the spatial
    expression of *Ultrabithorax. Cell* **47**, 311–21.
Wieschaus & Noell, E. (1986). Specificity of embryonic lethal mutations in *Drosophila*
    analysed in germ line clones. *Wilhelm Roux's Arch. Dev. Biol.* **195**, 63–73.
Wreggett, K. A., Hill, F., James, P. S., Hutchings, A., Butcher, G. W. & Singh, P. B.
    (1994). A mammalian homologue of *Drosophila* heterochromatin protein 1 (HP1) is a
    component of constitutive heterochromatin. *Cytogenet. Cell Genet.* **66**, 99–103.
Wu, C. (1993). Transvection, nuclear structure, and chromatin proteins. *J. Cell Biol.* **120**,
    587–90.
Zhang, C. C. & Bienz, M. (1992). Segmental determination in *Drosophila* conferred by
    hunchback (hb), a repressor of the homeotic gene *Ultrabithorax. Proc. Natl. Acad.
    Sci. USA* **89**, 7511–15.
Zink, B. & Paro, R. (1989). *In vivo* binding pattern of a *trans*-regulator of the homeotic
    genes in *Drosophila melanogaster. Nature* **337**, 468–71.
Zuckerkandl, E. (1974). Recherches sur les properties et l'activite biologique de la
    chromatine. *Biochimie* **56**, 937–54.

6

The biochemical basis of allele-specific gene expression in genomic imprinting and X inactivation

TIMOTHY H. BESTOR

Introduction

When considered in biochemical terms, genomic imprinting and X chromosome inactivation arc astonishing because they demand very unequal rates of transcription of similar or identical transcription units that are present in the same nucleus and exposed to the same set of regulatory factors. Inequalities of expression can persist for the life of the organism – decades in the case of X-linked genes in humans – and can even be transmitted through generations. What is it that prevents equilibrium of transcription factors between alleles in such a stable manner? At this time there seem to be two salient candidate mechanisms. The first depends on mitotic inheritance of allele-specific chromatin configurations in a manner that might share important characteristics with the Polycomb-group/trithorax-group (Pc-G/trx-G) regulatory system of *Drosophila*, and the second involves heritable covalent DNA modification mediated by DNA methyltransferases.

Heritable gene repression by the Pc-G/trx-G system and by cytosine methylation

Imprinting and X inactivation require that the inactive transcriptional state of genes be subject to clonal inheritance, and that only one of two alleles be affected. There are several experimental systems in which states of gene expression are heritable (some well-studied examples are transvection, position effect variegation, and telomere position effect; reviewed by Bestor *et al.*, 1994) but most of these affect both alleles and are observed only in organisms that bear gross chromosomal rearrangements, and are not thought to be involved in normal development. The epigenetic system perhaps most clearly involved in metazoan development is the Pc-G/trx-G system of *Drosophila*, in which the products of maternal-effect and segmentation genes catalyze the assembly of ubiquitous chromosomal proteins on and around homeotic selector genes (reviewed by Paro, 1993). These chromatin assemblies are replicated along with the DNA during S phase, and ensure the appropriate spatial pattern of homeotic gene expression several days after the decay of the spatially restricted maternal-effect and segmentation factors. Loss-of-function mutations in genes of the Pc-G lead to broadening of zones of expression of homeotic genes, while loss of function mutations in genes of the trx-G cause narrowed zones of homeotic gene expression. Such genetic data indicate that complexes of Pc-G proteins sustain the inactive state, and that complexes of trx-G proteins are stimulatory. It should be noted that most mutations that cause homeotic transformations in Drosophila affect genes that encode ubiquitous chromosomal proteins of the Pc-G/trx-G system rather than homeotic genes themselves.

Pc-G/trx-G proteins form very large complexes on the affected sequences, and loss-of-function mutations in any one of ten Pc-G genes have been shown to cause mis-expression of multiple homeotic genes (Simon et al., 1992). The Pc-G/trx-G proteins analyzed to date are highly heterogeneous, with little evidence of shared biochemical properties. Many members of the Pc-G are not thought to interact with DNA directly, and none has been shown to bind specific sequences in vitro (Paro, 1993; Orlando & Paro, 1993). The nature of the higher-order interactions among members of the Pc-G and trx-G are still unclear, although it is quite likely that the stability of the Pc-G and trx-G chromatin assemblies will be found to depend on extensive cooperative protein–protein and protein–DNA interactions. Although study of the biochemistry of the Pc-G/trx-G system is at an early stage, it does appear that development can depend on heritable gene repression mediated by mitotic inheritance of higher-order chromatin assemblies. The stability of this sort of repression is not known; non-covalent protein–protein and protein–DNA interactions must involve finite on and off rates, and some equilibration of factors between identical alleles must occur over time. The Pc-G/trx-G system functions over a period of about 10 days in the normal development of Drosophila (Simon et al., 1992); whether a system based on similar biochemistry might have sufficient stability to mediate imprinting and X inactivation in mammals is an open question. Furthermore, it has not been shown that allele-specific gene expression can be mediated by wholly non-covalent systems; the Pc-G/trx-G system affects both alleles.

The spontaneous off rate of a methyl substituent at the 5 position of cytosine (m^5C) is essentially zero; allele-specific gene expression could also be mediated by heritable patterns of methylated cytosine residues rather than heritable, non-covalent chromatin assemblies. The methylation of CpG dinucleotides within promoter regions strongly inhibits transcription of vertebrate genes both in vivo and *in vitro* (reviewed by Meehan *et al.*, 1992). The mechanism of inhibition may involve interference with the binding of transcription factors via interactions with the major groove methyl moieties of m^{5}C (Iguchi-Ariga & Schaffner, 1989), or methylation may target sequences for assembly into condensed, inactive chromatin during S phase (Keshet *et al.*, 1986; Hsieh & Lieber, 1992); this latter effect may be mediated by proteins that specifically bind to regions of DNA that contain methylated CpG dinucleotides. Two factors with this property have been characterized and termed MeCP-1 and MeCP-2 (reviewed by Meehan *et al.*, 1992). Although it is not certain whether the inhibitory effect of cytosine methylation is direct or indirect, or if the source of the effect differs among genes, it is clear that methylation of CpG sites within promoters strongly inhibits transcription.

It is also clear that methylation patterns are subject to clonal inheritance. When cultured cells were transfected with DNA molecules that had been methylated in predetermined but arbitrary patterns *in vitro*, the cellular DNA methylating system was found to maintain the methylation pattern of the integrated transforming DNA for many cell divisions (Wigler *et al.*, 1981). This is likely to be due in large part to the strong intrinsic preference of mammalian DNA methyltransferase for hemimethylated CpG sites (Bestor, 1992; reviewed by Bestor & Verdine, 1994), together with the coordination of DNA replication and DNA methylation in replication foci of S phase nuclei (Leonhardt *et al.*, 1992; Bestor & Verdine, 1994). Because cytosine methylation is heritable and introduces a chemical difference between alleles, the lack of equilibrium of factors between alleles is not so energetically problematic as in the case of purely non-covalent protein–DNA interactions. In short, the heritability of methylation patterns and their ability to extinguish transcription suits them for a role in allele-specific gene expression.

A shared sequence motif in DNA methyltransferase and mammalian *trithorax*

As discussed in the preceding section, cytosine methylation in vertebrates and the Pc-G/trx-G system in *Drosophila* can mediate the inheritance of states of gene expression, but until recently there was no perceptible relationship between the two systems. In 1992 a mammalian homolog of *trithorax* was identified as a gene that is frequently involved in translocations in childhood leukemias; it was cloned in several laboratories and named *HRX* (for human homolog of *trithorax*) (Tkachuk *et al.*, 1992) and *ALL-1* (for acute lymphocytic leukemia) (Gu *et al.*, 1992). The sequence of the HRX/ALL-1 protein and the murine homolog All-1 (Ma *et al.*, 1993) showed a surprising sequence motif: a novel cysteine-rich region that had been previously identified only in the N-terminal domain of DNA methyltransferase (Plate 1). This domain had previously been shown to bind Zn ions and to be involved in the discrimination of unmethylated and hemimethylated CpG sites (Bestor, 1992). It is also interesting to note that both trithorax and HRX/ALL-1 contain two clusters of canonical Zn finger sequences, but the Cys-rich region is absent from *Drosophila* trithorax, and *Drosophila* DNA does not contain detectable m^{5}C. For these and other reasons it was predicted that the Cys-rich region common to DNA methyltransferase and HRX/ALL-1 would be found to sense the methylation status of CpG dinucleotides (Ma *et al.*, 1993; Bestor & Verdine, 1994). Tests of this prediction are currently under way.

The Cys-rich sequence motif common to DNA methyltransferase and HRX/ALL-1 represents the first link between two important epigenetic regulatory systems; it is suggested that heritable methylation patterns might reinforce, and may have supplanted, regulation by heritable non-covalent chromatin configurations of the *Pc-G/trx*-G type (Bestor & Verdine, 1994). This suggestion is supported by considerations of comparative biology: vertebrates require greater stability in gene expression because of their long lives, very large size, and life-long persistence of numerous self-renewing stem cell populations (Bestor, 1990). Additional imperatives result from the very large size of the vertebrate genome (about 20 times that of the *Drosophila* genome) and the greater complexity of developmental decisions in vertebrates. The *Pc-G/trx*-G system alone might be capable of maintaining a given determined state for days or weeks (as in the case of homeotic gene regulation in *Drosophila*), but fail when the requirement is years or decades (as in humans). I suggest that regulation by heritable methylation patterns arose during evolution because of the stability of this type of marking, and non-covalent regulation may have been supplanted altogether in the case of genes subject to allele-specific repression. The ability to exercise this special form of gene control might yield a net selective advantage (Li *et al.*, 1992) even though cytosine methylation places a heavy mutational load on the mammalian genome (Bestor & Coxon, 1993).

Is methylation a primary or secondary effect in allele-specific gene repression?

The role of cytosine methylation in gene control has long been controversial. That methylation of promoter regions prevents transcription is well accepted, but it is widely felt that cytosine methylation stabilizes a silenced state after it is established by methylation-independent factors. However, experimental support of this conclusion is thin; it is based almost entirely on studies in which methylation of certain restriction sites was observed to lag behind gene inactivation (Lock *et al.*, 1987). This conclusion requires that the methylation status of all

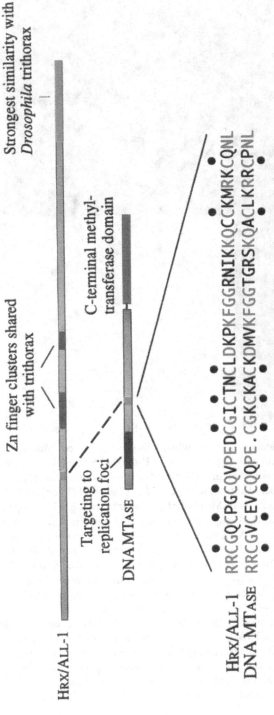

Strongest similarity with *Drosophila* trithorax

HRX/ALL-1

Zn finger clusters shared with trithorax

Targeting to replication foci

DNA MTASE

C-terminal methyl-transferase domain

HRX/ALL-1   RRCGQCPGCQVPEDCGICTNCLDKPKFGGRNIKKQCCKMRKCQNL
DNA MTASE   RRCGVCEVCQQPE . CGKCKACKDMVKFGGTGRSKQACLKRRCPNL

Plate 1. A sequence motif shared by DNA methyltransferase and HRX/ALL-1, a human homologue of *Drosophila* trithorax. A cysteine-rich sequence that was shown to bind Zn ions and to map to a region of DNA methyltransferase that suppresses *de novo* methylation (Bestor, 1992) was found to be present in HRX/ALL-1. The sequence of the shared motif is at the bottom of the figure; amino acid identities are in red, and the eight conserved cysteines are marked with bullets. The region of DNA methyltransferase that mediates interactions with replication foci is shown in black in the center of the figure; the protein can be seen to be composed of a C-terminal catalytic domain and an N-terminal regulatory domain. DNA methyltransferase consists of about 1500 amino acids. Shown to scale is a representation of HRX/ALL-1 (Gu *et al.*, 1992; Tkachuk *et al.*, 1992), which consists of about 4000 amino acids. The region of strongest similarity with *Drosophila* trithorax (also about 4000 amino acids) is near the C terminus; two clusters of Zn fingers are also shown. The cysteine-rich region is not discernible in the sequence of *Drosophila* trithorax, and *Drosophila* DNA has not been shown to contain m⁵C. It is suggested that the cysteine-rich region shown in the figure allows regulatory proteins to discriminate among DNA sequences on the basis of methylation status.

These images are available in colour as a download from www.cambridge.org/9780521179997

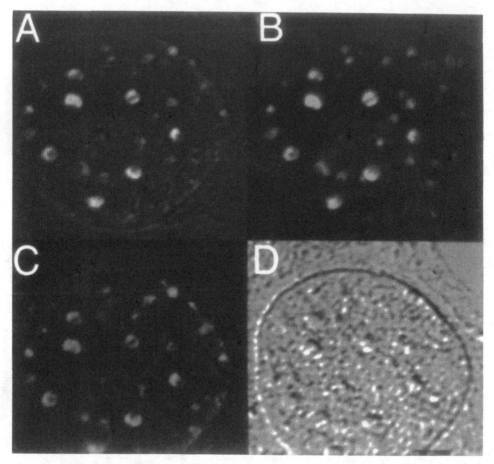

Plate 2. Visualization of the biochemical machines in which DNA is replicated. Mouse 3T3 fibroblasts were pulse-labeled for 5 min with 10 μM 5-bromo-2'-deoxyuridine (BrdU), then fixed with formaldehyde and stained with rhodamine-labeled antibodies to murine DNA methyltransferase and fluorescein-labeled antibodies to BrdU as described (Leonhardt *et al.*, 1992). The cells were examined with a Zeiss LSM410 confocal laser scanning microscope and equatorial optical sections were collected. A, superimposed staining pattern of BrdU (green) and DNA methyltransferase (red). B, DNA methyltransferase staining. C, sites of ongoing DNA replication as revealed by BrdU staining. D, phase-contrast image. The cell shown here was in mid to late S phase at the time of BrdU labeling and fixation. Note that DNA synthesis is occurring in two morphologically distinct classes of replication focus: large, toroidal foci that stain brightly for DNA methyltransferase, and small asymmetric foci that do not stain for DNA methyltransferase (compare B and C). The large, DNA methyltransferase-rich foci may be the site of replication of methylated sequences, and the small, DNA methyltransferase-poor foci may be the site of replication of the unmethylated portion of the genome. As discussed in the text, a major role of replication foci is the clonal transmission of methylation patterns and higher-order chromatin configurations during S phase; the morphological differences among replication foci must reflect biochemical differences that allow different foci to propagate different chromatin configurations.

These images are available in colour as a download from www.cambridge.org/9780521179997

CpG sites be accurately represented by the methylation status of the restriction sites tested, which are usually chosen on the basis of convenience. However, genomic sequencing has shown that changes in methylation status are not simultaneous across all sites, and the methylation status of arbitrarily chosen restriction sites is very unlikely to be an accurate representation of the methylation status of all CpG sites (Pfeifer *et al.*, 1990). Because of the fragmentary knowledge of methylation patterns in and around genes undergoing allele-specific inactivation, there does not seem to be a single case in which it can be regarded as proven that CpG methylation only stabilizes an inactive state established by other regulators.

Of course, there is no case in which methylation has been proven to be the primary event in gene silencing in a developmental process; the correlative nature of nearly all studies on the subject obviate such a conclusion. However, two robust lines of evidence indicate that allele-specific methylation is required for the maintenance of allele-specific gene expression. First, genes subject to imprinting or X inactivation show allele-specific methylation patterns, changes in methylation patterns accompany changes in rate of transcription, and methylation inhibitors and loss-of-function mutations in the DNA methyltransferase gene of mice cause a reversal of imprinting (reviewed by Efstratiadis, 1994; Surani, 1994). Second, chromosome inactivation and other forms of allele-specific gene inactivation are restricted to those organisms whose genomes contain m^5C (Bestor, 1990). (Parent-of-origin effects have been reported to occur in *Drosophila*, whose DNA lacks detectable m^5C. However, such effects seem to be rare, small and variable in magnitude, and are apparent only under special conditions; in no known case does an organism whose DNA lacks m^5C display allele-specific gene expression of a type or degree that can compare to that of many X-linked genes or the autosomal *H19* gene of mice or humans.)

What sort of evidence would be required to distinguish between primary and secondary roles for CpG methylation in allele-specific gene repression? The answer might come from examination of imprinting modifier loci (polymorphic loci that affect the methylation status of unlinked imprinted transgenes in mice) (Engler *et al.*, 1991; Forejt & Gregorová, 1992) and of human genetic diseases that are associated with abnormal methylation patterns and might involve genes similar to the imprinting modifier loci identified in mice (Jeanpierre *et al.*, 1993). It is suggested that if such modifier genes are found to encode developmentally regulated components of the DNA-methylating machinery (a stage-specific DNA methyltransferase or a factor that interacts with a DNA methyltransferase) then a causative rather than stabilizing role of DNA methylation could be inferred. Several imprinting modifier loci have been identified in the mouse (for examples, see Engler *et al.*, 1991; Forejt & Gregorová, 1992); cloning of the genes and biochemical characterization of the gene products may provide a means to distinguish between primary and secondary roles of CpG methylation in allele-specific gene inactivation. The characterization of genes that modify imprinting effects or methylation patterns appears at this time to be the most promising route towards identification of factors involved in the initial events of imprinting and X inactivation.

DNA replication and allele-specific gene inactivation

The epigenetic mark (whether covalent or non-covalent) that distinguishes imprinted and inactive X-linked genes is in many cases maintained with great fidelity over the life of the organism. This fact introduces two difficult questions: how can the mark be transmitted during cell proliferation in the absence of the chemical strand complementarity that underlies the replication of DNA, and what it is that prevents equilibrium of regulatory factors between the alleles?

Part of the answer to these questions may lie in the cell biology of DNA replication. It is now known that mammalian DNA is replicated not by soluble enzymes but by large biochemical machines, many of which are larger than an entire yeast nucleus (Plate 2). Each of these machines or replication foci contains many thousands of replication factors and tens to hundreds of replication forks (reviewed by Spector, 1993). Replication foci are assembled from pre-existing components at the beginning of S phase and are disassembled prior to G2; the number and morphology of replication foci changes in a characteristic manner during S phase (Nakamura *et al.*, 1986; Nakayasu & Berezney, 1989; O'Keefe *et al.*, 1992; Leonhardt *et al.*, 1992). Early foci are small (< 1 μm), numerous, and distributed through the nuclear volume, whereas in mid S phase the replication foci are larger and toroidal in shape; the interior of the toroids is occupied by centromeric satellite DNA (Leonhardt *et al.*, 1992). Late in S phase the large toroidal foci remain prominent, and smaller asymmetric foci appear throughout the nucleus and are especially numerous near the nuclear envelope (a mid or late S phase nucleus is shown in Plate 2). It should be noted that all extant data are derived from static images of fixed cells, and it is not known whether the morphology of replication foci changes during S phase or if new foci are assembled at different stages. In either case the conspicuous morphological changes suggest underlying differences in biochemical composition and function, and I propose that active and repressed genes are replicated in biochemically distinct replication foci; the methylation status and the higher-order chromatin structure of a particular sequence could be determined by the nature of the replication machine in which that sequence is replicated, and a pre-existing chromatin structure may target a chromosomal region for replication in a certain class of replication foci. According to this proposal most of the activity of the replication focus may be devoted to transmission of higher-order chromatin structures, methylation patterns, and patterns of protein modification such as histone phosphorylation, methylation, and acetylation. Actual DNA replication might occupy only a fraction of the factors in replication foci. It might also be noted that the formation of morphologically distinct replication foci in an ordered manner during S phase suggests a rationale for the differences in replication timing often observed for active and inactive genes (and recently observed for alleles of imprinted genes) (Kitsberg *et al.*, 1993; Knoll *et al.*, 1994); active and inactive genes may be replicated at different stages of S phase because replication foci that replicate particular chromatin configurations and methylation patterns are themselves assembled only at particular stages of S phase.

Acknowledgements

Angela Coxon, Michael Wyszynski, and Jeffrey Yoder made helpful comments on the manuscript. Work in the author's laboratory was supported by grants GM43565, CA60610 and GM00616 from the National Institutes of Health.

References

Bestor, T. H. (1990). DNA methylation: evolution of a bacterial immune function into a regulator of gene expression and genome structure in higher eukaryotes. *Phil. Trans. R. Soc. Lond.* B **326**, 179–87.

Bestor, T. H. (1992). Activation of mammalian DNA methyltransferase by cleavage of a Zn-binding regulatory domain. *EMBO J.* **11**, 2611–18.

Bestor, T. H., Chandler, V. & Feinberg, A. P. (1994). Epigenetic effects in eukaryotic gene expression. *Devel. Genet.* **15**, 458–62.

Bestor, T. H. & Coxon, A. (1993). The pros and cons of DNA methylation. *Curr. Biol.* **3**, 384–6.

Bestor, T. H. & Verdine, G. L. (1994). DNA methyltransferase. *Curr. Opin. Cell Biol.* **6**, 380–9.

Efstratiadis, A. (1994). Parental imprinting of autosomal mammalian genes. *Curr. Opin. Genet. Dev.* **4**, 265–80.

Engler, P., Haasch, C., Pinkert, C. A., Doglio, L., Glymour, M., Brinster, R. & Storb, U. (1991). A strain specific modifier on mouse chromosome 4 controls methylation of independent transgene loci. *Cell* **65**, 939–47.

Eversole-Cire, P., Ferguson-Smith, A. C., Sasaki, H., Brown, K. D., Cattanach, B. M., Gonzales, F. A., Surani, M. A. & Jones, P. A. (1993). Activation of an imprinted Igf-2 gene in mouse somatic cell cultures. *Molec. Cell Biol.* **13**, 4928–38.

Forejt, J. & Gregorová, S. (1992). Genetic analysis of genomic imprinting: An *Imprintor-1* gene controls inactivation of the paternal copy of the mouse *Tme* locus. *Cell* **70**, 443–50.

Gu, Y., Nakamura, T., Alder, H., Prasad, R., Canaani, O., Cimino, G., Croce, C. M. & Canaani, E. (1992). The t(4;11) chromosome translocation of human acute leukemias fuses the ALL-1 gene, related to *Drosophila* trithorax, to the AF-4 gene. *Cell* 71, 701–8.

Hsieh, C. L. & Lieber, M. (1992). CpG-methylated minichromosomes become inaccessible for V(D)J recombination after undergoing replication. *EMBO J.* 11, 315–25.

Iguchi-Ariga, S. M. & Schaffner, W. (1989). CpG methylation of the cAMP-responsive enhancer-promoter sequence TGACGTCA abolishes specific factor binding as well as transcriptional activation. *Genes Devel.* 3, 612–19.

Jeanpierre, M., Turleau, C., Aurias, A., Prieur, M., Ledeist, F., Fischer, A. & Viegas-Pequignot, E. (1993). An embryonic-like methylation pattern of classical satellite DNA is observed in ICF syndrome. *Hum. Molec. Genet.* 2, 731–5.

Keshet, I., Liemann-Hurwitz, J. & Cedar, H. (1986). DNA methylation affects the formation of active chromatin. *Cell* 44, 535–43.

Kitsberg, D., Selig, S., Brandeis, M., Simon, I., Keshet, I., Driscoll, D. J., Nicholls, R. D. & Cedar, H. (1993). Allele-specific replication timing of imprinted gene regions. *Nature* 364, 459–63.

Knoll, J. H. M., Cheng, S.-D. & Lalande, M. (1994). Allele-specificity of DNA replication timing in the Angelman/Prader-Willi syndrome imprinted region. *Nature Genet.* 6, 41–6.

Leonhardt, H., Page, A. W., Weier, H.-UI. & Bestor, T. H. (1992). A targeting sequence directs DNA methyltransferase to sites of DNA replication in mammalian nuclei. *Cell* 71, 865–74.

Li, E., Bestor, T. H. & Jaenisch, R. (1992). Targeted mutation of the DNA methyltransferase gene results in embryonic lethality. *Cell* 69, 915–26.

Lock, L. F., Takagi, N. & Martin, G. R. (1987). Methylation of the HPRT gene on the inactive X chromosome occurs after chromosome inactivation. *Cell* 48, 39–46.

Ma, Q., Alder H., Nelson, K. K., Chatterjee, D., Gu, Y., Nakamura, T., Canaani, E., Croce, C. M., Siracusa, L. D. & Buchberg, A. M. (1993). Analysis of the murine *All-1* gene reveals conserved domains with human *ALL-1* and identifies a motif shared with DNA methyltransferases. *Proc. Natl. Acad. Sci. USA* 90, 6350–4.

Meehan, R., Lewis, J., Cross, S., Nan, X. S., Jeppesen, P. & Bird, A. (1992). Transcriptional repression by methylation of CpG. *J. Cell Sci.* (Suppl. 16), 9–14.

Nakamura, H., Morita, T. & Sato, C. (1986). Structural organization of replicon domains during DNA synthetic phase in the mammalian nucleus. *Exp. Cell Res.* 165, 291–7.

Nakayasu, H. & Berezney, R. (1989). Mapping replication sites in the eukaryotic cell nucleus. *J. Cell Biol.* 108, 1–11.

O'Keefe, R. T., Henderson, S. C. & Spector, D. L. (1992), Dynamic organization of DNA replication in mammalian cell nuclei: spatially and temporally defined replication of chromosome-specific α satellite DNA sequences. *J. Cell Biol.* 116, 1095–110.

Orlando, V. & Paro, R. (1993). Mapping polycomb-repressed domains in the bithorax complex using *in vivo* formaldehyde cross-linked chromatin. *Cell* 75, 1187–98.

Paro, R. (1993). Mechanisms of heritable gene repression during development of *Drosophila. Curr. Opin. Cell Biol.* 5, 999–1005.

Pfeifer, G. P., Steigerwald, S. D., Hansen, R. S., Gartler, S. M. & Riggs, A. D. (1990). Polymerase chain reaction aided genomic sequencing of an X-chromosome linked CpG island: methylation patterns suggest clonal inheritance, CpG site autonomy, and explanation of activity state stability. *Proc. Natl. Acad. Sci. USA* 87, 8252–6.

Simon, J., Chiang, A. & Bender, W. (1992). Ten different Polycomb group genes are required for spatial control of the AbdA and abdB homeotic products. *Development* **114**, 493–505.

Spector, D. L. (1993). Macromolecular domains within the cell nucleus. *A. Rev. Cell. Biol.* **9**, 265–316.

Surani, M. A. (1994). Genomic imprinting: control of gene expression by epigenetic inheritance. *Curr. Opin. Cell Biol.* **6**, 390–5.

Tkachuk, D. C., Kohler, S. & Cleary, M. L. (1992). Involvement of a homolog of *Drosophila* trithorax by 11q23 chromosomal translocations in acute leukemias. *Cell* **71**, 691–700.

Wigler, M., Levy, D. & Perucho, M. (1981). The somatic inheritance of DNA methylation. *Cell* **24**, 33–40.

7

DNA methylation and mammalian development

RUDOLF JAENISCH, CAROLINE BEARD AND EN LI

Introduction

Approximately 60% of all CpG dinucleotides in the DNA of vertebrates are methylated at the C5 position, but the frequency with which the modified base is found at particular sites varies between cell types. These methylation patterns are transmitted by clonal inheritance (Bird, 1992; Eden & Cedar, 1994) through the strong preference of mammalian DNA (cytosine-5)-methyltransferase (DNA MTase) for hemimethylated DNA (Bestor & Ingram, 1983; Gruenbaum *et al.*, 1982). Methylation patterns are established during gametogenesis and early embryogenesis (Chaillet *et al.*, 1991; Jähner *et al.*, 1982), although little is known of the molecular mechanisms that control sequence-specific *de novo* methylation and demethylation. The cDNA coding for the murine MTase has been cloned, and sequence analysis (Bestor *et al.*, 1988) has shown that the enzyme contains a C-terminal catalytic domain of 500 amino acids (Lauster *et al.*, 1989; Posfai *et al.*, 1989) linked to an N-terminal regulatory domain of 1000 amino acids (Bestor, 1990). The enzyme is associated with the replication foci of S-phase cells (Leonhardt *et al.*, 1992); recent results have demonstrated that high levels of MTase are present in oocytes and preimplantation embryos (Carlson *et al.*, 1992).

Numerous studies have shown that the transcriptional control regions of genes are undermethylated in tissues where the gene is expressed relative to the same sequences in tissues where the gene is not expressed. Several lines of evidence support the notion that tissue-specific methylation patterns may be involved in the control of developmental gene regulation. (i) Changes in methylation status (usually the loss of methylated cytosines from promoter regions) are correlated with the activation of many tissue-specific genes during differentiation *in vivo* (Eden & Cedar, 1994). (ii) Gene reactivation occurs in certain cell types upon treatment with 5-azacytidine, an inhibitor of cytosine methylation (Jones *et al.*,

1983). (iii) Alleles on the inactive X chromosome are often methylated in promoter regions, whereas alleles on the active X chromosome are normally unmethylated (Grant & Chapman, 1988; Rastan, 1994). (iv) Allele-specific methylation has also been observed for many imprinted transgenes which are inherited in the unmethylated state from parents of one sex and in the methylated state from parents of the other sex (Hadchouel *et al.*, 1987; Reik *et al.*, 1987; Sapienza *et al.*, 1987; Sasaki *et al.*, 1991; Swain *et al.*, 1987). The functional role of DNA methylation in genomic imprinting was strengthened by the recent finding that three imprinted genes, *H19*, *Igf2*, and *Igf2r*, are differentially methylated depending on the parental origin of inheritance (Ferguson-Smith *et al.*, 1993; Sasaki *et al.*, 1992; Stöger *et al.*, 1993; for review see Efstratiadis, 1994; Reik & Allen, 1994).

We are interested in the role of DNA methylation in mammalian development. Using gene targeting in embryonic stem (ES) cells we have generated mice that are unable to maintain normal levels of CpG methylation owing to a defect in the DNA MTase gene. ES cells carrying two mutant MTase alleles are viable whereas mutant embryos die at midgestation with their genomic DNA substantially demethylated. To assess the role of DNA methylation in genomic imprinting, we have examined the expression of the three imprinted genes *H19, insulin-like growth factor 2 (Igf2)*, and *Igf2 receptor (Igf2r)* in mutant mice. Expression of all three imprinted genes was affected in mutant embryos, demonstrating that maintenance of DNA methylation is required for differential expression of imprinted genes during embryogenesis. The results summarized in this chapter have been published by Li *et al.* (1992, 1993).

DNA methylation is essential for embryonic development

ES cells carrying a mutant MTase gene are viable

The DNA MTase gene was disrupted by homologous recombination as described by Li *et al.* (1992) and ES cells carrying a single mutant allele were generated. In order to derive cells homozygous for the mutation, the remaining wild type (wt) allele was disrupted by a second round of gene targeting using a targeting vector carrying the hygromycin resistance gene as a selectable marker. The homozygous mutant cells showed normal morphology and growth rates in tissue culture with no discernible phenotype after more than 50 rounds of cell division. To assess whether the mutation affected the overall level of m^{5}C in genomic DNA, we analyzed endogenous retroviruses which are present in multiple copies and are known to be highly methylated. As summarized in Table 7.1, normal levels of methylation were detected in wt and heterozygous mutant

Table 7.1. *DNA MTase deficiency and survival of ES cells and embryos*

MTase genotype	ES cells		Embryos	
	m⁵C level	Proliferation	m⁵C level	Survival
+/+	normal	normal	normal	normal
+/−	normal	normal	normal	normal
−/−	reduced	normal	reduced	lethal

cell lines but significant demethylation was seen in homozygous mutant cells (Li *et al.*, 1992).

Mutant embryos die after gastrulation

Mice carrying the mutation in the germline were generated by injection of targeted ES cell clones into blastocysts. Whereas heterozygous animals were phenotypically normal, embryos that were homozygous for the mutation died by day 11 of gestation. When isolated at day 10.5, mutant embryos were stunted and of a developmental stage characteristic of normal embryos at day 9.5 or younger. The best-developed homozygous mutant embryos had about 20 somites, distinct forelimb buds, and a closed anterior neuropore. Histological analysis revealed that major organ rudiments were present but smaller than in wild type litter-mates. Close inspection revealed significantly increased numbers of dead or dying cells and considerably fewer mitotic figures in homozygous compared with wild type embryos (Li *et al.*, 1992). When the m⁵C content of DNA from homozygous and normal embryos was analyzed, no differences in methylation patterns were detected between heterozygous and wild type embryos. In contrast, genomic DNA from homozygous mutant embryos was substantially de-methylated (Table 7.1).

Embryonic lethality contrasts with the lack of a discernible mutant phenotype in homozygous ES cells, suggesting that a reduction in m⁵C might be cell-lethal in differentiated tissues but not in pluripotent ES cells. Homozygous embryos do, however, demonstrate significant morphogenesis and tissue differentiation prior to death, indicating that initial cellular differentiation is not affected by lack of methylation. The following hypothesis may explain the apparently normal development of homozygous embryos up to the stage of organogenesis. Sufficient genomic methylation might be maintained early in development by two sources of MTase activity.

(i) A *de novo* MTase might be specifically expressed during early development but inactive in differentiated cells. Indeed, such a *de novo* MTase has been detected previously in early development (Jähner *et al.*, 1982; Kafri *et al.*, 1992), during gametogenesis (Chaillet *et al.*, 1991) and in cultured embryonal carcinoma cells (Stewart *et al.*, 1982) but not in somatic cells. Such an enzyme would be able to maintain the reduced but stable level of DNA methylation in homozygous mutant ES cells, but be unable to sustain methylation patterns in differentiating somatic tissues of mutant embryos. In this context it is significant to note that the acquisition of adult levels of genomic m^{5}C by *de novo* methylation is achieved only at the time of gastrulation (Brandeis *et al.*, 1993; Monk *et al.*, 1987).

(ii) It has been shown that large maternal stores of methyltransferase are present in oocytes and blastocysts (Carlson *et al.*, 1992). Once the embryo has developed post gastrulation, the embryonic *de novo* MTase would be inactivated and the level of maternally derived MTase would become more limiting at each consecutive cell division. This would successively reduce genomic methylation to a level incompatible with cell survival.

DNA methylation and genomic imprinting

The observations summarized in the introduction correlate differential expression of imprinted genes with the inheritance of parental specific methylation patterns, but no direct evidence has been obtained so far linking the expression of imprinted genes with differential DNA methylation. We therefore examined the effect of reduced genomic methylcytosine levels on the expression of the *H19*, *Igf2* and *Igf2r* genes. Analysis of RNA from mutant embryos indicated that the expression of all three genes was altered (summarized in Table 7.2).

(i) *H19 gene:* Previous work has shown that the paternal allele of the *H19* gene is silent and the maternal allele is expressed in normal embryos (Bartolomei *et al.*, 1991). The comparison of wt and mutant embryos indicated that the typically inactive paternal allele was activated in homozygous embryos; this result is consistent with the notion that normal levels of DNA methylation are essential for gene inactivity.

(ii) *Igf2 gene:* The *Igf2* gene is closely linked to the *H19* gene but reciprocally imprinted, i.e. expressed only from the paternal allele (DeChiara *et al.*, 1991). In contrast to *H19*, no *Igf2* expression was seen in homozygous mutant embryos. These results, therefore, suggest that, in contrast to *H19*, a normal level of DNA methylation is required for the expression of the active paternal allele.

(iii) *Igf2r gene:* It has been shown that the *Igf2r* gene, which is located on chromosome 17, is expressed exclusively from the maternal allele (Barlow *et al.*, 1991). Similarly to *Igf2*, the mutation of the MTase gene resulted in silencing of the normally active maternal allele.

Table 7.2. *DNA methylation and genomic imprinting*

MTase genotype	H19		Igf2		Igf2r	
	P[a]	M[a]	P	M	P	M
+/+	−	+	+	−	−	+
+/−	−	+	+	−	−	+
−/−	+	+	−	−	−	−

[a]P, expression of paternal allele; M, expression of maternal allele.

Although numerous experiments have correlated DNA methylation with gene repression and demethylation with gene activation (Bird, 1986; Eden & Cedar, 1994), experimental proof that DNA methylation controls the activity of cellular genes *in vivo* has been lacking. The activation of the normally silent paternal *H19* allele in DNA MTase-deficient embryos provides the first *in vivo* evidence for a causal link between DNA methylation and gene activity. It has been shown recently that the CpG island in the promoter region of the paternal *H19* allele becomes methylated *de novo* after fertilization (Bartolomei *et al.*, 1993; Ferguson-Smith *et al.*, 1991). The simplest interpretation of our results is that interference with the maintenance of this CpG island methylation leads to activation of the gene and loss of the imprint.

In contrast to the activation of the *H19* gene, it is less clear how genomic DNA demethylation could lead to the inactivation of the expressed *Igf2* and *Igf2r* alleles. Unlike *H19*, the closely linked *Igf2* gene shows no obvious parental-origin-specific methylation of the promoter CpG island (Sasaki *et al.*, 1992). It has been proposed that expression of the two reciprocally imprinted genes *H19* and *Igf2* is functionally and/or mechanistically related and that the imprinting of a single chromosomal site might control the activity of both genes (Bartolomei *et al.*, 1993). Our results are consistent with the possibility that *H19* is the 'primary' imprinted gene whose activity is directly controlled by the parental-specific methylation. *H19* transcription may, in turn, suppress in *cis* the expression of the closely linked *Igf2* gene by either competing for a common set of regulatory elements shared by the *Igf2* gene or directly inhibiting the transcription of the *Igf2* gene. Mutually exclusive expression is also seen in X chromosome inactivation, where the *Xist* gene, located at the X inactivation center, is expressed exclusively from the inactive X chromosome (Norris *et al.*, 1994). It has been suggested that the *Xist* mRNA, which lacks a conserved open reading frame (as does the *H19* mRNA), may act in *cis* to cause X chromosome inactivation (Rastan, 1994).

It is interesting to consider the repression of the *Igf2r* gene in MTase mutant embryos in relation to a recently proposed model, which identified a downstream CpG island as the 'imprinting box' (Stöger *et al.*, 1993). It was shown that this island becomes specifically methylated in the expressed maternal allele during oogenesis. Stöger *et al.* hypothesized that the maternal-specific methylation of this box may represent the primary imprinting signal for the maternal *Igf2r* allele and that the CpG island may act as a 'gene silencer', for example by binding a repressor protein when not methylated and thus inhibiting expression of the paternal allele. Methylation of CpG islands may play a crucial role in establishing and maintaining genomic imprinting patterns (Bird, 1993). Methylated CpG islands have also been detected on the inactive X chromosome and have been suggested to stabilize repression (Riggs & Pfeifer, 1992). Methylation of CpG islands may be a general mechanism to control differential expression of identical alleles of genes such as imprinted and X-linked genes.

Our results clearly establish that DNA methylation plays a critical role in genomic imprinting. More specifically, DNA methylation is required for maintaining monoallelic expression of three imprinted genes, *H19*, *Igf2* and *Igf2r*, during embryonic development. It will be particularly interesting to study whether methylation changes are involved in the formation of Wilms' tumors, which in some cases show biallelic expression of the *H19* and *Igf2* genes (Ogawa *et al.*, 1993; Rainier *et al.*, 1993).

DNA methylation has been hypothesized to be involved in numerous processes, which include X inactivation, genomic imprinting, virus latency, carcinogenesis, aging, and the regulation of tissue-specific gene expression during development. The mutant ES cells and animals described here make possible rigorous tests of these hypotheses. The mutant ES cells may also aid in isolating other methyltransferases whose function might be to establish the methylation patterns in early development and to set up genomic imprints in the gametes.

Acknowledgements

Supported by NIH grant R35 CA 44339.

References

Barlow, D. P., Stöger, R., Herrmann, B. G., Saito, K. & Schweifer, N. (1991). The mouse insulin-like growth factor type-2 receptor is imprinted and closely linked to the *Tme* locus. *Nature* **349**, 84–7.

Bartolomei, M. S., Webber, A. L., Brunkow, M. E. & Tilghman, S. M. (1993). Epigenetic mechanisms underlying the imprinting of the mouse *H19* gene. *Genes Devel.* **7**, 1663–73.

124 R. Jaenisch, C. Beard & E. Li

Bartolomei, M. S., Zemel, S. & Tilghman, S. M. (1991). Parental imprinting of the mouse *H19* gene. *Nature* **351**, 153–5.

Bestor, T. (1990). DNA methylation: evolution of a bacterial immune function into a regulator of gene expression and genome structure in higher eukaryotes. *Phil. Trans. R. Soc. Lond.* B**326**, 179–87.

Bestor, T. H. & Ingram, V. M. (1983). Two DNA methyltransferases from murine erythroleukemia cells: purification, sequence specificity, and mode of interaction with DNA. *Proc. Natl. Acad. Sci. USA* **80**, 559–63.

Bestor, T. H., Laudano, A. P., Mattaliano, R. & Ingram, V. M. (1988). Cloning and sequencing of a cDNA encoding DNA methyltransferase of mouse cells. The carboxyl-terminal domain of the mammalian enzymes is related to bacterial restriction methyltransferases. *J. molec. Biol.* **203**, 971–83.

Bird, A. (1986). CpG rich islands and the function of DNA methylation. *Nature* **321**, 209–13.

Bird, A. (1992). The essentials of DNA methylation. *Cell* **70**, 5–8.

Bird, A. (1993). Imprints on islands. *Curr. Biol.* **3**, 275–7.

Brandeis, M., Kafri, T., Ariel, M., Chaillet, J. R., McCarrey, J., Razin, A. & Cedar, H. (1993). The ontogeny of allele-specific methylation associated with imprinted genes in the mouse. *EMBO J.* **12**, 3669–77.

Carlson, L. L., Page, A. W. & Bestor, T. H. (1992). Properties and localization of DNA methyltransferase in preimplantation mouse embryos: implications for genomic imprinting. *Genes Devel.* **6**, 2536–41.

Chaillet, J. R., Vogt, T. F., Beier, D. R. & Leder, P. (1991). Parental-specific methylation of an imprinted transgene is established during gametogenesis and progressively changes during embryogenesis. *Cell* **66**, 77–83.

DeChiara, T., Robertson, E. & Efstratiadis, A. (1991). Parental imprinting of the mouse insulin-like growth factor II gene. *Cell* **64**, 849–59.

Eden, S. & Cedar, H. (1994). Role of DNA methylation in the regulation of transcription. *Curr. Opin. Genet. Devel.* **4**, 255–9.

Efstratiadis, A. (1994). Parental imprinting of autosomal mammalian genes. *Curr. Opin. Genet. Devel.* **4**, 265–80.

Ferguson-Smith, A. C., Cattanach, B. M., Barton, S. C., Beechey, C. V. & Surani, M. A. (1991). Embryological and molecular investigations of parental imprinting on mouse chromosome 7. *Nature* **351**, 667–71.

Ferguson-Smith, A. C., Sasaki, H., Cattanach, B. M. & Surani, M. A. (1993). Parental-origin-specific epigenetic modification of the mouse *H19* gene. *Nature* **362**, 751–5.

Grant, S. G. & Chapman, V. M. (1988). Mechanisms of X-chromosome regulation. *A. Rev. Genet.* **22**, 199–233.

Gruenbaum, Y., Cedar, H. & Razin, A. (1982). Substrate and sequence specificity of a eukaryotic DNA methylase. *Nature* **295**, 620–2.

Hadchouel, M., Farza, H., Simon, D., Tiollais, P. & Pourcel, C. (1987). Maternal inhibition of hepatitis B surface antigen gene expression in transgenic mice correlates with de novo methylation. *Nature* **329**, 454–6.

Jähner, D., Stuhlmann, H., Stewart, C. L., Harbers, K., Lohler, J., Simon, I. & Jaenisch, R. (1982). *De novo* methylation and expression of retroviral genomes during mouse embryogenesis. *Nature* **298**, 623–8.

Jones, P. A., Taylor, S. M. & Wilson, V. L. (1983). Inhibition of DNA methylation by 5-azacytidine. *Rec. Results Cancer Res.* **84**, 202–11.

Kafri, T., Ariel, M., Brandeis, M., Shemer, R., Urven, L., McCarrey, J., Cedar, H. & Razin, A. (1992). Developmental pattern of gene-specific DNA methylation in the mouse embryo and germ line. *Genes Devel.* **6**, 705–14.

Lauster, R., Trautner, T. A. & Noyer-Widner, M. (1989). Cytosine-specific type II DNA methyltransferases. A conserved enzyme core with variable target-recognizing domains. *J. molec. Biol.* **206**, 305–12.

Leonhardt, H., Page, A. W., Weier, H.-U. & Bestor, T. H. (1992). A targeting sequence directs DNA methyltransferase to sites of DNA replication in mammalian nulcei. *Cell* **71**, 865–73.

Li, E., Beard, C. & Jaenisch, R. (1993). Role for DNA methylation in genomic imprinting. *Nature* **366**, 362–5.

Li, E., Bestor, T. H. & Jaenisch, R. (1992). Targeted mutation of the DNA methyltransferase gene results in embryonic lethality. *Cell* **69**, 915–26.

Monk, M., Boubelik, M. & Lehnert, S. (1987). Temporal and regional changes in DNA methylation in the embryonic, extraembryonic and germ cell lineages during mouse embryo development. *Development* **99**, 371–82.

Norris, D. P., Patel, D., Kay, G. F., Penny, G. D., Brockdorff, N., Sheardown, S. A. & Rastan, S. (1994). Evidence that random and imprinted Xist expression is controlled by preemptive methylation. *Cell* **77**, 41–51.

Ogawa, O., Eccles, M. R., Szeto, J., NcNoe, L. A., Yun, K., Maw, M. A., Smith, P. J. & Reeve, A. E. (1993). Relaxation of insulin-like growth factor II gene imprinting implicated in Wilms tumor. *Nature* **362**, 749–51.

Posfai, J., Bhagwat, A. S., Posfai, G. & Roberts, R. J. (1989). Predictive motifs derived from cytosine methyltransferases. *Nucleic Acids Res.* **17**, 2421–35.

Rainier, S., Johnson, L. A., Dobry, C. J., Ping, A. J., Grundy, P. E. & Feinberg, A. P. (1993). Relaxation of imprinted genes in human cancer. *Nature* **362**, 747–9.

Rastan, S. (1994). X chromosome inactivation and the *Xist* gene. *Cur. Opin. Genet. Devel.* **4**, 292–7.

Reik, W. & Allen, N. D. (1994). Imprinting with and without methylation. *Curr. Biol.* **4**, 145–7.

Reik, W., Collick, A., Norris, M., Barton, S. & Surani, A. (1987). Genomic imprinting determines methylation of parental alleles in transgenic mice. *Nature* **328**, 248–51.

Riggs, A. D. & Pfeifer, G. P. (1992). X-chromosome inactivation and cell memory. *Trends Genet.* **8**, 169–74.

Sapienza, C., Peterson, A., Rossant, J. & Balling, R. (1987). Degree of methylation of transgenes is dependent on gamete of origin. *Nature* **328**, 251–4.

Sasaki, H., Hamada, T., Ueda, T., Seki, R., Higashinakagawa, T. & Sakaki, Y. (1991). Inherited type of allele methylation variations in a mouse chromosome region where an integrated transgene shows methylation imprinting. *Development* **111**, 573–81.

Sasaki, H., Jones, P., Chaillet, R., Ferguson-Smith, A., Barton, S., Reik, W. & Surani, A. (1992). Parental imprinting: potentially active chromatin of the repressed maternal allele of the mouse insulin-like growth factor II (*Igf2*) gene. *Genes Devel.* **6**, 1843–56.

Stewart, C., Stuhlmann, H., Jähner, D. & Jaenisch, R. (1982). *De novo* methylation, expression, and infectivity of retroviral genomes introduced into embryonal carcinoma cells. *Proc. Natl. Acad. Sci. USA* **79**, 4098–102.

Stöger, R., Kubicka, P., Liu, C.-G., Kafri, T., Razin, A., Cedar, H. & Barlow, D. P. (1993). Maternal-specific methylation of the imprinted mouse *Igf2r* locus identifies the expressed locus as carrying the imprinting signal. *Cell* **73**, 61–71.

Swain, J., Stewart, T. & Leder, P. (1987). Parental legacy determines methylation and expression of an autosomal transgene: a molecular mechanism for parental imprinting. *Cell* **50**, 719–27.

III

Mechanisms of imprinting

8

X chromosome inactivation and imprinting

MARY F. LYON

Introduction

Dosage compensation for X-linked genes in mammals is brought about by inactivation of one X chromosome in the somatic cells of females, with the result that XY males and XX females both effectively have a single dosage of X-linked gene products (reviewed by Lyon, 1992, 1994; Gartler *et al.*, 1992). Typically, in eutherian mammals either of the two X chromosomes is inactivated in different cells of the same animal. This leads to females heterozygous for X-linked genes having a characteristic variegated phenotype, such as that seen in the tortoiseshell cat, heterozygous for orange and black or tabby fur color. However, marsupials also exhibit X chromosome inactivation and in these the picture is different, with the paternally derived X chromosome being preferentially inactivated in all cells of the animal (reviewed by Cooper *et al.*, 1993). In addition, in mice and rats similar preferential inactivation of the paternally derived X chromosome is seen in two extraembryonic cell lineages, the trophectoderm and primitive endoderm (Takagi & Sasaki, 1975). Whether or not similar non-random inactivation occurs in human extraembryonic tissues is a controversial point (Harrison, 1989). Thus, imprinting is an important component in X chromosome inactivation. In order to attempt to understand something of the association of the two phenomena, one has to consider the mechanism of X inactivation.

Mechanism of X chromosome inactivation

In the very early female embryo, both X chromosomes in each cell are active (Epstein *et al.*, 1978). Inactivation is first initiated in the mouse embryo in trophectoderm and primitive endoderm, the two lineages that show imprinting, at the late blastocyst stage (Fig. 8.1) (Monk & Harper, 1979). Somewhat later, at

129

the egg cylinder stage, inactivation takes place in the primitive ectoderm, which gives rise to the embryo proper, where the choice of X chromosome is random. Once inactivation has occurred it remains stable throughout all further cell divisions in the lifetime of the animal, except in the female germ cell, where reactivation occurs around the time of meiosis.

According to present thinking, the mechanism of X inactivation has three parts, the first of which is initiation of inactivation in the early embryo. The second component is spreading of the inactivation to cover the whole, or almost the whole, chromosome; the third is the maintenance of inactivation throughout all subsequent cell divisions.

X inactivation center

Initiation of X inactivation is thought to be brought about by the X inactivation center (XIC) located on the X chromosome. Evidence for the existence of this center came originally from mouse X autosome translocations. When an X chromosome is broken into two segments by such a translocation, only one segment undergoes inactivation; the other remains active in all cells. The interpretation is that the segment that remains active lacks an inactivation center (reviewed by Lyon, 1988; Rastan & Brown, 1990). In individuals with supernumerary X chromosomes, e.g. XXY, XXXX, a single X chromosome remains active and all others become inactive. Thus there is considered to be a counting mechanism such that one X chromosome remains active per two autosome sets; this mechanism is thought to act on the X inactivation center. One XIC receives some blocking factor, and the chromosome with the blocked center remains active (reviewed by Rastan, 1994). All other XICs in the cell (normally one) then initiate inactivation, which spreads in a *cis*-limited manner along the chromosome in both directions. Segments without an XIC remain active.

By study of different translocations and deletions it has been possible to map the XIC to band XD in mouse and band Xq13 in humans. From the relevant region a human gene was cloned, with the unique property of being expressed from the inactive but not the active X chromosome (Brown *et al.*, 1991). The gene was termed *XIST* (*X Inactive Specific Transcript*). A homologous gene (*Xist*) with the same properties of expression was cloned from the region of the XIC in the mouse (Borsani *et al.*, 1991; Brockdorff *et al.*, 1991). From the combination of its location and its unique pattern of expression, *XIST/Xist* is a strong candidate for a role in the X inactivation center; the first hypothesis would be that the imprinting seen in X chromosome inactivation is mediated through the *Xist* locus. The suggestion would be that some imprint on *Xist* affects its probability of expression and hence of involvement in initiating X inactivation or not.

Evidence concerning the role of the Xist *gene*

Before considering the imprinting of *Xist* it is important to deal with the evidence that it may indeed be part of the XIC. For *Xist* to have a causal role in X inactivation it must be expressed at appropriate stages in development. Kay *et al.* (1993) studied the expression of *Xist* in the very early mouse embryo. No expression was seen in 2-cell embryos, but by the 8-cell and morula stages expression was already present, and continued through the blastocyst and egg cylinder stages. X chromosome inactivation first occurs in the trophectoderm at the late blastocyst stage, at least a day later than the first appearance of *Xist* expression (Fig. 8.1) (Takagi *et al.*, 1982). By breeding embryos in which the two parentally derived alleles of *Xist* were distinguishable, Kay *et al.* (1993) also showed that when *Xist* expression first appeared only the activity of the paternally derived allele (X^P) was seen. Expression of the maternally derived allele (X^m) was not conclusively seen until the egg cylinder stage. Thus, *Xist* is expressed before the time of initiation of X inactivation; its first expression is imprinted, but random expression occurs later. In all these aspects, the pattern of expression of *Xist* is such that it could have a causal role in X inactivation rather than being a consequence of this phenomenon. However, since expression was seen as early as the 8-cell stage by Kay *et al.* (1993) and even earlier at the 4-cell stage by Kay *et al.* (1994), when both X chromosomes are active, expression of *Xist* is clearly not sufficient for X inactivation. Some other factor must also be involved.

As already mentioned, X chromosome activity in germ cells differs from that in somatic cells. In precursors of female germ cells, inactivation occurs normally, as in somatic tissue, but reactivation of the inactive X chromosome occurs at around the time of onset of meiosis. Conversely, in male germ cells the single X chromosome becomes inactive early in spermatogenesis (reviewed by Lyon, 1994). These changes in X chromosome activity are accompanied by changes in expression of *Xist*. Various groups of authors have studied *Xist* expression in the male. By contrast to the female, in which *Xist* is expressed in all adult tissues, in the male no expression of *Xist* is seen except in the testis (McCarrey & Dilworth, 1992; Richler *et al.*, 1992; Salido *et al.*, 1992). Isolation and fractionation of germ cells, and studies of testes of young animals, in which germ cells are undergoing development, have shown that the expression is in germ cells, rather than somatic cells, of the testis. In the female, McCarry & Dilworth (1992) showed that *Xist* expression disappeared from germ cells at around the time of reactivation of the X chromosome. Thus, as in the embryo, the expression of *Xist* is appropriate for it to have a causal role in the change of X chromosome activity, but the evidence that it in fact has such a role is not yet complete.

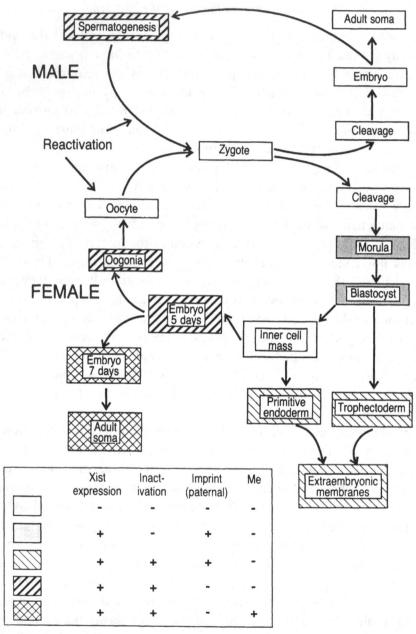

Fig. 8.1. Changes in X chromosome activity during the life cycle of the mouse. The diagram shows the correlation of *Xist* expression with inactivation, and with the presence of imprinting. Me, methylation. This refers to methylation of CpG islands of genes on the inactive X chromosome (not to methylation of the *Xist* gene). Reprinted with permission from Lyon (1993).

A further situation in which *Xist* expression changes with X chromosome activity is in embryonic stem cells (ES cells). In some XX embryocarcinoma (EC) and also in ES cell lines, both X chromosomes are active while the cells are maintained in a totipotent state, but if the cells are allowed to differentiate X chromosome inactivation occurs (Martin *et al.*, 1978; Rastan & Robertson, 1985). Kay *et al.* (1993) showed that differentiation of such an XX ES cell line was accompanied by *Xist* expression. This is a point of considerable interest: it implies that ES cells constitute a suitable system for studying the role of *Xist* in X inactivation.

Imprinting of the Xist gene

Rastan and colleagues (Kay *et al.*, 1994; Norris *et al.*, 1994) have carried out two series of experiments on the imprinting of the *Xist* gene. In the first they considered the possible role of DNA methylation in imprinting and expression of *Xist*. DNA methylation has been proposed as a possible mechanism of imprinting (reviewed by Bird, 1993). The inactive X chromosome is known to show differential methylation of CpG islands (Riggs & Pfeifer, 1992), and hence the question of methylation of the *Xist* gene in different cell types is highly relevant. Norris *et al.* (1994) found that in adult male mice, where the *Xist* gene on the single active X chromosome is not expressed, it was fully methylated at sites in the promoter and 5' region of the body of the gene. Conversely, in the female both methylated and unmethylated forms of the corresponding sites were present (Fig. 8.2). In order to find which X chromosome carried the unmethylated *Xist*, Norris *et al.* studied females heterozygous for the translocation T16H. In these females the randomness of X inactivation is lost, and the translocated X remains active in all cells. By breeding such females with a distinguishable *Xist* allele on each X chromosome, Norris *et al.* showed that the translocated active X chromosome carried a fully methylated *Xist* gene, whereas the *Xist* allele on the normal inactive X chromosome was completely unmethylated at the same sites.

Norris *et al.* also studied yolk sac endoderm tissue of normal females, in which the paternal X chromosome is preferentially inactivated, in contrast to the random inactivation in the embryo itself. Again having bred females with distinguishable alleles of *Xist* on the two X chromosomes, they found that the paternal, expressed, allele of *Xist* was completely unmethylated and the maternal allele fully methylated (Fig. 8.2).

These results indicated that methylation was associated with lack of transcription of *Xist*. In order to test whether methylation might also be associated with imprinting of *Xist*, Norris *et al.* studied male germ cells. They found that

		Me	Transcript	XCI
Female soma	X^I	−	+	+
	X^A	+++	−	−
Male soma	X^A	+++	−	−
Sperm	X^I	−	+	+
Yolk sac endoderm	X^M	+++	−	−
	X^P	−	+	+
ES cells totipotent	X^M	+	−	−
	X^P	+	−	−
ES cells differentiated	X^I	−	+	+
	X^A	++	−	−

Fig. 8.2. Methylation of the 5' region of the *Xist* gene, and its association with transcription of the gene, and with X chromosome inactivation. Me, methylation of the *Xist* gene; XCI, X chromosome inactivation; X^A, active X chromosome; X^I, inactive X chromosome. Data from Norris *et al.* (1994).

methylation of *Xist* was lost at around the time of entry into meiosis. This was shown by study of mice with impaired spermatogenesis, arrested at around the pachytene stage, and of young mice in which the first wave of spermatogenesis was occurring. A characteristic feature of the demethylation of *Xist* in male germ cells was that a small group of sites, which the authors named 'the *Mlu*I cluster', remained fully methylated. This was not seen in the demethylated *Xist* of the inactive X chromosome of females, but as yet its significance is not clear; the authors consider the general demethylation to be the important feature. This demethylated state of *Xist* was retained in mature sperm. Hence, the paternal gamete entering the new zygote was presumably also demethylated, and thus differential methylation could constitute the parental imprint on the *Xist* gene. The state of methylation of *Xist* in female germ cells is not yet known, but as both X chromosomes are active and the *Xist* locus inactive, as shown by McCarrey & Dilworth (1992), it seems reasonable to surmise that the gene is methylated.

In order to study whether differential methylation of *Xist* in female embryos could be a cause rather than a consequence of changes in its expression, Norris *et al.* (1994) studied a line of XX ES cells in which X chromosome inactivation occurred on differentiation. In a control XY cell line the single *Xist* allele was fully methylated both before and after differentiation. In the XX cells before differentiation both a methylated and an unmethylated allele were present, although methylation was not complete (Fig. 8.2). As differentiation proceeded, methylation became more complete. Thus, in both male and female ES cells methylation of *Xist* preceded the time of its first transcription. The ES cells used carried distinguishable alleles of *Xist* and hence it was possible to show that these cells had lost the parental imprint on *Xist*. Either allele of *Xist* was expressed in different cells, and equal amounts of isozymes of the X-linked PGK1 enzyme were produced, indicating random X inactivation. The results thus suggest that in the undifferentiated ES cells, where *Xist* is not transcribed and both X chromosomes are active, differential methylation of *Xist* (marking it as the future active or inactive allele) had already occurred. It is possible, however, that these ES cells were not representative of all such cells: Tada *et al.* (1993a), using ES cells in which the X chromosomes were distinguishable by translocations, found that the parental imprint was still retained, at least in cells forming the mural region of embryoid bodies.

Further insight into the imprinting of *Xist* has come from studies of androgenotes, gynogenotes and parthenogenotes. Earlier work on parthenogenotes had shown that the counting mechanism maintaining one X chromosome active per two autosome sets can override the parental origin of chromosomes. Thus, in diploid parthenogenotes with two maternally derived X chromosomes, inactivation of one X chromosome still occurs, even in extra-embryonic tissues (Rastan *et al.*, 1980; Rastan & Robertson, 1985), and in XO females with a paternally derived X chromosome this remains active in extra-embryonic as well as embryonic tissues (Papaioannou & West, 1981).

Kay *et al.* (1994) studied the expression of *Xist* in parthenogenetic and gynogenetic embryos with two maternally derived X chromosomes. Whereas in normal female embryos *Xist* expression first appeared at the 4-cell stage, in parthenogenotes and gynogenotes it was delayed, first appearing at the morula and the blastocyst stages, respectively (Fig. 8.3). In embryos with distinguishable alleles of *Xist*, cells expressing one or other occurred equally. By contrast, in androgenotes with only X^P chromosomes, and therefore unmethylated *Xist* alleles, expression of *Xist* began at the 4-cell stage. This evidence suggests that the parental imprints on *Xist* indeed determine its expression in the early embryo, and the imprint appears to be lost by the blastocyst stage.

The androgenetic embryos yielded further interesting results. Whereas all gynogenetic embryos are XX, androgenetic embryos can be chromosomally of three types: X^PX^P, X^PY and YY. The YY embryos would be expected to be eliminated early. The results suggested that all the remaining embryos, both

		Embryonic stage		
		4-cell	8-cell to morula	blastocyst
Androgenotes	$X^P X^P$	+	±	−
	$X^P Y$	+	±	−
Normal embryo	$X^M X^P$	+	+	+
	$X^M Y$	−	−	−
Gynogenotes	$X^M X^M$	−	−	+
Parthenogenotes	$X^M X^M$	−	−	+

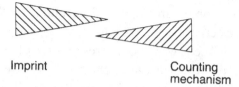

Imprint   Counting mechanism

Fig. 8.3. Transcription of the *Xist* gene in normal embryos, androgenotes, gynogenotes and parthenogenotes. The results indicate that the parental imprint is lost before the blastocyst stage, and that the counting mechanism for X chromosomes is not present in early cleavage and morula stages. Data from Kay *et al.* (1994).

$X^P X^P$ and $X^P Y$, were expressing *Xist* (Fig. 8.3). Thus, the counting mechanism maintaining one *Xist* allele inactive was apparently not functional. A further difference from normal embryos lay in the duration of expression of *Xist*. Whereas normally *Xist* expression is first seen at the 4-cell stage and then persists, in the androgenetic embryos down-regulation began at the late 8-cell stage and expression had disappeared by the blastocyst stage in both $X^P X^P$ and $X^P Y$ embryos. The authors conclude that in normal embryos some other maternally inherited factor maintains the expression of *Xist*, and that this is missing in androgenetic embryos.

Thus, this work has provided evidence that differential methylation of the promoter and 5′ region of the *Xist* gene could be itself the imprint. This imprint could then lead to differential expression of X^m and X^P alleles of *Xist* in the early embryo, and this in turn to preferential inactivation of the X^P. There is also evidence that the imprint on *Xist* is lost early in development, in line with the random inactivation of either X chromosome in the embryo proper. This contrasts with the situation in some autosomal cases where the imprint apparently persists late into development. The counting mechanism for X chromosomes is not functional when *Xist* is first expressed. This first expression of *Xist* is well before the inactive X chromosome first appears; some other, as yet unidentified, factor is needed to trigger inactivation. Furthermore, another imprinted and maternally expressed factor is apparently needed to maintain transcription of *Xist* after the morula stage.

Possible method of spreading of X chromosome inactivation

If differential methylation forms the imprint on *Xist*, it is interesting to consider the role of methylation in the X inactivation process. The suggestion was put forward by various authors that methylation might form the mechanism of spreading of inactivation along the chromosome (Riggs, 1975; Holliday & Pugh, 1975). It is now known that CpG islands in the 5′ region of genes on the inactive X chromosome are heavily methylated, in contrast to their unmethylated state in the genome generally (Gartler *et al.*, 1992; Riggs & Pfeifer, 1992). However, this methylation is not seen in all types of X inactivation, being absent in marsupials (Cooper *et al.*, 1993), in mouse germ cells (Grant *et al.*, 1992) and possibly also in extraembryonic lineages (Kratzer *et al.*, 1983; Grant *et al.*, 1992). In addition, it appears after the first initiation of inactivation (Lock *et al.*, 1987; Grant *et al.*, 1992). It is therefore thought to be part of the mechanism stabilizing inactivation, rather than the spreading mechanism. Recently, another type of differential methylation has been found, in which certain sites in the body of the gene are differentially methylated on the active, rather than inactive, X chromosome, but the role of this is not yet known (Piper *et al.*, 1993).

If differential methylation is not the spreading mechanism, other possibilities include some change in the structure of the chromatin fiber or in the binding of proteins to chromatin. The sequence of the *Xist* gene has been determined with a view to understanding its role in spreading inactivation. The structure of the gene is well conserved among mammals (Brockdorff *et al.*, 1992; Brown *et al.*, 1992). In both human and mouse the gene has no substantial open reading frame, and the gene product is retained in the nucleus. Thus, the gene may act through RNA, possibly by preventing the binding of proteins or by altering the chromatin configuration in the region.

Evolution of X chromosome imprinting and inactivation

A further question concerns the association of imprinting and X inactivation in evolution. An early suggestion was that in primitive mammals X inactivation in somatic cells of females had evolved from an earlier inactivation of the X chromosome in male germ cells (Cooper, 1971; Lifschytz & Lindsley, 1972). Inactivation of heteromorphic sex chromosomes during meiosis is seen in various animal groups in which the male is the heterogametic sex (Jablonka & Lamb,

1988) and clearly has some selective advantage, possibly in protecting unsaturated pairing sites. The suggestion was that inactivation of the paternal X chromosome in spermatogenesis was carried over into the embryo and provided a starting point for somatic X inactivation. The discovery of the demethylation imprint on the *Xist* gene in sperm, leading to the differential expression of the paternal allele of *Xist* in the early embryo, provides evidence in favor of this suggestion.

In the very early embryo the mechanism for counting X chromosomes is apparently not functional. In a normal animal imprinting would be enough to give the observed single X chromosome activity, without the need for a counting mechanism. The single X^m in X^mY males would be active and the X^P of X^mX^P females inactive. In eutherians, from observation of X chromosome aneuploids and polyploids, it is known that there is a counting mechanism. In triploids either one or two (Endo *et al.*, 1982) and in tetraploids two X chromosomes are active (Webb *et al.*, 1992). The mechanism is present in the extraembryonic lineages in which imprinting is seen: one X^m of X^mX^m parthenogenotes can become inactive and the X^P of X^PO females can remain active. However, it appears in some way less effective, as the second X^m of X^mX^m parthenogenotes (Endo & Takagi, 1981) and of X^mX^mY females does have a tendency to remain active (Tada *et al.*, 1993b). In marsupials it is not really clear if a counting mechanism is present, since far fewer sex chromosome aneuploids are available for study (Cooper *et al.*, 1993).

It may be that the primitive form of X inactivation was the imprinted type and that the counting mechanism only arose with the switch to random inactivation. The imprinted type of X inactivation is less stable than the random type. In marsupials, reactivation of the paternal allele of X-linked genes may occur in cultured cells or in some tissues *in vivo* (Cooper *et al.*, 1993). It is possible that there is some feature of imprinted X inactivation that makes instability inherent and that the selective advantage that led to the evolution of random inactivation lay in its providing more stable inactivation and hence better dosage compensation. However, at present it is not known if there is any causal connection between the imprint and lower stability; the association could be merely fortuitous.

Thus, the hypothetical picture would be that in evolution the inactivation of the primitive X chromosome first took place in male germ cells, as the X and Y began to differentiate. This resulted in differential methylation of the *Xist* locus, which when carried over into the very early embryo led to differential expression of the X chromosome. In present-day mammals the function of X inactivation seems clearly to be dosage compensation. Activity of additional X chromosome material in aneuploids and translocation heterozygotes is clearly harmful (Shao

& Takagi, 1990; Tada *et al.*, 1993b). Dosage compensation is also seen in *Drosophila* and *Caenorhabditis elegans*; thus, this phenomenon has evolved at least three times and must be selectively advantageous. However, it is possible that dosage compensation was not the original function of X inactivation. In mouse embryos with activity of supernumerary X chromosomes, the extra-embryonic tissues are poorly developed, as in parthenogenotes (Tada *et al.*, 1993b). It is possible that in evolution the inactivation of the paternal X chromosome favored the development of the extraembryonic tissues and thus was involved in the evolution of viviparity. It may be that the function of dosage compensation was added only later, and that this was still later associated with the development of a random, more stable type of X inactivation in eutherians.

References

Bird, A. P. (1993). Imprints on islands. *Curr. Biol.* **3**, 275–7.

Borsani, G., Tonlorenzi, R., Simmler, M. C., Dandolo, L., Arnaud, D., Capra, V., Grompe, M., Pizzuti, A., Muzny, D., Lawrence, C., Willard, H. F., Avner, P. & Ballabio, A. (1991). Characterization of a murine gene expressed from the inactive X chromosome. *Nature* **351**, 325–9.

Brockdorff, N., Ashworth, A., Kay, G. F., Cooper, P., Smith, S., McCabe, V. M., Norris, D. P., Penny, G. D., Patel, D. & Rastan, S. (1991). Conservation of position and exclusive expression of mouse *Xist* from the inactive X chromosome. *Nature* **351**, 329–31.

Brockdorff, N., Ashworth, A., Kay, G. F., McCabe, V. M., Norris, D. P., Cooper, P. J., Swift, S. & Rastan, S. (1992). The product of the mouse *Xist* gene is a 15 kb inactive X-specific transcript containing no conserved ORF and located in the nucleus. *Cell* **71**, 515–26.

Brown, C. J., Ballabio, A., Rupert, J. L., Lafreniere, R. G., Grompe, M., Tonlorenzi, R. & Willard, H. F. (1991). A gene from the region of the human X inactivation centre is expressed exclusively from the inactive X chromosome. *Nature* **349**, 38–44.

Brown, C. J., Hendrich, B. D., Rupert, J. L., Lafreniere, R. G., Xing, Y., Lawrence, J. & Willard, H. F. (1992). The human *Xist* gene; analysis of a 17 kb inactive X-specific RNA that contains conserved repeats and is highly localized within the nucleus. *Cell* **71**, 527–42.

Cooper, D. W. (1971). A directed genetic change model for X chromosome inactivation in eutherian mammals. *Nature* **231**, 292–4.

Cooper, D. W., Johnston, P. G., Watson, J. M. & Graves, J. A. M. (1993). X-inactivation in marsupials and monotremes. *Semin. Devel. Biol.* **4**, 117–28.

Endo, S. & Takagi, N. (1981). A preliminary cytogenetic study of X chromosome inactivation in diploid parthenogenetic embryos from LT/Sv mice. *Jap. J. Genet.* **56**, 349–56.

Endo, S., Takagi, N. & Sasaki, M. (1982). The late-replicating X chromosome in digynous mouse triploid embryos. *Devel. Genet.* **6**, 137–43.

Epstein, C. J., Smith, S., Travis, B. & Tucker, G. (1978). Both X chromosomes function before visible X chromosome inactivation in female mouse embryos. *Nature* **274**, 500–3.

Gartler, S. M., Dyer, K. A. & Goldman, M. A. (1992). Mammalian X-chromosome inactivation. In *Molecular Genetic Medicine*, vol. 2, ed. T. Friedman, pp. 121–60. New York: Academic Press.

Grant, M., Zuccotti, M. & Monk, M. (1992). Methylation of CpG sites of two X-linked genes coincides with X-inactivation in the female mouse embryo but not in the germ line. *Nature Genet.* **2**, 161–6.

Harrison, K. B. (1989). X-chromosome inactivation in the human cytotrophoblast. *Cytogenet. Cell Genet.* **52**, 37–41.

Holliday, R. & Pugh, J. E. (1975). DNA modification mechanisms and gene activity during development. *Science* **187**, 226–32.

Jablonka, E. & Lamb, M. J. (1988). Meiotic pairing constraints and the activity of sex chromosomes. *J. theor. Biol.* **133**, 23–36.

Kay, G. F., Barton, S. C., Surani, M. A. & Rastan, S. (1994). Imprinting and X chromosome counting mechanisms determine *Xist* expression in early mouse development. *Cell* **77**, 639–50.

Kay, G. F., Penny, G. D., Patel, D., Ashworth, A., Brockdorff, N. & Rastan, S. (1993). Expression of *Xist* during mouse development suggests a role in the initiation of X chromosome inactivation. *Cell* **72**, 171–82.

Kratzer, P. G., Chapman, V. M., Lambert, H., Evans, R. E. & Liskay, R. M. (1983). Differences in the DNA of the inactive X chromosomes of fetal and extraembryonic tissues of mice. *Cell* **33**, 37–42.

Lifschytz, E. & Lindsley, D. L. (1972). The role of X-chromosome inactivation during spermatogenesis. *Proc. Natl. Acad. Sci. USA* **69**, 182–6.

Lock, L. F., Takagi, N. & Martin, G. R. (1987). Methylation of the *Hprt* gene on the inactive X occurs after chromosome inactivation. *Cell* **48**, 39–46.

Lyon, M. F. (1988). The William Allan memorial award address: X-chromosome inactivation and the location and expression of X-linked genes. *Am. J. Hum. Genet.* **42**, 8–16.

Lyon, M. F. (1992). Some milestones in the history of X-chromosome inactivation. *A. Rev. Genet.* **26**,. 15–27.

Lyon, M. F. (1993). Epigenetic inheritance in mammals. *Trends Genet.* **9**, 123–8.

Lyon, M. F. (1994). X-chromosome inactivation. In *Molecular Genetics of Sex Determination*, ed. S. S. Wachtel, pp. 123–42. San Diego: Academic Press.

Martin, G. R., Epstein, C. J., Travis, B., Tucker, G., Yatziv, S., Martin, D. W., Clift, S. & Cohen, S. (1978). X-chromosome inactivation during differentiation of female teratocarcinoma stem cells *in vitro*. *Nature* **271**, 329–33.

McCarrey, J. R. & Dilworth, D. D. (1992). Expression of *Xist* in mouse germ cells correlates with X-chromosome inactivation. *Nature Genet.* **2**, 200–3.

Monk, M. & Harper, M. I. (1979). Sequential X chromosome inactivation coupled with cellular differentiation in early mouse embryos. *Nature* **281**, 311–13.

Norris, D. P., Patel, D., Kay, G. F., Penny, G. D., Brockdorff, N., Sheardown, S. A. & Rastan, S. (1994). Evidence that random and imprinted *Xist* expression is controlled by preemptive methylation. *Cell* **77**, 41–51.

Papaioannou, V. E. & West, J. D. (1981). Relationship between the parental origin of the X chromosomes, embryonic cell lineage and X chromosome expression in mice. *Genet. Res., Camb.* **37**, 183–97.

Piper, A. A., Bennett, A. M., Noyce, L., Swanton, M. K. & Cooper, D. W. (1993). Isolation of a clone partially encoding hill kangaroo X-linked hypoxanthine phosphoribosyltransferase; sex differences in methylation in the body of the gene. *Somat. cell. molec. Genet.* **19**, 141–59.

Rastan, S. (1994). X chromosome inactivation and the *Xist* gene. *Curr. Opin. Genet. Devel.* **4**, 292–7.

Rastan, S. & Brown, S. D. M. (1990). The search for the mouse X-chromosome inactivation centre. *Genet. Res.* **56**, 99–106.

Rastan, S., Kaufman, M. H., Handyside, A. & Lyon, M. F. (1980). X-chromosome inactivation in the extraembryonic membranes of diploid parthenogenetic mouse embryos demonstrated by differential staining. *Nature* **288**, 172–3.

Rastan, S. & Robertson, E. J. (1985). X-chromosome deletions in embryo-derived (EK) cell lines associated with lack of X-chromosome inactivation. *J. Embryol. exp. Morphol.* **90**, 379–88.

Richler, C., Soreq, H. & Wahrman, J. (1992). X inactivation in mammalian testis is correlated with inactive X-specific transcription. *Nature Genet.* **2**, 192–5.

Riggs, A. D. (1975). X inactivation, differentiation and DNA methylation. *Cytogenet. Cell Genet.* **14**, 9–25.

Riggs, A. D. & Pfeifer, G. P. (1992). X-chromosome inactivation and cell memory. *Trends Genet.* **8**, 169–74.

Salido, E. C., Yen, P. H., Mohandas, T. K. & Shapiro, L. J. (1992). Expression of the X-inactivation-associated gene *Xist* during spermatogenesis. *Nature Genet.* **2**, 196–9.

Shao, C. & Takagi, N. (1990). An extra maternally derived X chromosome is deleterious to early mouse development. *Development* **110**, 969–75.

Tada, T., Tada, M. & Takagi, N. (1993a). X chromosome retains the memory of its parental origin in murine embryonic stem cells. *Development* **119**, 813–21.

Tada, T., Takagi, N. & Adler, I.-D. (1993b). Parental imprinting on the mouse X chromosome: effects on the early development of XO, XXY and XXX embryos. *Genet. Res., Camb.* **62**, 139–48.

Takagi, N. & Sasaki, M. (1975). Preferential inactivation of the paternally derived X chromosome in the extraembryonic membranes of the mouse. *Nature* **256**, 640–2.

Takagi, N., Sugawara, O. & Sasaki, M. (1982). Regional and temporal changes in the pattern of X-chromosome replication during the early post-implantation development of the female mouse. *Chromosoma* **85**, 275–86.

Webb, S., De Vries, T. J. & Kaufman, M. H. (1992). The differential staining pattern of the X chromosome in the embryonic and extraembryonic tissues of postimplantation homozygous tetraploid mouse embryos. *Genet. Res., Camb.* **59**, 205–14.

9

Imprinting of H19 and Xist in uniparental embryos

M. AZIM SURANI, ANNE C. FERGUSON-SMITH, HIROYUKI
SASAKI AND SHEILA C. BARTON

Summary

A comparative analysis of epigenetic modifications and expression of the mammalian genes *H19* (on chromosome 7) and *Xist* (on the X chromosome) was carried out. The key differences are, firstly, that the *Xist* gene is expressed when paternally inherited whereas the *H19* gene is expressed when maternally inherited. Secondly, the *Xist* gene shows transient monoallelic expression lasting only a few cleavage divisions but the *H19* gene shows a highly stable monoallelic expression in most tissues following blastocyst implantation. Both the long- and short-term imprinting of the two genes probably involves DNA methylation at some stage. Epigenetic modifications and expression of the two genes were examined, particularly in uniparental embryos, to gain further insights into the regulation of their expression.

The paternal *H19* gene is apparently methylated after fertilization both in the normal and in androgenetic embryos. Both paternal copies of the gene were methylated and repressed in androgenones; both maternal copies were unmethylated and expressed in parthenogenetic embryos. The exception was found in the androgenetic trophoblast, where the *H19* gene was relatively unmethylated and expressed. This suggests that either the maternal genome is necessary to achieve the appropriate repression of *H19* in the trophoblast or this reflects lineage-specific variations in the *H19* methylation.

In *Xist*, the paternal copy was expressed in X^mX^p embryos throughout the preimplantation development, but expression was never observed in X^mY. In the X^mX^m gynogenones, and X^pX^p and X^pY androgenones, all the maternal copies of *Xist* were repressed whereas the paternal copies were expressed. It is possible that methylation differences between the parental copies of *Xist* inherited directly from the germline are responsible for this bias in the expression of the paternal gene. At the compacting morula stage, the parental imprints are apparently erased: one copy of *Xist* in X^mX^m embryos was selected at random and expressed. At the same time, inappropriate *Xist* expression in X^PY androgenones was extinguished. However, expression was also unexpectedly lost in the majority of the X^PX^P embryos. This suggests that expression of *Xist* may also require a gene product from the maternal genome, implicating a novel imprinted gene that regulates *Xist* expression.

Introduction

Genetic imprinting starts in the germline when homologous chromosomes are physically segregated. This process is responsible for the monoallelic expression of imprinted genes in embryos, which is both time- and tissue-specific (see Surani & Reik, 1992). The extent to which parental imprints undergo additional modifications postzygotically is unknown. It is possible that interactions between parental genomes, including oocyte cytoplasm, as well as products of modifier genes may have a role in this process.

   The purpose of this chapter is to consider aspects of genetic imprinting of *H19* and *Xist* and in particular to determine whether imprinting occurs appropriately in uniparental embryos. This is interesting in the context of the role of the genotype-specific modifiers that are known to affect imprinting of some transgene loci, and because such modifier(s) may themselves be subject to a parental origin effect (Allen *et al.*, 1990; Surani *et al.*, 1990; Chaillet, 1992; Peterson & Sapienza, 1993). These and other investigations suggest that parental imprinting may be a multistep process that begins in the germline; further postfertilization events then follow to achieve time- and tissue-specific monallelic expression of imprinted genes.

Imprinting of the *H19* gene

In postimplantation embryos, the mouse *H19* gene is imprinted so that the paternal copy is both methylated and repressed, at least from midgestation onwards (Bartolomei *et al.*, 1991, 1993; Ferguson-Smith *et al.*, 1993; Brandeis *et al.*, 1993). However, because critical sites in the *H19* promoter are not methylated in sperm, these modifications must therefore occur postzygotically (Ferguson-Smith *et al.*, 1993). The *H19* gene is first expressed in the trophectoderm of late blastocysts and subsequently in a wide variety of tissues of both endodermal and mesodermal origins at around day 8.5 of gestation (d8.5) (Poirier *et al.*, 1991). Both *H19* and *Xist* lack a conserved open reading frame between the mouse and human genes, suggesting that the product may be RNA (Pachnis *et al.*, 1988; Brannan *et al.*, 1990; Brown *et al.*, 1991; Brockdorff *et al.*, 1992). There is some evidence suggesting that dosage control of *H19* is crucial for normal development (Brunkow & Tilghman, 1991).

Methylation of the paternal H19 gene

The inactive paternal *H19* copy is hypermethylated at its CpG island promoter and in the 5′ flanking region; the active maternal copy is unmethylated in these regions (Ferguson-Smith *et al.*, 1993; Brandeis *et al.*, 1993; Bartolomei *et al.*, 1993). In addition, the chromatin of the inactive paternal promoter is more resistant to nucleases, suggesting a closed chromatin configuration (Ferguson-Smith *et al.*, 1993; Bartolomei *et al.*, 1993). Thus methylated CpGs and/or condensed chromatin structure are likely to prevent initiation complex formation at the paternally derived *H19* promoter. However, CpG islands such as the CpG island promoters of the *H19* gene are usually unmethylated in sperm DNA, although some differentially modified sites located 5′ to this region are methylated (Bird, 1986; Ferguson-Smith *et al.*, 1993). This suggests that the *H19* paternal promoter is likely to act postzygotically and therefore that modifiers could influence this event.

The results of one study show that for at least one *Hp*II site at the 5′ end of *H19* gene, neither of the parental copies is fully methylated in both morulae and blastocysts (Brandeis *et al.*, 1993). Our preliminary studies show that on d4.5 blastocysts cultured *in vitro*, the paternal promoter may be unmethylated, but it is methylated in almost all the sites examined after implantation (H.S., A.C. F.-S., A. Shum, S.C.B. & M.A.S., unpublished). The progression of methylation apparently differs between different portions of the egg cylinders, the paternal copy being almost fully methylated at 6.5 dpc in the embryonic portion but not in the trophoblast. Our preliminary results show that both parental copies were nearly equally expressed in embryos cultured *in vitro* to the fully expanded blastocyst stage at 4.5 dpc. Because blastocysts express the *H19* gene in the trophectoderm cells only (Poirier *et al.*, 1991), this biallelic expression may be confined to these cells. The principal point, then, is to consider whether *H19* imprinting occurs appropriately in androgenones and parthenogenones and determine whether interactions between parental genomes play an important role in the process.

Methylation and expression of H19 in androgenones and parthenogenones

To establish whether methylation of the paternal copy can occur appropriately when one of the parental genomes is absent, we examined methylation and expression of *H19* in androgenones and parthenogenones that lack the maternal and paternal genomes, respectively. In embryos at 9.5 dpc, both the *H19* copies were fully methylated in the androgenetic embryo although *H19* in the trophoblast was clearly less methylated. Trophoblast material from parthenogenetic embryos cannot be analyzed because this tissue develops particularly poorly in these embryos (Surani *et al.*, 1990).

Analysis of *H19* expression was therefore carried out by *in situ* hybridization using, as a control, insulin-like growth factor II gene (*Igf2*), which is imprinted reciprocally to the *H19* gene, with the paternally derived copy being active and the maternal copy being inactive (DeChiara *et al.*, 1991; Ferguson-Smith *et al.*, 1991). In control conceptuses, both *H19* and *Igf2* were expressed in all the extraembryonic and embryonic tissues except for the neuroepithelium where the expression of both genes was close to the background level of transcript. By contrast, androgenetic embryos at a comparable developmental stage showed *Igf2* expression identical with that in the control embryos, whereas *H19* expression was detected in the trophoblast only, with virtually no expression seen in the embryo and the yolk sac (Walsh *et al.*, 1994). These results suggest that there is specific repression of *H19* in androgenetic embryos, as *Igf2* is expressed apparently normally. The expression of the paternal *H19* gene in the androgenetic trophoblast is inconsistent with the parental imprinting of this gene. It is possible that the androgenetic trophoblast may require the presence of maternally encoded factor to down-regulate paternally expressed *H19*. Alternatively, these results may represent an example of tissue-specific imprinting. A precedent for this is the biallelic expression of the otherwise monoallelically expressed *Igf2* gene in the choroid plexus and leptomeninges of the brain (De Chiara *et al.*, 1991; Ohlsson *et al.*, 1994). Two studies in humans have also indicated that the *H19* gene is biallelically expressed in the human fetal placenta (Zhang & Tycko, 1992) and the completely androgenetic hydatidiform moles (Mutter *et al.*, 1993).

Parthenogenetic conceptuses were examined in a manner similar to that described for androgenones. Methylation analysis in the embryo showed that both the copies of *H19* were unmethylated. We have previously shown that both the copies of *H19* are expressed and the levels of transcript *H19* are two-fold higher than in controls (Ferguson-Smith *et al.*, 1993).

Initiation of methylation of the paternally derived *H19* promoter at around the time of implantation coincides with the onset of *de novo* methylation of the bulk genome (Monk, 1990). CpG islands of X-linked genes also become methylated at similar developmental stages (Lock *et al.*, 1987; Singer-Sam *et al.*, 1990; Grant *et al.*, 1992). Furthermore, the relative undermethylation of the paternal *H19* copy in the extraembryonic lineages compared with the embryonic lineages agrees well with the previous observations on non-imprinted sequences and X-linked genes (Sanford *et al.*, 1985; Monk, 1990). Thus it appears that the occurrence of the overall hypermethylation of the paternal *H19* copy follows the general rules of DNA methylation in mouse development.

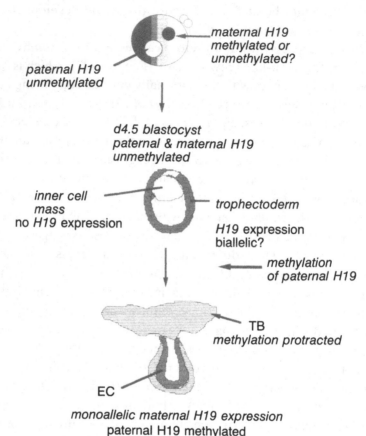

paternal H19
unmethylated

maternal H19
methylated or
unmethylated?

d4.5 blastocyst
paternal & maternal H19
unmethylated

inner cell
mass
no H19 expression

trophectoderm

H19 expression
biallelic?

methylation
of paternal H19

TB
methylation protracted

EC

monoallelic maternal H19 expression
paternal H19 methylated
maternal H19 unmethylated

Fig. 9.1. A summary of events controlling imprinting and expression of the *H19* gene. TB, trophoblast; EC, egg cylinder. See text for details.

Germline imprint, DNA methylation and H19 expression

The relationship between the germline imprint, methylation and gene silencing is still not entirely clear (see Fig. 9.1). It is possible that the germline imprint and allele inactivation may be two distinct steps of the parental imprinting process. Based on studies with imprinted transgenes, it appears that parental imprinting could be a multistep process in which the modifiers identified in different genetic backgrounds may have a role (Allen *et al.*, 1990; Surani *et al.*, 1990; Surani, 1991; Chaillet, 1992; Peterson & Sapienza, 1993). However in the *H19* gene, it appears that appropriate methylation does occur in androgenetic embryos without a maternal genome. By contrast, both of the maternal *H19* genes in par-thenogenones were unmethylated. This suggests that whatever steps are involved in the methylation, they do not involve imprinted modifiers, at least for the *H19* gene and possibly for *Igf2* and *Igf2r* (Walsh *et al.*, 1994). However, there is some evidence suggesting that both parental alleles of *Igf2*, *Igf2r* (Latham *et al.*, 1994) and *H19* (H.S., A.C. F.-S., A. Shum, S.C.B. & M.A.S., unpublished) are expressed in preimplantation embryos irrespective of their parental origin. In addition, for some genes such as *Ins-2*, the paternal gene only is expressed in the yolk sac whereas both parental genes are expressed in the pancreas (Giddings *et al.*, 1994), confirming that the germline imprinting is followed by subsequent steps to confer tissue- and time-specific monoallelic expression. Therefore it is possible that postzygotic modifications of imprinted genes could have an important role in imprinting.

One of the key questions is the nature of the germline imprint. There is no doubt that DNA methylation is an important component of the parental-origin-specific activity of imprinted genes: embryos with the null mutation in the DNA methyltranferase gene show deregulation of expression of imprinted genes (Li *et al.*, 1993). Stöger *et al.* (1993) have suggested that differential DNA methylation, found in an intron of *Igf2r*, constitutes such a germline imprint because this modification was inherited from the egg, thus marking the maternal allele for activity. However, as both paternal alleles of *Igf2r* are active in the androgenetic blastocyst (presumably devoid of this intron methylation) (Latham *et al.*, 1994) then this germline-specific methylation is not a prerequisite for activity. If DNA methylation can act as a germline imprint, only a few DNA modifications at selective 'key' CpG sites in the *H19* locus may serve as the imprinting signal, since the promoter region is unmethylated in sperm. Therefore, such key sites in the *H19* locus may be distinct from the sites that are critical for transcriptional activity. Nevertheless, it still remains to be demonstrated whether DNA methylation is the germline imprint or not. Biallelic expression of imprinted genes, including *H19*, has been reported in several human cancers (Rainier *et al.*, 1993; Ogawa *et al.*, 1993). It will be interesting to ask whether this is caused by the erasure of the imprint or by the cancer cells' inability to respond to the imprint.

Imprinting of the *Xist* gene

The *Xist* locus is a candidate for the X inactivation center and is expressed exclusively from the inactive X chromosome (Brown *et al.*, 1991; Brockdorff *et al.*, 1991). Like *H19*, the *Xist* gene product is untranslated (Brown *et al.*, 1991; Brockdorff *et al.*, 1992). Because *Xist* expression precedes X inactivation, it is assumed that *Xist* may play an early role in the process. Of particular significance in the context of this chapter is that the earliest *Xist* expression is subject to parental imprinting: only the paternal *Xist* is expressed during preimplantation development, whereas the maternal *Xist* is first detected shortly before gastrulation (Kay *et al.*, 1993).

There are apparently two principal control mechanisms that govern expression of *Xist* during preimplantation development. The initial expression of *Xist* is due to parental imprinting; recent evidence has shown that the paternal copy of *Xist* is unmethylated at the onset of meiosis and when it enters the zygote it is expressed preferentially (Kay *et al.*, 1993, 1994; Norris *et al.*, 1994). Later there is loss of parental imprints, and a counting mechanism ensures *Xist* expression is appropriate for the number of X chromosomes in the embryo (Rastan, 1983). Additional features of *Xist* regulation are the lineage-specific regulation and the likely involvement of a maternally encoded factor (Kay *et al.*, 1994).

A number of important questions arise concerning the role of imprinting for the expression of *Xist* during preimplantation development. Firstly, there is an apparent change from initial parental *Xist* expression to random *Xist* expression. Therefore the parental imprints may be either labile or lineage-specific; if the former applies than it is important to determine whether the imprints are erased. Normal X^mX^p embryos express the paternal *Xist*, but the normal X^mY embryos never express *Xist*. Hence, the X^mX^p embryos express *Xist* because they carry the paternal *Xist*, whereas the normal X^mY carries the maternal *Xist* that may be repressed. To assess the relationship between the parental origin of the X chromosome, expression of *Xist* and chromosome counting, androgenones (X^pX^p, X^pY) containing all paternally inherited *Xist* and gynogenones (X^mX^m) containing only maternally inherited *Xist* were examined during preimplantation development.

Xist *expression in gynogenones*

Gynogenones were constructed containing both a (C57B1 × CBAF)$_1$ and a 129/ Sv pronucleus so that allele-specific expression of both alleles (X^mX^m) could be distinguished (Barton & Surani, 1993; Kay *et al.*, 1994). Unlike the expression of *Xist* in normal embryos, expression of *Xist* was delayed in gynogenones until the late morula or blastocyst stage (Fig. 9.2). Indeed all the blastocysts expressed *Xist*. Furthermore, both copies of *Xist* were expressed in individual blastocysts. Because the relative proportion of expression of the two alleles differed in individual blastocysts, it is most likely that the individual cells expressed either one or the other copy of *Xist* and that expression was unlikely to be biallelic.

One possibility is that, in the gynogenetic X^mX^m embryos, *Xist* is programmed by imprinting to be silent; expression at the late morula/blastocyst stage occurred following the erasure of imprints. Although this would allow expression of the maternal copy of *Xist* for the first time, the loss of imprints would require

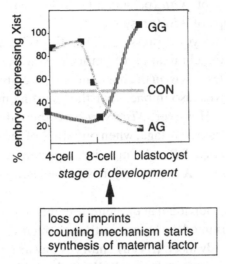

Fig. 9.2. *Xist* expression in the control (CON), androgenetic (AG) and gynogenetic (GG) embryos during preimplantation development. Control embryos will
typically consist of an equal number of X^mX^p and X^mY embryos; only the 50% of
the latter will express *Xist*. Gynogenones will all be X^mX^m, whereas the androgenones will initially be $X^pX^p : X^pY : YY$ in the Mendelian ratio of 1 : 2 : 1.
The results are discussed in the text. The major point of transition in the
expression of *Xist* is indicated by 'loss of imprints'. This coincides with the
initiation of two groups of cells: outer (putative trophectoderm) and inner
(putative inner cell mass) cells. It is suggested that only the outer cells may express
Xist; in these cells the proposed maternal factor essential for *Xist* expression will
be synthesized.

alternative constraints for expression to be restricted to one copy of *Xist* only.
This could be achieved by the X chromosome counting mechanism if it became
effective at this time, allowing only one *Xist* allele to be expressed.

Xist *expression in androgenones*

As with gynogenones, androgenetic zygotes were constructed with 129/Sv and
PGK pronuclei to allow detection of allele-specific expression of *Xist* (Barton &
Surani, 1993; Kay *et al.*, 1994). In contrast to gynogenones, which are all X^mX^m,
androgenetic embryos before any selection will be X^pX^p, X^pY, or YY in the
Mendelian ratio of 1 : 2 : 1. In these androgenetic embryos, *Xist* expression was
first detected at the 4-cell stage, just as in normal embryos. Indeed, nearly 75%
of the embryos expressed *Xist*. Because YY embryos will not express *Xist*, it is
most likely that all the X^pX^p and X^pY embryos express *Xist*. Indeed, allele-
specific RT–PCR analysis showed that at least some embryos at the 4-cell stage

expressed both copies of *Xist* (presumably X^PX^P) whereas other embryos expressed only one copy of *Xist* (presumably X^PY).

The proportion of embryos expressing *Xist* at the 5–7 cell stage rose to 90%, presumably owing to the elimination of embryos with a YY constitution. The expression of both copies of *Xist* in the presumed X^PX^P embryos and of the single copy in the X^PY embryos also implies that the counting mechanism is not yet functional at this stage. However, *Xist* expression thereafter declined progressively through to the blastocyst stage, when only 16% of the embryos were found with *Xist* expression (Fig. 9.2). As may be expected, most of the embryos expressed only one copy of *Xist* (the majority of the embryos are expected to be X^PY).

In a further analysis, individual androgenetic embryos were sexed and expression of *Xist* was determined as before, although such analysis could only be performed from more advanced (8-cell) embryos onwards. This study revealed that the X^PY embryos outnumbered X^PX^P embryos by 3 : 1, suggesting a selection against X^PX^P embryos. These results show that in the androgenetic blastocyst *Xist* expression was evidently down-regulated after the initial expression of all the copies of *Xist*. A few X^PY morulae, but no blastocysts, were found that expressed *Xist*. More surprising, perhaps, was the finding that the *Xist* expression was extinguished in the majority of the X^PX^P embryos as well. Because both the X^PY and X^PX^P embryos start to lose the expression of *Xist* at the later morula stage, it seems possible that androgenones lack a factor needed to sustain expression of *Xist*.

Regulation of *Xist* by imprinting and counting mechanisms

The control of *Xist* expression by imprinting is apparently short-lived. The second mechanism regulating *Xist* expression becomes evident at the morula stage. Expression of *Xist* in androgenones and gynogenones strengthens the case for the early regulation of *Xist* by imprinting. Not only are both copies of *Xist* initially expressed in the androgenetic X^PX^P embryos, but androgenetic X^PY also showed *Xist* expression. This is particularly striking, as *Xist* expression is never seen in the normal X^mY fertilized embryo (Kay *et al.*, 1993). The lack of *Xist* expression in early gynogenones is equally compatible with the role of parental imprinting, since X^mX^m embryos failed to express this gene. This situation persists until about the compacting morula stage.

Recent evidence has shown that there is major genome-wide demethylation during preimplantation development so that, by the morula stage, many of the methylated sites that enter the zygote at fertilization become demethylated (Monk, 1990; Kafri *et al.*, 1992). It is possible that at this time the *Xist* gene also loses its methylation imprints and becomes free from the constraints on its expression imposed by parental imprinting. However, it is important to note that in gynogenones, only one of the two alleles is randomly expressed. Because there are no inherent differences between the expressed and inactive copies of *Xist*, a mechanism for counting the number of X chromosomes may ensure that only one copy of *Xist* is expressed. Evidently, sometime at the morula stage this mechanism may also account for the repression of *Xist* in androgenetic XPY embryos, indicating that this is indeed a powerful mechanism for regulating *Xist* expression. However, unexpectedly, there was also a loss of *Xist* in the majority of the XPXP embryos. This suggests a requirement for a maternal genome to allow *Xist* expression once the early imprinted regulation is replaced by random expression (Figs. 9.2 and 9.3). The loss of *Xist* expression in androgenones would not compromise XPY embryos greatly but would affect XPXP embryos (Figs. 9.2 and 9.3). Interestingly, in one study on postimplantation androgenetic embryos, all nine androgenetic egg cylinders were found to be of XY genotype (Kaufman *et al.*, 1989). The proposed key events controlling *Xist* expression during preimplantation development are summarized in Fig. 9.3.

Loss of imprints and starting to count

It is possible that a *trans*-acting factor is needed for the continued expression of *Xist*. If this factor is expressed by the maternal genome then loss of *Xist* in androgenetic embryos will be predicted. Therefore, continued expression of *Xist* may require a *trans*-acting factor encoded by the maternal genome; the gene encoding this factor would therefore itself be imprinted. It is possible that initially a maternal product essential for *Xist* expression is present in the oocyte. Later, this factor may be synthesized by the maternal genome but only when embryonic cells leave the pluripotential lineage and start to undergo differentiation. If so, then the outer cells destined to become trophectoderm (Johnson & Ziomek, 1981) would be the first cells to synthesize this gene product, rather than the inner cells destined to become inner cell mass cells. Hence the inner cell mass cells should lose *Xist* expression and the trophectoderm should express *Xist*.

Embryonic and extraembryonic lineages

In normal embryos the paternal copy of *Xist* is expressed throughout preimplantation development, but preferential inactivation of the paternal X chromosome is seen only in the trophoblast and primitive endoderm lineage and not in the primitive ectoderm that gives rise to the embryo (see Lyon, this volume). In fact, there is apparently random X inactivation in embryonic tissues at gastrulation.

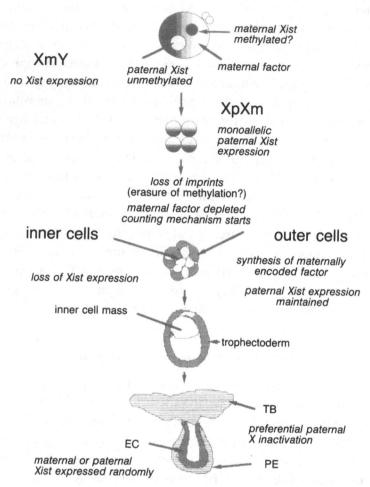

XmY

no Xist expression

maternal Xist
methylated?

paternal Xist   maternal factor
unmethylated

XpXm

monoallelic
paternal Xist
expression

loss of imprints
(erasure of methylation?)
maternal factor depleted
counting mechanism starts

inner cells   **outer cells**

synthesis of maternally
encoded factor

loss of Xist expression

paternal Xist expression
maintained

inner cell mass

trophectoderm

TB

preferential paternal
X inactivation

EC

maternal or paternal   PE
Xist expressed randomly

Fig. 9.3. A summary of the control of *Xist* expression in normal XY and XX
embryos.

Based on our observations of *Xist* expression in gynogenones, the parental
imprint is apparently erased at the morula–blastocyst stage' and the counting
mechanism establishes expression of a single *Xist* locus in XX embryos. This
makes it possible for random inactivation to occur in the embryo.

    There are a number of possible mechanisms to account for the differences
between the embryonic and extraembryonic lineages concerning X inactivation.
One obvious possibility is that in normal embryos *Xist* expression is controlled by
tissue-specific imprinting. In the inner population of cells destined to become
epiblast and embryonic tissue, the early expression of the paternal *Xist* is
extinguished and then this is followed by random expression of *Xist* before
gastrulation. This study demonstrates that parental imprints could be lost at the

morula stage except in the cells destined to form the trophectoderm, where *Xist* expression of the paternal gene may be maintained. When expression occurs in the embryonic tissue at gastrulation, the postulated maternal factor will be synthesized and either of the two copies of *Xist* should activate, as is observed. With the counting mechanism in force, only one allele is activated. It is possible that the inactive copy succumbs to remethylation at a subsequent stage.

Conclusions

These studies show that the initial imprinted expression of *Xist* is likely to be controlled by a germline imprint, possibly a differential methylation of the parental copies of *Xist*. However, these imprints are apparently erased after a few cleavage divisions. The later expression of *Xist* may require a factor that is encoded by the maternal genome and therefore by another unidentified imprinted gene. The identification of this gene and its role, if any, as the imprinted X-chromosome counting controller should be informative on some of these complexities.

It is not clear whether the absence of a maternal genome is responsible for the expression of *H19* in the androgenetic trophoblast. Alternatively, this may simply be a lineage-specific difference. There is evidence to show that the paternal *H19* gene acquires full methylation shortly after blastocyst implantation. The paternal *H19* promoter is apparently unmethylated in sperm. The long-term monoallelic expression of the maternal *H19* gene implicates DNA methylation to ensure stable silencing of the paternal copy. Whether DNA methylation is the key germline imprint for the *H19* gene is unclear at present. It is also important to note that most of the imprinted genes show time- and tissue-specific monoallelic expression, which argues for the ability to manipulate the germline imprint during development. It is likely that this process takes a variety of different forms, as illustrated by these studies on *H19* and *Xist*.

Acknowledgements

Our special thanks to Sohaila Rastan and Graham Kay, with whom the collaborative work on the *Xist* gene was carried out. The comments from all the members of our group have proved invaluable. The work was supported by grants from the Wellcome Trust (Grant nos. 036481 and 035634) and from the Human Frontiers Science Program.

References

Allen, N. D., Norris, M. L. & Surani, M. A. (1990). Epigenetic control of transgene expression and imprinting by genotype-specific modifiers. *Cell* **61**, 853–61.

Bartolomei, M. S., Webber, A. L., Brunkow, M. E. & Tilghman, S. M. (1993). Epigenetic mechanisms underlying the imprinting of the mouse *H19* gene. *Genes Devel.* **7**, 1663–73.

Bartolomei, M. S., Zemel, S. & Tilghman, S. M. (1991). Parental imprinting of the mouse *H19* gene. *Nature* **351**, 153–5.

Barton, S. C. & Surani, M. A. (1993). Manipulations of genetic constitution by nuclear transplantation. *Meth. Enzymol.* **225**, 732–44.

Bird, A. (1986). CpG-rich island and the function of DNA methylation. *Nature* **321**, 209–13.

Brandeis, M., Kafri, T., Ariel, M., Chaillet, J. R., McCarrey, J., Razin, A. & Cedar, H. (1993). The ontogeny of allele-specific methylation associated with imprinted genes in the mouse. *EMBO J.* **12**, 3669–77.

Brannan, C. I., Dees, E. C., Ingram, R. S. & Tilghman, S. M. (1990). The product of the *H19* gene may function as an RNA. *Molec. Cell Biol.* **10**, 28–36.

Brockdorff, N., Ashworth, A., Kay, G. F., Cooper, P., Smith, S., McCabe, V. M., Norris, D. P., Penny, G. D., Patel, D. & Rastan, S. (1991). Conservation of position and exclusive expression of mouse *Xist* from the inactive X chromosome. *Nature* **351**, 329–31.

Brockdorff, N., Ashworth, A., Kay, G. F., McCabe, V. M., Norris, D. P., Cooper, P. J., Swift, S. & Rastan, S. (1992). The product of the mouse *Xist* gene is a 15 kb inactive X-specific transcript containing no conserved ORF and located in the nucleus. *Cell* **71**, 515–26.

Brown, C. J., Ballabio, A., Rupert, J. L., Lafreniere, R. G., Grompe, M., Tonlorenzi, R. & Willard, H. F. (1991). A gene from the region of the human X-inactivation centre is expressed exclusively from the inactive X chromosome. *Nature* **349**, 38–44.

Brunkow, M. E. & Tilghman, S. M. (1991). Ectopic expression of the *H19* gene in mice causes prenatal lethality. *Genes Devel.* **5**, 1092–101.

Chaillet, J. R. (1992). DNA methylation and genomic imprinting in the mouse. *Semin. devel. Biol.* **3**, 99–105.

DeChiara, T. M., Robertson, E. L. & Efstratiadis, A. (1991). Parental imprinting of the mouse insulin-like growth factor II gene. *Cell* **64**, 849–59.

Ferguson-Smith, A. C., Cattanach, B. M., Barton, S. C., Beechey, C. V. & Surani, M. A. (1991). Embryological and molecular investigations of parental imprinting on mouse chromosome 7. *Nature* **351** 667–70.

Ferguson-Smith, A. C., Sasaki, H., Cattanach, B. M. & Surani, M. A. (1993). Parental-origin-specific modification of the mouse *H19* gene. *Nature* **362**, 751–5.

Giddings, S. T., King, C. D., Harman, K. W., Flood, J. F. & Carnaghi, L. R. (1994). Allele specific inactivation of insulin 1 and 2 in the mouse yolk sac indicates imprinting. *Nature Genet.* **6**, 310–13.

Grant, M., Zuccotti, M. & Monk, M. (1992). Methylation of CpG sites of two X-linked genes coincides with X-inactivation in the female mouse embryo but not in the germ line. *Nature Genet.* **2**, 161–6.

Johnson, M. H. & Ziomek, C. A. (1981). The foundation of two distinct cell lineages within the mouse morula. *Cell* **24**, 71–80.

Kafri, T., Ariel, M., Brandeis, M., Schemer, R., Urven, L., McCarrey, J., Cedar, H. & Razin, A. (1992). Development pattern of gene-specific DNA methylation in the mouse embryo and germ line. *Genes Devel.* **6**, 705–14.

Kafri, T., Gao, X. & Razin, A. (1993). Mechanistic aspects of genome-wide demethylation in the preimplantation mouse embryo. *Proc. Natl. Acad. Sci. USA* **90**, 10558–62.

Kaufman, M. H., Lee, K. K. & Spiers, S. (1989). Post-implantation development and cytogenetic analysis of diandric heterozygous diploid mouse embryos. *Cytogenet. Cell Genet.* **52**, 15–18.

Kay, G. F., Penny, G. D., Patel, D., Ashworth, A., Brockdorff, N. & Rastan, S. (1993). Expression of *Xist* during mouse development suggests a role in the initiation of X chromosome inactivation. *Cell* **72**, 171–82.

Kay, G. G., Barton, S. C., Surani, M. A. & Rastan, S. (1994). Imprinting and X chromosome counting mechanisms determine Xist expression in early mouse development. *Cell* **77**, 639–50.

Latham, K. E., Doherty, A. S., Scott, C. D. & Schultz, R. M. (1994). *Igf2r* and *Igf2* gene expression in androgenetic, gynogenetic and parthenogenetic preimplantation mouse embryos: Absence of regulation by genomic imprinting. *Genes Devel.* **8**, 290–9.

Li, E., Beard, C. & Jaenisch, R. (1993). Role for DNA methylation in genomic imprinting. *Nature* **366**, 362–5.

Lock, L. F., Takagi, N. & Martin, G. R. (1987). Methylation of the *Hprt* gene on the inactive X occurs after chromosome inactivation. *Cell* **48**, 39–46.

Monk, M. (1990). Changes in DNA methylation during mouse embryonic development in relation to X chromosome activity and imprinting. *Phil. Trans. R. Soc. Lond.* B **326**, 179–87.

Mutter, G. L., Stewart, C. L., Chaponot, M. L. & Pomponio, R. J. (1993). Oppositely imprinted genes *H19* and insulin-like growth factor 2 are coexpressed in human and androgenetic trophoblast. *Am. J. Hum. Genet.* **53**, 1906–11.

Norris, D. P., Patel, D., Kay, G. F., Penny, G. D., Brockdorff, N., Sheardown, S. A. & Rastan, S. (1994). Evidence that random and imprinted *Xist* expression is controlled by preemptive methylation. *Cell* **77**, 41–51.

Ogawa, O., Eccles, M. R., Szeto, J., McNoe, L. A., Yun, K., Maw, M. A., Smith, P. J. & Reeve, A. E. (1993). Relaxation of insulin-like growth factor II gene imprinting implicated in Wilms' tumor. *Nature* **362**, 749–51.

Ohlsson, R., Hedborg, F., Holmgren, L., Walsh, C. & Ekstrom, T. J. (1994). Overlapping patterns of *IGF2* and *H19* expression during human development: biallelic *IGF2* expression correlates with lack of *H19* expression. *Development* **120**, 361–8.

Pachnis, V., Brannan, C. I. & Tilghman, S. M. (1988). The structure and expression of a novel gene activated in early mouse embryogenesis. *EMBO J.* **7**, 673–81.

Peterson, K. & Sapienza, C. (1993). Imprinting the genome: imprinted genes, imprinting genes, and a hypothesis for their interaction. *A. Rev. Genet.* **27**, 7–31.

Poirier, F., Chan, C.-T.J., Timmons, P. M., Robertson, E. J., Evans, M. J. & Rigby, P. W. J. (1991). The murine *H19* gene is activated during embryonic stem cell differentiation in vitro and at the time of implantation in the developing embryo. *Development* **113**, 1105–14.

Rainier, S., Johnson, L. A., Dobry, C. J., Ping, A. J., Grundy, P. E. & Feinberg, A. P. (1993). Relaxation of imprinted genes in human cancer. *Nature* **362**, 747–9.

Rastan, S. (1983). Non-random X chromosome inactivation in mouse X:autosome translocation: location of the inactivation center. *J. Embryol. exp. Morphol.* **78**, 1–22.

Sanford, J. P., Chapman, V. M. & Rossant, J. (1985). DNA methylation in extraembryonic lineages of mammals. *Trends Genet.* **1**, 89–93.

Singer-Sam, J., Grant, M., LeBon, J. M., Okuyama, K., Chapman, V., Monk, M. & Riggs, A. D. (1990). Use of a HpaII-polymerase chain reaction assay to study DNA methylation in the *Pgk-1* CpG island of mouse embryos at the time of X-chromosome inactivation. *Molec. Cell Biol.* **10**, 4987–9.

Stöger, R., Kubicka, P., Liu, C.-G., Kafri, T., Razin, A., Cedar, H. & Barlow, D. P. (1993). Maternal-specific methylation of the imprinted mouse *Igf2r* locus identifies the expressed locus as carrying the imprinting signal. *Cell* **73**, 61–71.

Surani, J. A. (1991). Genomic imprinting: developmental significance and molecular mechanism. *Curr. Opin. Genet. Devel.* **1**, 241–6.

Surani, M. A., Kothary, R., Allen, N. D., Singh, P. B., Fundele, R., Ferguson-Smith, A. C. & Barton, S. C. (1990). Genomic imprinting and development in the mouse. *Development* (Suppl.), 89–98.

Surani, M. A. & Reik, W. (1992). Genomic imprinting in mouse and man. *Semin. devel. Biol.* **3**, 73–160.

Walsh, C., Glaser, A., Fundele, R., Ferguson-Smith, A. C., Barton, S. C., Surani, M. A. & Ohlsson, R. (1994). The non-viability of uniparental conceptuses correlates with the loss of the products of imprinted genes. *Mech. Devel.* **46**, 55–62.

Zemel, S., Bartolomei, M. S. & Tilghman, S. M. (1992). Physical linkage of two mammalian imprinted genes, *H19* and insulin-like growth factor 2. *Nature Genet.* **2**, 61–5.

Zhang, Y. & Tycko, B. (1992). Monoallelic expression of the human *H19* gene. *Nature Genet.* **1**, 40–3.

10

Imprinted genes, allelic methylation, and imprinted modifiers of methylation

WOLF REIK, ROBERT FEIL, NICHOLAS D. ALLEN, THOMAS F.
MOORE AND JÖRN WALTER

Introduction

The past couple of years have witnessed substantial progress in the molecular genetic analysis of parental imprinting in mammals. A number of imprinted genes have been identified, and their phenotypic effects are being elucidated by genetic analysis (Bartolomei, 1994). Epigenetic modifications of DNA and chromosomes that are specific for parental origin have been detected in all imprinted genes examined. Hence, differences in allelic methylation, allelic chromatin structure, and allele-specific timing of DNA replication have been found to be associated with imprinted genes, and are thought to be molecular components of the imprinting process (Kitsberg *et al.*, 1993; Surani, 1993; Barlow, 1993; Reik & Allen 1994; Bartolomei, 1994; Efstratiadis, 1994). Genetic analysis is beginning to define the *cis*-acting sequence requirements for imprinting; it appears that a variety of different sequence requirements exist for different imprinted genes, which act at different stages of development. Diverse sequence elements may also be involved in germline reprogramming and initiation, as well as somatic maintenance and potential loss of imprints.

The next step in our understanding of the molecular basis of imprinting will come from the identification of *trans*-acting factors which are involved in the mechanism of imprinting. One gene has already been shown to affect imprinting in *trans*: in embryos that are deficient in methyltransferase enzyme, expression of a number of imprinted genes is aberrant, thus demonstrating that DNA methylation is necessary at least for the somatic maintenance of imprinting (Li *et al.*, 1993). Evidence is also accumulating for the existence of modifier genes that affect epigenetic modification of specific targets such as transgenes, although a role for these modifiers in the parental imprinting of endogenous genes is as yet unproven.

In this chapter, we discuss the various patterns of allelic methylation that have been described in imprinted genes. Specifically, we describe different genetic

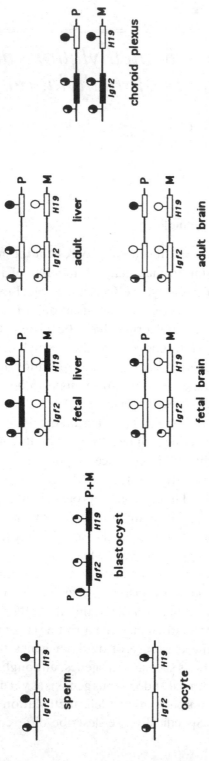

Fig. 10.1. Summary of allelic methylation in the mouse *Igf2* and *H19* genes. In the *Igf2* gene two regions are allele-specifically methylated: one of *ca.* 3 kb upstream of the gene (see also Fig. 10.2), and one in the intron-4–exon-6 part of the gene. The region of allelic methylation in the *H19* gene includes the body of the gene as well as upstream and downstream sequences except in adult choroid plexus, where the indicated level of methylation refers to the body of the gene and 3 kb of downstream sequences (the allele-specific methylation of the *H19* promoter has not been determined). Methylation in the two genes, on both maternal (M) and paternal (P) alleles, is indicated, with the degree of methylation varying between absence of methylation (open circles) and complete methylation (filled circles). The two genes are shown as open (no or very low expression) or dark (expression) boxes. (Data are from Sasaki *et al.*, 1992; Ferguson-Smith *et al.*, 1993; Bartolomei *et al.*, 1993; Brandeis *et al.*, 1993; Feil *et al.*, 1994). In the blastocyst, *Igf2* may be expressed from both parental alleles (Latham *et al.*, 1994), although it is not known at what level. Since this is a summary of a large body of data, lollipops cannot be equated with individual methylation sites, and sometimes the behaviour of individual sites may be slightly different from the 'lollipop average'.

elements in the mouse *Igf2* gene that show allelic differences in epigenetic modification, and elucidate some of the developmental and tissue-specific factors involved. We briefly consider the relevance of allelic methylation of the human *IGF2* and *H19* genes to the fetal overgrowth syndrome, Beckwith–Wiedemann syndrome. Finally, we describe a genetic system for the mapping and identification of modifiers of transgene methylation; these and other genes may be involved in the control of allele-specific methylation at endogenous imprinted loci.

Structural aspects of allelic methylation

Two regions of allelic methylation have been identified so far in and around the mouse *Igf2* gene (Fig. 10.1). Both are paternally methylated, i.e. methylation occurs in the expressed copy of the gene (Sasaki *et al.*, 1992; Brandeis *et al.*, 1993; Feil *et al.*, 1994). A structural analysis by bisulfite genomic sequencing of the most upstream of the two regions (approximately 3 kb upstream of the first promoter) was carried out. This region was the first allelic methylation difference identified in an autosomal gene in the mouse (Sasaki *et al.*, 1992). A detailed structural analysis was performed to determine the methylation status of CpG dinucleotides that could not be analyzed by restriction enzymes, and to determine the methylation patterns on individual maternal and paternal chromosomes. Most importantly, we were interested in the clonality or otherwise of allelic methylation patterns. This is a crucial question, since the simple view of heritability of CpG methylation by faithful maintenance of a pre-established pattern might suggest that allelic differences, once introduced into chromosomes at an early embryonic stage, are retained on the majority of parental chromosomes in fetal and adult tissues. Clearly, functional imprints that influence gene expression allele-specifically must have a high degree of clonal stability.

This simple view of allelic methylation is not supported by our analysis (Feil *et al.*, 1994). Individual chromosome analysis in the *Igf2* upstream region in the fetus (in which parental chromosomes could be identified by polymorphisms), and in mature spermatozoa, revealed an unpredictable and not very orderly pattern where individual chromosomes are concerned, but a highly predictable and consistent pattern when the whole population of chromosomes is examined (Fig. 10.2 gives a few representative examples of fetal maternal, fetal paternal, and sperm chromosomes). A number of points are of interest here. First, there is a gradient of methylation with high levels in the most upstream CpGs and low levels of methylation in the more downstream CpGs. Second, overall there is more methylation on paternal than on maternal chromosomes, especially in the five most upstream CpGs. However, there is not a single CpG that is methylated

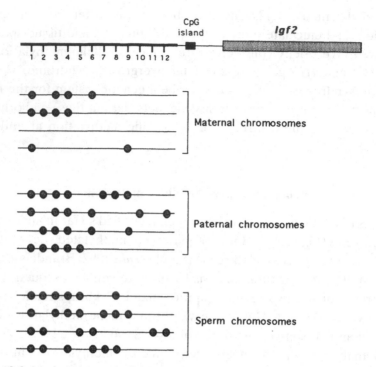

Fig. 10.2. Methylation on individual parental chromosomes in the *Igf2* upstream region. A region at *ca*. 3 kb upstream of the *Igf2* gene, comprising 12 CpG dinucleotides (1–12), is more methylated on the expressed paternal than on the repressed maternal allele in the embryo (Sasaki *et al.*, 1992). Methylation on individual fetal and sperm chromosomes was analyzed by genomic bisulfite sequencing (Feil *et al.*, 1994). Representative methylation patterns for maternal, paternal and sperm chromosomes are shown. Methylated CpGs on the individual chromosomes are shown as filled circles.

on the majority of paternal but on the minority of maternal alleles. In addition, in the 36 chromosomes sequenced, most individual patterns only occurred once, and there were only two patterns that were found three times (one of which was that of a 'methylation empty' chromosome, which only occurred in the maternal alleles). Thus, overall there is little evidence of simple clonality. In addition, individual sperm chromosomes exhibit quite different patterns (Fig. 10.2). Because only one sperm chromosome contributes to an individual embryo, these patterns subsequently have to be altered in the embryo (with presumably both increase and decrease in methylation).

Our single-chromosome analysis gives the impression of a far more dynamic balance between *de novo* methylation and demethylation than was hitherto suspected, at least in the early mammalian embryo. This may involve active demethylases (Jost, 1993; Kafri *et al.*, 1993) as well as chromatin components that would contribute to the overall heritability of a pattern. Recently, single-chromosome analysis of methylation in *Neurospora crassa* (Selker *et al.*, 1993) and in *Petunia* (Meyer *et al.*, 1994) has also demonstrated diverse patterns at the level of the individual chromosome, which are, however, predictable on a population basis. In these cases, lack of simple clonality is even more obvious because asymmetric (non-CpG) methylation was also detected. Together, these observations suggest that inheritance of methylation involves *trans*-acting factors, which may interact with a variety of *cis*-acting sequence elements.

Developmental and tissue-specific control of allelic methylation

Allelic methylation in the region upstream of *Igf2* is present in all fetal and adult tissues, irrespective of whether or not they express the gene (with one exception; see below). This is also the case for paternal-allelic methylation of the neighboring and reciprocally imprinted *H19* gene (although there may be some increase from fetal to adult stages) (Ferguson-Smith *et al.*, 1993; Brandeis *et al.*, 1993; Bartolomei *et al.*, 1993). By contrast, the second region of paternal methylation in *Igf2*, which is in the intron-4–exon-6 part of the gene, is highly tissue-specific and correlates with *Igf2* expression (Fig. 10.1). In fetal liver, a major site of IGF-II production, the paternal allele is highly methylated, whereas in fetal brain, where little IGF-II is produced, both parental alleles are undermethylated (Feil *et al.*, 1994). This is similar to the situation in the paternally imprinted *Igf2r* gene, where intron methylation is found on the expressed (maternal) allele, although in this instance tissue specificity has not been demonstrated (Stöger *et al.*, 1993). An imprinted keratin-promoter–*lacZ* transgene also exhibits tissue-specific methylation of the expressed allele (Thorey *et al.*, 1992). These findings indicate that there may be 'silencer' sequences that are suppressible by epigenetic modification, and that (at least for the *Igf2* gene) this suppression may occur in a highly tissue-specific fashion. Epigenetic modifications (increased sensitivity to DNase-I) are associated with silencer elements in the chicken lysozyme and ovalbumin genes (Gross & Garrard, 1988). Epigenetic influences on silencer sequences have also been reported in yeast, *Saccharomyces cerevisiae*, where intriguingly, the silencer elements associated with mating type genes also act as origins of replication (Laurenson & Rine, 1992).

Another striking example of the tissue-specificity of allelic methylation in the *Igf2* gene occurs in the choroid plexus epithelium, where *Igf2* is expressed from both paternal alleles and *H19* is not expressed (at least not in the adult). Here, both regions in *Igf2* become methylated, as does the body of the *H19* gene and 3 kb of downstream sequences (but not the downstream enhancer region). The *Igf2* and *H19* genes therefore adopt a largely bipaternal pattern of methylation

(Feil *et al.*, 1994). A requirement for biallelic expression of *Igf2* in the choroid plexus in later development is perhaps one of the reasons why the *Igf2* promoters do not become extensively methylated on the inactive allele (in contrast to *H19* and *Igf2r*). The absence of methylation on the maternal allele may, however, occasionally lead to biallelic expression in situations where it normally does not occur (see below).

Studies so far have shown that the allele-specific patterns of methylation in *Igf2* and *H19* are not present in parental germ cells, but instead arise in the early embryo in a lineage- and tissue-specific fashion (Fig. 10.1) (Brandeis *et al.*, 1993; Szabó & Mann, 1994; Feil *et al.*, 1994). Indeed, *Igf2* as well as *Igf2r* may be expressed biallelically at the blastocyst stage (Latham *et al.*, 1994), and *H19* expression may be biallelic in the early extraembryonic tissues (Walsh *et al.*, 1994). It is nevertheless interesting that all three regions of paternal methylation described here are also highly methylated in spermatozoa. In *H19* and the *Igf2* 3' region, this is followed by a loss of methylation during preimplantation development, and subsequent remethylation of the paternal allele (Brandeis *et al.*, 1993; T. Kafri, A. Razin, W. Dean, R.F. & W.R., unpublished). The allelic pattern of the *Igf2* upstream region is at least partly established in blastocysts (Brandeis *et al.*, 1993). These observations suggest that germline-specific methylation on its own is unlikely to provide the primary imprinting signal for *Igf2* and *H19*. This may be in contrast to the *Igf2r* gene, where allele-specific methylation in an intronic region on the expressed maternal allele is already present in the mature oocyte, whereas sperm are unmethylated in this region (Stöger *et al.*, 1993). The same is true for some imprinted transgenes that are methylated upon maternal transmission (Chaillet *et al.*, 1991; Ueda *et al.*, 1992). Overall, we note that paternal methylation is significantly altered and re-established after fertilization, whereas in all instances where allelic methylation patterns are already observed in the germline, it concerns methylation in the egg and on the maternal allele in the embryo.

It appears that tissue-specific factors influence the somatic patterns of allelic methylation of imprinted genes in fetal and adult tissues. Different elements in these genes can behave differently (as shown here for the *Igf2* upstream and 3' regions) and may have different roles in the imprinting process, from reversal and initiation in germ cells, to somatic maintenance and potential loss in specific tissues and in disease.

Allelic methylation in the Beckwith–Wiedemann syndrome

The human imprinted *IGF2* and *H19* genes are both implicated in this fetal overgrowth syndrome and its associated embryonal tumors. Most BWS cases are sporadic, but familial cases occur in which there is linkage to chromosome 11p15 (syntenic with distal chromosome 7 in the mouse, where *Igf2* and *H19* are located). A minority of sporadic BWS patients have uniparental paternal disomy (UPD) of chromosome 11p15; paternal disomy is invariably mosaic, with a normal cell lineage also being present (Henry *et al.*, 1991; Slatter *et al.*, 1994). This means that lack of *H19* and overexpression of *IGF2* (as occurs in the disomic lineage) is not cell-lethal at any stage of development. In a proportion of non-disomic sporadic BWS cases, biallelic expression of the otherwise maternally imprinted *IGF2* gene has been observed, and this clearly implicates excess *IGF2* expression in the disease (Weksberg *et al.*, 1993a; Ogawa *et al.*, 1993). There may, however, be differences in phenotype between UPD and non-UPD cases, certainly with respect to hemihypertrophy, and possibly also with a higher incidence of tumors in the UPD cases (Slatter *et al.*, 1994). The absence of *H19* could contribute to this phenotype since it has been demonstrated that it may have proliferation-suppressing activity (Hao *et al.*, 1993). Other imprinted genes (*Insulin*, *WT1*, etc.) in this region could also contribute to the phenotype.

Loss of imprinting of *IGF2*, resulting in biallelic expression, could arise from a number of mutational or non-mutational mechanisms. In the previous section we described a developmentally regulated instance of biallelic expression in the choroid plexus. We sought to determine whether there are any similarities between physiological and pathological instances of biallelic expression. We therefore examined a group of sporadic BWS patients (including some mosaic UPD cases) for allele-specific methylation of *IGF2* and *H19* (Reik *et al.*, 1994). In all cases it was found that allelic methylation of both genes was normal in non-disomic BWS, with the paternal allele being methylated, and was increased in UPD cases in proportion with the disomic lineage (the *IGF2* assay examines allelic methylation in the ninth-exon region, which corresponds to the 3' part of mouse *Igf2* described earlier). We do not know, however, whether we are actually looking at biallelically expressing tissue: most of our analysis was on peripheral blood DNA, where allele-specific expression was not analyzed. Nevertheless, the findings suggest the possibility that loss of suppression of the maternal *IGF2* allele may be achieved without major alteration of allelic methylation patterns, suggesting that this situation could be quite different from the developmentally regulated expression in choroid plexus. Interestingly, this may suggest that although methylation may be involved in somatic maintenance of imprinting, additional factors are also required to keep the maternal *IGF2* allele silent.

Allele-specific expression may also become disrupted in BWS cases with translocations in 11p15, which are invariably maternally inherited (Weksberg *et al.*, 1993b). There are different clusters of translocation breakpoints (which are possibly associated with different phenotypes), the nearest to *IGF2/H19* being about 400 kb 5' of *IGF2* (Weksberg *et al.*, 1993b). Translocations may derepress the maternal *IGF2* allele by a position-effect type of mechanism, or alternatively they may disrupt (imprinted) genes that are required for silencing of the maternal *IGF2* allele. So far there is no information about maintenance or otherwise of allelic methylation in these BWS cases.

A curious finding in our study was a distortion in the frequency of particular alleles (in the ninth exon, where allelic methylation occurs) at the *IGF2* locus, exclusively in UPD Beckwith–Wiedemann cases. Hence, the frequency of the allele that is rare in the normal population, as well as in the non-UPD Beckwith–Wiedemann cases, was found to be greatly increased in disomic BWS (Reik *et al.*, 1994). Because of the presence of putative regulatory elements in this region (as gleaned from mouse studies) it is conceivable that variant alleles in this region could result in different levels of *IGF2* transcription. In this case the phenotype of the two types of disomy (for the one or the other allele) could be slightly different and hence lead to differential intrauterine loss or diagnosis.

A class of paternally imprinted modifiers?

The results presented above may suggest that imprinted genes have a variety of *cis*-acting sequence elements which may be used to control different aspects of imprinting at different stages of development, as well as tissue-specifically. Clearly, this implies the existence of a number of *trans*-acting factors that are necessary to keep the imprints intact and functional at various stages of development. As mentioned previously, the methyltransferase gene is one such example.

The existence of other *trans*-acting factors is implied by two observations. First, experiments investigating *Xist* expression in androgenetic embryos suggest that a gene with exclusive maternal expression is required to maintain expression of the paternal *Xist* allele (Kay *et al.*, 1994). Second, the rescue of embryos with a maternally transmitted T^{hp} deletion by a paternal *Mus m. musculus* genome may also involve modifiers of parental imprinting; in this case they may be paternally expressed (Forejt & Gregorová, 1992; Allen & Reik, 1992). It is intriguing that these modifiers, which act on imprinted genes, seem to be themselves imprinted.

More generally, a class of modifier genes which alter methylation of transgenic DNA has also been described (Sapienza *et al.*, 1989; Allen *et al.*, 1990; Reik *et al.*, 1990; Engler *et al.*, 1991). Different alleles of these modifier genes are present in different inbred mouse strains, thus allowing their genetic characterization. Although to date one such modifier, *Ssm1*, has been chromosomally mapped, the molecular basis of the action of these genes is unknown. However, certain similarities with modifiers of position-effect variegation in *Drosophila* have been noted. Whether or not such modifiers act on imprinted genes is unknown at present; again, however, we note that some of them are themselves imprinted.

We are interested in a modifier gene that acts on the transgenic locus *TKZ751* (Allen *et al.*, 1990). The BALB/c allele of the modifier increases methylation at this locus, whereas the DBA/2 allele does not increase methylation. Intriguingly, the BALB/c allele has to be maternally inherited in order to increase transgene methylation in the offspring. The parental origin of the transgene itself does not influence its methylation (Fig. 10.3). The mechanism of action of this modifier gene is unknown, but the available evidence suggests that it may act early in development (around the blastocyst stage; Allen & Mooslehner, 1992), and may act specifically in the embryonic lineages (J. Walter *et al.*, in preparation). Backcross analysis of the *TKZ751* modifier shows segregation of methylation phenotypes in the offspring. Detailed analysis of phenotype distribution suggests that apart from the major, imprinted modifier gene, a small number of minor loci are involved as well, which potentially act additively or substitutively with the major gene. Mapping with microsatellite markers has localized the major gene to the proximal part of chromosome 17, and one of the minor additive loci may be on distal chromosome 4 (J. Walter *et al.*, in preparation). It remains to be seen whether the substitutive loci are imprinted as well.

Another possible example of a paternally imprinted modifier gene is the one affecting methylation of the E36 transgene. This transgene exhibits increased methylation when maternally transmitted, but can also become methylated when paternally transmitted, if exposed to a maternally inherited BALB/c modifier (but not with DBA/2; Wu *et al.*, 1992; C. Pourcel, personal communication). An intriguing question is whether imprinted modifier genes that are active in the somatic tissues of the embryo post-fertilization are also expressed in the maternal germline before fertilization, thus leading to methylation of the transgene in the maternal germline.

Why should modifier genes be imprinted? From the genetic conflict theory of imprinting (Haig & Westoby, 1989; Moore & Haig, 1991; Haig, 1992), a gene that either influences the expression of imprinted genes or acts independently on fetal growth (or other aspects of parental–allelic conflict) will be under selective pressure to become imprinted. It is therefore possible that imprinted modifiers of DNA methylation may act to influence gene expression at other imprinted loci. Identification and cloning of imprinted modifiers of DNA methylation will allow these interesting questions to be addressed.

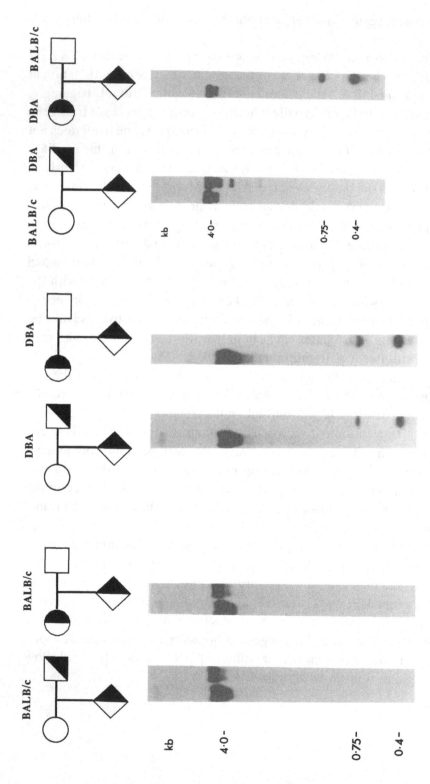

Fig. 10.3. Paternal imprinting of modifier genes. The *TKZ751* transgene is highly methylated on a BALB/c inbred background, but undermethylated on a DBA/2 background. Parental transmission of the transgene has no effect on methylation. When a transgenic male (with a low degree of transgene methylation) is crossed with a BALB/c female, methylation is increased in the offspring, suggesting a dominant action of the BALB/c modifier alleles. If, however, a transgenic female is crossed with a BALB/c male, methylation in the offspring remains low, suggesting that the modifier genes are imprinted and expressed when maternally transmitted (data from Allen *et al.*, 1990).

Conclusions

Imprinted genes may have a variety of different sequence elements that are required at different stages of development and in different tissues. Such elements may have diverse roles in initiation, maintenance, and reversal of imprinting, and are likely to be targets for epigenetic modification. A number of modifier genes, including the methyltransferase gene, may therefore act to initiate and maintain imprints and allele-specific expression by acting on these elements. A particularly intriguing class of modifier genes are themselves imprinted, and it is important to determine whether other imprinted loci are among their targets.

References

Allen, N. D. & Mooslehner, K. A. (1992). Imprinting, transgene methylation and genotype-specific modification. *Semin. devel. Biol.* **3**, 87–98.

Allen, N. D., Norris, M. L. & Surani, M. A. (1990). Epigenetic control of transgene expression and imprinting by genotype-specific modifiers. *Cell* **61**, 853–60.

Allen, N. D. & Reik, W. (1992). Imprinter or Imprinted? *BioEssays* **14**, 857–9.

Barlow, D. P. (1993). Methylation and imprinting: from host defense to gene regulation. *Science* **260**, 309–10.

Bartolomei, M. S. (1994). The search for imprinted genes. *Nature Genet.* **6**, 220–1.

Bartolomei, M. S., Webber, A. L., Brunkow, M. E. & Tilghman, S. M. (1993). Epigenetic mechanisms underlying the imprinting of the mouse *H19* gene. *Genes Devel.* **7**, 1663–73.

Brandeis, M., Kafri, T., Ariel, M., Chaillet, J. R., Razin, A. & Cedar, H. (1993). The ontogeny of allele-specific methylation associated with imprinted genes in the mouse. *EMBO J.* **12**, 3669–77.

Chaillet, J. R., Vogt, T. F., Beier, D. R. & Leder, P. (1991). Parental-specific methylation of an imprinted transgene is established during gametogenesis and progressively changes during embryogenesis. *Cell* **66**, 77–83.

Efstratiadis, A. (1994). Parental imprinting of autosomal mammalian genes. *Curr. Opin. Genet. Devel.* **4**, 265–80.

Engler, P., Haasch, D., Pinkert, C. A., Doglio, L., Glymour, M., Brinster, R. & Storb, U. (1991). A strain-specific modifier on mouse chromosome 4 controls the methylation of independent transgenic loci. *Cell* **65**, 939–47.

Feil, R., Walter, J., Allen, N. D. & Reik, W. (1994). Developmental control of allelic methylation in the imprinted mouse *Igf2* and *H19* genes. *Development* **120**, 2933–43.

Ferguson-Smith, A. C., Sasaki, H., Cattanach, B. M. & Surani, M. A. (1993). Parental-origin-specific epigenetic modification of the mouse *H19* gene. *Nature* **362**, 751–4.

Forejt, J. & Gregorová, S. (1992). Genetic analysis of genomic imprinting: An *Imprintor-1* gene controls inactivation of the paternal copy of the mouse *Tme* locus. *Cell* **70**, 443–50.

Gross, D. S. & Garrard, W. T. (1988). Nuclease hypersensitive sites in chromatin. *A. Rev. Biochem.* **57**, 159–97.

Haig, D. (1992). Genomic imprinting and the theory of parent-offspring conflict. *Semin. devel. Biol.* **3**, 153–60.

Haig, D. & Westoby, M. (1989). Parent-specific gene expression and the triploid endosperm. *Am. Nat.* **134**, 147–55.

Hao, Y., Crenshaw, T., Moulton, T., Newcomb, E. & Tycko, B. (1993). Tumour suppressor activity of *H19* RNA. *Nature* **365**, 764–7.

Henry, I., Bonaiti-Pellie, C., Chehensse, V., Beldjord, C., Schwartz, C., Utermann, G. & Junien, C. (1991). Uniparental paternal disomy in a genetic cancer-predisposing syndrome. *Nature* **351**, 665–7.

Jost, J.-P. (1993). Nuclear extracts of chicken embryos promote an active demethylation of DNA by excision repair of 5-methyldeoxycytidine. *Proc. Natl. Acad. Sci. USA* **90**, 4684–8.

Kafri, T., Gao, X. & Razin, A. (1993). Mechanistic aspects of genome-wide demethylation in the preimplantation mouse embryo. *Proc. Natl. Acad. Sci. USA* **90**, 10558–62.

Kay, G. F., Barton, S. C., Surani, M. A. & Rastan, S. (1994). Imprinting and X-chromosome counting mechanisms determine *Xist* expression in early mouse development. *Cell* **7**, 639–50.

Kitsberg, D., Selig, S., Brandeis, M., Simon, I., Keshet, I., Driscoll, D. J., Nicholls, R. D. & Cedar, H. (1993). Allele-specific replication timing of imprinted gene regions. *Nature* **364**, 459–63.

Latham, K. E., Doherty. A. S., Scott, C. D. & Schultz, R. M. (1994). *Igf2r* and *Igf2* gene expression in androgenetic and parthenogenetic preimplantation mouse embryos: absence of regulation by genomic imprinting. *Genes Devel.* **8**, 290–9.

Laurenson, P. & Rine, J. (1992). Silencers, silencing and heritable transcriptional states. *Microbiol. Rev.* **56**, 543–60.

Li, E., Beard, C. & Jaenisch, R. (1993). Role for DNA methylation in genomic imprinting. *Nature* **366**, 362–5.

Meyer, P., Niedenhof, I. & Lohuis, M. (1994). Evidence for cytosine methylation of non-symmetrical sequences in transgenic *Petunia hybrida*. *EMBO J.* **13**, 2084–8.

Moore, T. & Haig, D. (1991). Genomic imprinting in mammalian development: a parental tug-of-war. *Trends Genet.* **7**, 45–9.

Ogawa, O., Becroft, D. M., Morison, I. M., Eccles, M. R., Skeen, J. E., Mauger, D. C. & Reeve, A. E. (1993). Constitutional relaxation of insulin-like growth factor II gene imprinting associated with Wilms' tumour and gigantism. *Nature Genet.* **5**, 408–12.

Reik, W. & Allen, N. D. (1994). Imprinting with and without methylation. *Curr. Biol.* **4**, 145–7.

Reik, W., Brown, K., Slatter, R., Sartori, P., Elliott, M. & Maher, E. R. (1994). Allelic methylation of *H19* and *IGF2* in the Beckwith–Wiedemann syndrome. *Hum. molec. Genet.* **3**, 1297–301.

Reik, W., Howlett, S. K. & Surani, M. A. (1990). Imprinting by DNA methylation: from transgenes to endogenous gene sequences. *Development* (Suppl.), 99–106.

Sapienza, C., Paquette, J., Tran, T. H. & Peterson, A. (1989). Epigenetic and genetic factors affect transgene methylation imprinting. *Development* **107**, 165–73.

Sasaki, H., Jones, P. A., Chaillet, J. R., Ferguson-Smith, A. C., Barton, S. C., Reik, W. & Surani, M. A. (1992). Paternal imprinting: potentially active chromatin of the repressed maternal allele of the mouse insulin-like growth factor II (*Igf2*) gene. *Genes Devel.* **6**, 1843–56.

Selker, E. U., Fritz, D. Y. & Singer, M. J. (1993). Dense nonsymmetrical DNA methylation resulting from repeat-induced point mutation in *Neurospora. Science* **262**, 1724–8.

Slatter, R. S., Elliott, M., Welham, K., Carrera, M., Schofield, P. N., Barton, D. E. & Maher, E. R. (1994). Mosaic uniparental disomy in Beckwith Wiedemann syndrome. *J. med. Genet.* **31**, 749–53.

Stöger, R., Kubicka, P., Liu, C.-G., Kafri, T., Razin, A., Cedar, H. & Barlow, D. P. (1993). Maternal-specific methylation of the imprinted mouse *Igf2r* locus identifies the expressed locus as carrying the imprinting signal. *Cell* **73**, 61–71.

Surani, M. A. (1993). Genomic imprinting: silence of the genes. *Nature* **366**, 302–3.

Szabó, P. & Mann, J. R. (1994). Expression and methylation of imprinted genes during in vitro differentiation of mouse parthenogenetic and androgenetic stem cell lines. *Development* **120**, 1651–60.

Thorey, I. S., Pedersen, R. A., Linney, E. & Oshima, R. G. (1992). Parent-specific expression of a human keratin 18/β-galactosidase fusion gene in transgenic mice. *Devel. Dynamics* **195**, 100–12.

Ueda, T., Yamazaki, K., Suzuki, R., Fujimoto, H., Sasaki, H., Sasaki, Y. & Higashinakagawa, T. (1992). Parental methylation patterns of a transgenic locus in adult somatic tissues are imprinted during gametogenesis. *Development* **116**, 831–9.

Weksberg, R., Shen, D. R., Fei, Y. L., Song, Q. L. & Squire, J. (1993a). Disruption of insulin-like growth factor 2 imprinting in Beckwith Wiedemann syndrome. *Nature Genet.* **5**, 143–50.

Weksberg, R., Teshima, I., Williams, B., Greenberg, C., Pueschel, S., Chernos, J., Fowlow, S., Hoyme, E., Anderson, I., Whiteman, D., Fisher, N. & Squire, J. (1993b). Molecular characterisation of cytogenetic alterations associated with the Beckwith Wiedemann syndrome phenotype refines the localisation and suggests the gene for BWS is imprinted. *Hum. molec. Genet.* **2**, 549–56.

Wu, X., Hadchouel, M., Farza, H., Amar, L. & Pourcel, C. (1992). Sex-dependent *de novo* methylation of the transgene and its insertional locus on mouse chromosome 13. In *Mechanisms of Eukaryotic DNA Recombination*, pp. 69–73. Academic Press.

11

Genomic imprinting of the H19 and Igf2 genes in the mouse

SHIRLEY M. TILGHMAN, MARISA S. BARTOLOMEI, ANDREA L. WEBBER, MARY E. BRUNKOW, JENNIFER SAAM, PHILIP A. LEIGHTON AND KARL PFEIFER

The reciprocal imprinting of *Igf2* and *H19*

A long-standing assumption of Mendelian genetics was that autosomal genes, present in two copies in diploid organisms, were functionally equivalent. That this is not always the case in mammals has now been firmly established with the discovery of the phenomenon of parental or genomic imprinting. The first imprinted gene identified in mammals was the gene encoding insulin-like growth factor 2 (*Igf2*), a mitogenic polypeptide that is thought to have an important role in regulating growth during embryogenesis (DeChiara *et al.*, 1990, 1991). This gene, whose expression was shown to be almost entirely derived from the paternal chromosome, mapped to the distal end of mouse chromosome 7, a region that had been implicated by genetic analysis in genomic imprinting (Searle & Beechey, 1990).

The next gene in this region whose imprinting was uncovered was the *H19* gene. It maps just 90 kilobases (kb) of DNA 3′ of the *Igf2* gene, but somewhat surprisingly, its expression is entirely maternal (Bartolomei *et al.*, 1991). Thus *Igf2* and *H19* are imprinted in opposite directions. The *H19* gene is an unusual gene of no known function. It is transcribed by RNA polymerase II, processed by splicing and polyadenylation, yet it does not appear to encode a protein (Pachnis *et al.*, 1988; Brannan *et al.*, 1990).

Recently, a third imprinted gene has been identified in the cluster 15 kb upstream of *Igf2*, the *insulin-2* gene (*Ins-2*). Although normally expressed in pancreatic islet cells in the adult where it is expressed from both alleles, it is also expressed in the extraembryonic membranes of mouse embryos, but in this tissue the expression is entirely paternal (Giddings *et al.*, 1994). *Ins-2* is not the only conditionally imprinted gene. In fact, *Igf2* is also expressed from both chromosomes in the choroid plexus and leptomeninges, two non-neuronal tissues in the brain (DeChiara *et al.*, 1991).

The physical linkage of the *Ins-2*, *Igf2* and *H19* genes suggested that their imprinting was coupled in some manner, although their expression from different chromosomes eliminated the most straightforward models for *cis*-acting regulators of imprinting, akin to the mechanisms thought to act in X chromosome inactivation. This possibility of a functional connection was greatly strengthened by the observation that at least two of the genes, *Igf2* and *H19*, are expressed in a very similar, if not identical, pattern during development (Lee *et al.*, 1990; Poirier *et al.*, 1991). Both genes are activated at the time of implantation in extraembryonic tissues and by day 7.5 in the embryo proper. Expression of both genes persists in a wide array of tissues of endoderm and mesoderm origin, with no detectable expression in the central and peripheral nervous system. We proposed several years ago that the reciprocal imprinting of the *Igf2* and *H19* genes may be mediated by their competition in *cis* for common regulatory elements (Fig. 11.1) (Bartolomei & Tilghman, 1992; Bartolomei *et al.*, 1993). The competition is set up by different epigenetic markings on one or both of the two chromosomes, presumably placed there during gametogenesis.

Two important requirements of this model need to be identified functionally: the regulatory elements for which the genes compete, and the mark(s) that bias the competition.

DNA methylation as the mark

From the outset, the likeliest candidate for the epigenetic mark to bias transcription of *H19* and *Igf2* differently on the two parental chromosomes was DNA methylation. We explored the allele-specific DNA methylation of the *H19* gene using F_1 hybrids between two different subspecies of mice, the *Mus musculus domesticus* strain C57BL/6J and *M. musculus castaneus*. These experiments, as well as those of others, demonstrated that in most somatic cells, the inactive paternal allele of the *H19* gene was hypermethylated relative to the active maternal allele, in a region that spanned approximately 5 kb of the 5′ flanking region and the gene itself (Bartolomei *et al.*, 1993; Brandeis *et al.*, 1993; Ferguson-Smith *et al.*, 1993). This nicely coincided with expectation, in that methylation was generally considered to act negatively to repress transcription. The surprise came, however, when the only allele-specific methylation of the *Igf2* gene was found on the *active* paternal allele, upstream of its most proximal promoter (Sasaki *et al.*, 1992). So if this is also a mark, it must act positively, possibly preventing a repressor from binding or facilitating the binding of an activator (Fig. 11.1).

Although the presence of parental-specific domains of DNA methylation within these imprinted genes was suggestive of a mark, it did not prove that methylation *per se*, or these methyl groups in particular, functioned in that

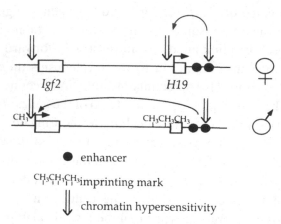

Fig. 11.1. The enhancer competition model to explain the opposite imprinting of *H19* and *Igf2*. The *H19* and *Igf2* genes are indicated by the boxes, with the horizontal arrows indicating the transcribed alleles. The two *H19* enhancers are designated by filled circles. The positions of allele-specific methylation of the paternal chromosome are indicated by the CH_3 symbols. The double-lined arrows indicate sites of restriction enzyme or DNase I hypersensitivity. The single-lined arrows leading from the enhancers indicate the engagement of the enhancers with the *H19* gene on the maternal allele and the *Igf2* gene on the paternal allele. The data for the methylation at *Igf2* are taken from Sasaki *et al.* (1992) and the data for *H19* from Bartolomei *et al.* (1993).

capacity. That issue was resolved when Li *et al.* (1992, 1993) generated a mouse containing a targeted mutation in the DNA methyltransferase gene, the gene responsible for maintaining the presence of methyl groups in DNA. In homozygous mutant embryos, transcription of the normally silent paternal *H19* gene is activated at the same time that all *Igf2* expression is lost. This important result is the first to directly implicate DNA methylation in the mechanism of parental imprinting and confirms the fact that the direction of the mark is different for the two genes.

Is DNA methylation sufficient to fully explain imprinting? The answer to that question depends on whether the methylation patterns are inherited from the appropriate gamete, in this case from sperm, and whether they survive a genome-wide demethylation event which occurs between the 8- and 32-cell stage of embryogenesis in mice (Monk *et al.*, 1987; Kafri *et al.*, 1992). The first requirement is clearly met, as at least a subset of the methylation domain at *H19* and *Igf2* is present in sperm DNA (Bartolomei *et al.*, 1993). Whether these persist in early development, however, is still being investigated. Brandeis *et al.* (1993) used a very sensitive PCR-based assay to show that at least one site of the *Igf2* promoter remains methylated throughout embryogenesis on some chromosomes, whereas none of the three methylation sites examined at *H19* did so.

Although further work is necessary to assay all the relevant sites at both genes, the initial results suggest that the extensive methylation domains in differentiated somatic tissue are largely acquired after the early stages of embryogenesis. As to whether there are key 'nucleation' methylation sites, which are established and maintained in the required manner, this remains to be determined.

The role of the *H19* enhancers in the imprinting of *H19* and *Igf2*

The second part of the enhancer competition model requires the existence of regulatory elements for which the genes compete in *cis*. Very little is known about the regulatory elements that govern expression of either *Igf2* or *H19*. Only two enhancers have been identified to date; both lie 3' of the *H19* gene, and have been shown to activate its transcription in tissue culture cells derived from the liver and gut (Yoo-Warren *et al.*, 1988), as well as in transgenic mice (Brunkow & Tilghman, 1991). These two enhancers may represent only a subset of the enhancers that govern expression of *H19*, as they are not sufficient to direct expression of the *H19* transgene in a number of tissues of mesodermal origin.

To ask whether the '*H19*' enhancers participate in the expression of the *Igf2* gene, 100 kb further upstream, we tested whether both parental copies of one of the enhancers were in an open conformation, as judged by whether a restriction enzyme could gain access to their DNA in chromatin. In fact, they exhibited identical hypersensitivities, indicating that both copies were in an open conformation (Bartolomei *et al.*, 1993). Several groups have provided evidence in support of the notion that enhancers only adopt open conformations when they are engaged in transcription (Jenuwein *et al.*, 1993; Reitman *et al.*, 1993), leading to the conclusion that the *H19* enhancers are actively involved in transcription on both alleles. Thus the paternal '*H19*' enhancers are likely to be active in transcription. Whether it is the *Igf2* gene that they activate remains to be established.

The relative roles of the *Igf2* and *H19* genes in reciprocal imprinting

The picture that emerges from Fig. 11.1 is that the inhibition of *H19* transcription by the allele-specific DNA methylation domain on the paternal chromosome allows the '*H19*' enhancers to engage in *Igf2* transcription. On the apparently unmarked maternal chromosome, the relative strength of the accessible *H19* promoter, its proximity to the enhancers, and/or the absence of methylation at the *Igf2* locus biases the competition in *H19*'s direction.

Whatever the relative importance of the methylation at *H19* versus that at *Igf2* to their overall imprinting, there appears to be a different consequence of the methylation in the assembly of an active chromatin conformation at the pro-moters. Once again, using the access of a restriction enzyme or the sequence non-specific enzyme DNase I to sequences at the promoters of the genes, several groups have shown that whereas the active maternal promoter of the *H19* gene is an open conformation, the methylated paternal promoter is inaccessible to these enzymes (Bartolomei *et al.*, 1993; Ferguson-Smith *et al.*, 1993). In contrast, both parental *Igf2* promoters are in equivalently open conformation, irrespective of their degree of methylation (Sasaki *et al.*, 1992).

A second difference between the apparent consequences of the methylation imprints on the two genes is their effects in transgenic mice. In the *H19* gene, transgenic mice carrying a 14 kb transgene that encompasses approximately 4 kb of 5′ and 8 kb of 3′ flanking sequence, along with an internally deleted structural gene, is correctly imprinted in heterologous chromosomal positions (Bartolomei *et al.*, 1993). As expected, the paternally inherited copy of the transgene is heavily methylated, whereas the maternally inherited copy is unmethylated. The same has not proven to be the case for *Igf2* transgenes, however, configured as a 5′ flanking sequence driving β-galactosidase reporter expression (Lee *et al.*, 1993). One possible conclusion from these observations is that the *H19* and *Igf2* genes share a common signal for imprinting and that signal lies proximal to the *H19* gene. Alternatively, there may be *Igf2*-specific imprinting elements that were not contained within the transgene.

A role for the *H19* gene in imprinting?

The enhancer competition model does not require that the product of the *H19* gene play any role in the imprinting itself, only that its transcriptional apparatus participate in a competition with that of the *Igf2* gene. However, the model could suggest one resolution to the mystery of the unusual nature of the *H19* gene product as a non-coding RNA. That is, the sole function of the *H19* gene may be to act as the transcriptional 'foil' to facilitate the imprinting of *Igf2*. Put another way, the only important domain of the *H19* gene would be its transcriptional regulatory apparatus. This suggestion, however, is difficult to reconcile with the evolutionary conservation of both the *H19* gene's primary and secondary struc-tures (Brannan *et al.*, 1990; Tilghman *et al.*, 1992). If the gene was only acting as a transcription unit, presumably what was being transcribed would not be con-served.

Another scenario is suggested by the similarities between *H19* and *XIST*, a gene that is expressed in an allele-specific manner in the X chromosome (Brockdorff, *et al.*, 1991; Brown *et al.*, 1991; Pizzuti *et al.*, 1991). Like *H19*, the *XIST* gene does not encode an open reading frame that is conserved between humans and mice (Brockdorff *et al.*, 1992; Brown *et al.*, 1992). Thus both *H19* and *XIST* encode RNAs with no known protein products, and are expressed in an allele-specific manner from chromosomes on which the neighboring genes are selectively silent.

XIST maps to the X inactivation center of the mammalian X chromosome, and is exclusively expressed from the inactive X chromosome (Brockdorff *et al.*, 1991; Brown *et al.*, 1991; Pizzuti *et al.*, 1991). Based on its map position and its exclusive transcription from the inactive X chromosome, several investigators have suggested that *XIST* could be the long-sought-after X chromosome inactivation center. Circumstantial evidence in favor of a role for *XIST* in X chromosome inactivation has been steadily mounting. *XIST* is not transcribed in XY males, which do not undergo X chromosome inactivation (Brockdorff *et al.*, 1991; Brown *et al.*, 1991; Pizzuti *et al.*, 1991). Allelic differences at the X chromosome inactivation center in mice (*Xce*) can affect the likelihood that an X chromosome will be chosen for inactivation in XX female cells (Cattanach *et al.*, 1969; Cattanach & Papworth, 1981; Johnson & Cattanach, 1981). X chromosomes with 'strong' *Xce* alleles are more likely to remain active than those with 'weak' alleles. Those allelic differences inversely correlate with levels of *Xist* RNA expression, in that the X chromosome with strong *Xce* alleles express less *Xist* than those with weak alleles (Brockdorff *et al.*, 1991). Finally, the activation of *Xist* precedes X chromosome inactivation in mouse embryos, and therefore its expression is not a consequence of the process (Kay *et al.*, 1993).

Table 11.1 contains a comparison between the properties of *Xist* and *H19* RNAs, and the mechanisms by which each gene is regulated in an allele-specific way. The *XIST* RNA in humans and its counterpart, *Xist* RNA in mice, are localized to the nucleus, and possibly even to the inactive X chromosome, although at the moment the *in situ* hybridization studies on which this conclusion is based cannot distinguish between the inactive X as the site of *XIST* transcription, versus its localization (Brockdorff *et al.*, 1992; Brown *et al.*, 1992). Biochemical fractionation studies, on the other hand, place both the human and mouse *H19* RNAs in comparable 28–30 S cytoplasmic particles (Brannan *et al.*, 1990).

At first glance, the sizes of the genes and their transcripts are quite different (Fig. 11.2). The *H19* gene is composed of five exons, separated by four very small intervening sequences, and codes for a 2.5 kb transcript in both humans and mice (Pachnis *et al.*, 1988; Brannan *et al.*, 1990). *Xist/XIST*, on the other hand, is a large gene, with a transcript approximately 17 kb in length (Brockdorff *et al.*, 1992; Brown *et al.*, 1992). The number of exons of the *Xist* gene is not conserved in mammals, as the human gene has two extra exons at its 3' end, which are differentially spliced. What is similar between the overall structures of *H19* and

Table 11.1. *A comparison between* H19 *and* Xist

Property	*H19*	*Xist*
Protein coding capacity	no conserved ORFs	no conserved ORFs
Size of RNA	2387 bases	14 739 bases
Size of gene	3 kilobases	19 kilobases
Number of exons	5	6
Mouse/human conservation	77% (optimized)[a]	47.8% (unoptimized)[a]
Conserved secondary structure	yes	yes
Tandem repeats	no	yes
Location of RNA	cytoplasmic particle	nuclear
Allele specificity	maternal expression	paternal expression[b]
DNA methylation	paternal allele	maternal allele[b]

[a] The *H19* gene alignment was first obtained using the GAP program in the GCG Sequence Analysis Package, then optimized further. The *Xist* gene comparison was not optimized.
[b] The *Xist* gene is expressed exclusively from the paternal allele only in early development in the mouse. Thereafter its expression is monoallelic, but the choice is random.
Sources of data: Brannan *et al.* (1990), Brockdorff *et al.* (1992), Bartolomei *et al.* (1993), Kay *et al.* (1993) and Norris *et al.* (1994).

Xist is the placement of large outside exons that are separated by very small exons.

Both *Xist* and *H19* are modestly conserved at the primary sequence level. The overall degree of sequence identity between mouse and human *H19* is only 77% (Brannan *et al.*, 1990). For *XIST*, the overall degree of conservation is even less although, as is the case for *H19*, there are regions such as exon 4 that are relatively well conserved (Hendrich *et al.*, 1993). However, there is significant evolutionary conservation at the level of secondary structure throughout the sequence of both RNAs. This is evident in the presence of long, energetically favorable stem–loop structures, which are conserved between homologs by virtue of compensatory base substitutions in the stems. A particularly noteworthy example within *H19* is shown in Fig. 11.3. When the *XIST/Xist* RNAs were examined for similar structures, several were detected. As was the case for *H19*, the longest of these coincided with the most conserved region of the RNA. However, when the primary sequences of these two regions were compared between the gene families, no similarities were apparent.

Both human and mouse *XIST/Xist* contain a numer of short tandem repeats throughout their lengths (Brockdorff *et al.*, 1992; Brown *et al.*, 1992). Although

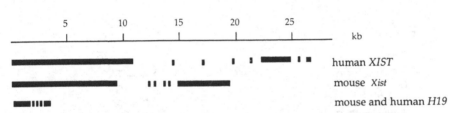

Fig. 11.2. The structures of the *H19* and *XIST* genes. The exons of the human *XIST*, mouse *Xist* and *H19* genes are indicated by the black boxes, with the spaces between representing the introns. (Taken from Brockdorff *et al.*, 1992; Brown *et al.*, 1992; Pachnis *et al.*, 1988; Brannan *et al.*, 1990.)

the repeat lengths vary in number between *XIST* and *Xist*, their positions and sequence motifs are conserved. There is no comparable extensive pattern of simple sequence repeats in *H19*, but a short region at the 5' end of both the human and mouse *H19* RNAs contains the sequence TGGGGG repeated 8–10 times. In neither gene is the significance of these repeats clear.

Like *H19*, there is evidence for a central role for DNA methylation in at least the early stages of *Xist* expression (Norris *et al.*, 1994). The choice of which X chromosome to inactivate in eutherian mammals is a random one in most somatic cells, with the exception of the endodermal cells in the extraembryonic membranes, which are among the first cells to differentiate in early embryos. There the choice is paternal inactivation, and in that case X chromosome inactivation can be considered to be imprinted (Takagi & Sasaki, 1975; West *et al.*, 1977). Norris *et al.* (1994) have recently shown that the paternal *Xist* allele becomes demethylated during meiosis and remains so until fertilization. They argue that the hypomethylation permits paternal-specific *Xist* expression by the 4-cell stage, and thereby directs paternal-specific X chromosome inactivation in the earliest tissues to differentiate. Between the morula and blastocyst stages, the genome-wide demethylation presumably erases the paternal methylation in all other uncommitted embryonic cells, and the counting mechanism that inactivates all but one X chromosome with random choice is initiated. Even in these cells, the pattern of DNA methylation around the *Xist* gene is again consistent with a negative role for methylation, as demonstrated by methylation over the silent allele on the active X chromosome (Norris *et al.*, 1994).

It remains to be seen whether either of these two genes that reside within imprinted domains and encode RNAs have some functional role to play, either in their own imprinting or in the imprinting of neighboring genes. The attractiveness of considering RNA as a regulatory molecule for imprinting is its ability to act in *cis*, unlike proteins, which must be translated in the cytoplasm before returning to the nucleus.

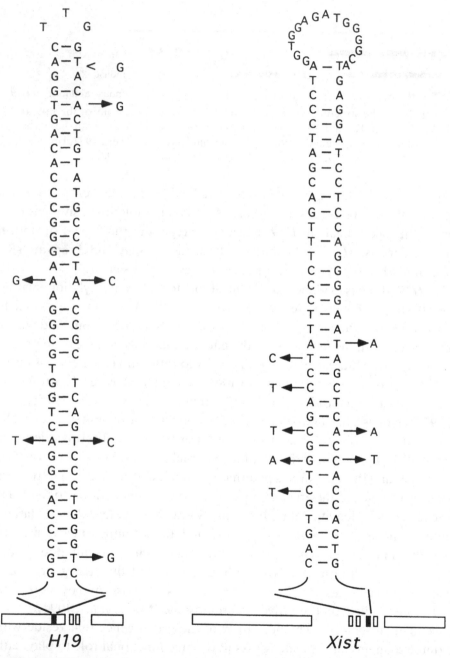

Fig. 11.3. Conserved stem–loop structures in the *H19* and *Xist* genes. The most conserved region of the mouse *H19* gene, within exon 1, is drawn in an extended stem–loop. The bases that differ between the mouse and human genes are indicated by the arrows. The most conserved region of the mouse *Xist* gene, within exon 4, is drawn similarly, with the base differences in the human gene indicated by the arrows.

Acknowledgements

This work was supported by a grant from the National Cancer Institute (CA44976). S.M.T. is an Investigator of the Howard Hughes Medical Institute; M.S.B. was supported by a Postdoctoral Fellowship from the Public Health Service; J.S. was supported by a NSF Predoctoral Fellowship, and K.P. by a Damon Runyon–Walter Winchell Postdoctoral Fellowship.

References

Bartolomei, M. & Tilghman, S. M. (1992). Parental imprinting of mouse chromosome 7. *Semin. devel. Biol.* **3**, 107–17.

Bartolomei, M. S., Webber, A. L., Brunkow, M. E. & Tilghman, S. M. (1993). Epigenetic mechanisms underlying the imprinting of the mouse *H19* gene. *Genes Devel.* **7**, 1663–73.

Bartolomei, M. S., Zemel, S. & Tilghman, S. M. (1991). Parental imprinting of the mouse H19 gene. *Nature* **351**, 153–5.

Brandeis, M., Kafri, T., Ariel, M., Chaillet, J. R., McCarrey, J., Razin, A. & Cedar, H. (1993). The ontogeny of allele-specific methylation associated with imprinted genes in the mouse. *EMBO J.* **12**, 3669–77.

Brannan, C. I., Dees, E. C., Ingram, R. S. & Tilghman, S. M. (1990). The product of the H19 gene may function as an RNA. *Molec. Cell Biol.* **10**, 28–36.

Brockdorff, N., Ashworth, A., Kay, G. F., Cooper, P., Smith, S., McCabe, V. M., Norris, D. P., Penny, G. D., Patel, D. & Rastan, S. (1991). Conservation of position and exclusive expression of mouse *Xist* from the inactive X chromosome. *Nature* **351**, 329–31.

Brockdorff, N., Ashworth, A., Kay, G. F., McCabe, V. M., Norris, D. P., Cooper, P. J., Swift, S. & Rastan, S. (1992). The product of the mouse *Xist* gene is a 15 kb inactive X-specific transcript containing no conserved ORF and located in the nucleus. *Cell* **71**, 515–26.

Brown, C. J., Ballabio, A., Rupert, J. L., Lafreniere, R. G., Grompe, M., Tonlorenzi, R. & Willard, H. F. (1991). A gene from the region of the human X chromosome inactivation centre is expressed exclusively from the inactive X chromosome. *Nature* **349**, 38–44.

Brown, C. J., Hendrich, B. D., Rupert, J. L., Lafreniere, R. G., Xing, Y., Lawrence, J. & Willard, H. F. (1992). The human *XIST* gene: analysis of a 17 kb inactive X-specific RNA that contains conserved repeats and is highly localized within the nucleus. *Cell* **71**, 527–42.

Brunkow, M. E. & Tilghman, S. M. (1991). Ectopic expression of the *H19* gene in mice causes prenatal lethality. *Genes Devel.* **5**, 1092–101.

Cattanach, B. M. & Papworth, D. (1981). Controlling elements in the mouse. V. Linkage tests with X-linked genes. *Genet. Res.* **38**, 57–70.

Cattanach, B. M., Pollard, C. E. & Peres, J. N. (1969). Controlling elements in the mouse X chromosome. I. Interaction with X-linked genes. *Genet. Res.* **14**, 233–5.

DeChiara, T. M., Efstratiadis, A. & Roberston, E. J. (1990). A growth-deficiency phenotype in heterozygous mice carrying an insulin-like growth factor II gene disrupted by targeting. *Nature* **345**, 78–80.

DeChiara, T. M., Robertson, E. J. & Efstratiadis, A. (1991). Parental imprinting of the mouse insulin-like growth factor II gene. *Cell* **64**, 849–59.

Ferguson-Smith, A. C., Sasaki, H., Cattanach, B. M. & Surani, M. A. (1993). Parental-origin-specific epigenetic modifications of the mouse *H19* gene. *Nature* **362**, 751–5.

Giddings, S. J., King, C. D., Harman, K. W., Flood, J. F. & Carnaghi, L. R. (1994). Allele specific inactivation of insulin 1 and 2, in the mouse yolk sac, indicates imprinting. *Nature Genet.* **6**, 310–13.

Hendrich, B. D., Brown, C. J. & Willard, H. F. (1993). Evolutionary conservation of possible functional domains of the human and murine *XIST* genes. *Hum. molec. Genet.* **2**, 663–72.

Jenuwein, T., Forrster, W. C., Qui, R.-G. & Grosschedl, R. (1993). The immunoglobulin u enhancer core establishes local factor access in nuclear chromatin independent of transcriptional stimulation. *Genes Devel.* **7**, 2016–32.

Johnson, P. G. & Cattanach, B. M. (1981). Controlling elements in the mouse. IV. Evidence of non-random X-inactivation. *Genet. Res.* **37**, 151–60.

Kafri, T., Ariel, M., Brandeis, M., Shemer, R., Urven, L., McCarrey, J., Cedar, H. & Razin, A. (1992). Developmental pattern of gene-specific DNA methylation in the mouse embryo and germ line. *Genes Devel.* **6**, 705–14.

Kay, G. F., Penny, G. D., Patel, D., Ashworth, A., Brockdorff, N. & Rastan, S. (1993). Expression of *Xist* during mouse development suggests a role in the initiation of X chromosome inactivation. *Cell* **72**, 171–82.

Lee, J. E., Pintar, J. & Efstratiadis, A. (1990). Pattern of the insulin-like growth factor II gene expression during early mouse embryogenesis. *Development* **110**, 151–9.

Lee, J. E., Tantravahi, U., Boyle, A. L. & Efstratiadis, A. (1993). Parental imprinting of an *Igf2* transgene. *Molec. Reprod. Devel.* **35**, 382–90.

Li, E., Beard, C. & Jaenisch, R. (1993). The role of DNA methylation in genomic imprinting. *Nature* **366**, 362–5.

Li, E., Bestor, T. H. & Jaenisch, R. (1992). Targeted mutation of the DNA methyltransferase gene results in embryonic lethality. *Cell* **69**, 915–26.

Monk, M., Boubelik, M. & Lehnert, S. (1987). Temporal and regional changes in DNA methylation in the embryonic, extraembryonic and germ cell lineages during mouse embryo development. *Development* **99**, 371–82.

Norris, D. P., Patel, D., Kay, G. F., Penny, G. D., Brockdorff, N., Sheardown, S. A. & Rastan, S. (1994). Evidence that random and imprinted *Xist* expression is controlled by preemptive methylation. *Cell* **77**, 41–51.

Pachnis, V., Brannan, C. I. & Tilghman, S. M. (1988). The structure and expression of a novel gene activated in early mouse embryogenesis. *EMBO J.* **7**, 673–81.

Pizzuti, A., Muzny, D., Lawrence, C., Willard, H. F., Avner, P. & Ballabio, A. (1991). Characterization of a murine gene expressed from the inactive X chromosome. *Nature* **351**, 325–8.

Poirier, F., Chan, C.-T. J., Timmons, P. M., Robertson, E. J., Evans, M. J. & Rigby, P. W. J. (1991). The murine *H19* gene is activated during embryonic stem cell differentiation in vitro and at the time of implantation in the developing embryo. *Development* **113**, 1105–14.

Reitman, M., Lee, E., Westphal, H. & Felsenfeld, G. (1993). An enhancer/locus control region is not sufficient to open chromatin. *Molec. Cell Biol.* **13**, 3990–8.

Sasaki, H., Jones, P. A., Chaillet, J. R., Ferguson-Smith, A. C., Barton, S., Reik, W. & Surani, M. A. (1992). Parental imprinting: potentially active chromatin of the repressed maternal allele of the mouse insulin-like growth factor (*Igf2*) gene. *Genes Develop.* **6**, 1843–56.

Searle, A. G. & Beechey, C. V. (1990). Genome imprinting phenomena on mouse chromosome 7. *Genet. Res.* **56**, 237–44.

Takagi, N. & Sasaki, M. (1975). Preferential inactivation of the paternally derived X chromosome in the extraembryonic membranes of the mouse. *Nature* **256**, 640–2.

Tilghman, S. M., Brunkow, M. E., Brannan, C. I., Dees, C., Bartolomei, M. S. & Phillips, K. (1992). The mouse *H19* gene: its structure and function in mouse development. In *Nuclear Processes and Oncogenes*, ed. P. A. Sharp, pp. 188–200. New York: Academic Press.

West, J. D., Frels, W. I. & Chapman, V. M. (1977). Preferential expression of the maternally derived X chromosome in the mouse yolk sac. *Cell* **12**, 873–82.

Yoo-Warren, H., Pachnis, V., Ingram, R. S. & Tilghman, S. M. (1988). Two regulatory domains flank the mouse *H19* gene. *Molec. Cell Biol.* **8**, 4707–15.

12

Plasticity of imprinting

ROLF OHLSSON, TOMAS EKSTRÖM, GARY FRANKLIN, SUSAN
PFEIFER-OHLSSON, HENGMI CUI, STEPHEN MILLER,
ROSEMARY FISHER AND COLUM WALSH

Introduction

When the phonemenon of parental imprinting was first discovered, it was assumed that the monoallelic expression of imprinted genes would be manifested in every tissue at all developmental stages. Many of the genes now characterized, however, show monoallelic expression only in certain tissues (DeChiara *et al.*, 1991; Giddings *et al.*, 1994), at certain developmental stages (Kay *et al.*, 1993), or within a subgroup of the population (Forejt & Gregorová, 1992; Jinno *et al.*, 1994). The normally repressed maternal allele of *Igf2*, for instance, has been found to be active in the choroid plexus and leptomeninges of mice (DeChiara *et al.*, 1991) and humans (Ohlsson *et al.*, 1994), giving biallelic expression in this tissue alone. Similarly, the mouse *Ins1* and *Ins2* genes are expressed in a parent-of-origin-specific manner in the mouse yolk sac, but not in the pancreas (Giddings *et al.*, 1994). Temporal variation is seen at the mouse *Xist* locus, which is paternally expressed in morulae and blastocysts but which is monoallelically expressed from a randomly chosen parental allele from gastrulation onwards (Kay *et al.*, 1993; Lyon, this volume). Some reports also suggest that the ability to be imprinted may depend on the primary sequence of the gene, so that only certain alleles of a polymorphic gene can undergo imprinting. This phenomenon may be seen at the *Tme* locus in mice, a locus tightly linked to *Igf2r* and expressed primarily from the maternal allele (Barlow *et al.*, 1991). Genetic studies have suggested that the *Tme* locus is only imprinted in certain species of inbred mice (Forejt & Gregorová, 1992), although a final verdict on this has not yet been reached. Such a polymorphism has also been suggested for the *WT1* gene in humans, which is biallelically expressed in kidney and some placentae, but is active from the paternally derived allele only in some placental and brain tissues (Jinno *et al.*, 1994). The human *IGF2R* gene also appears to be imprinted in only a fraction of the population (Xu *et al.*, 1993). Such variation in the manifestation of the imprint may also reflect incomplete penetrance or indeed the presence of modifier loci, which affect the epigenetic mark and/or its interpretation. Such modifier genes have been shown to affect the expression of transgenes in mice in a strain-specific fashion (Allen *et al.*, 1990; Engler *et al.*, 1991; Sapienza *et al.*, 1989). These observations point to a certain plasticity in the interpretation of the imprint, to allow tissue- and stage-specific reprogramming of the allelic usage of the gene.

Here we describe and discuss some novel results with respect to the allelic usage of the *IGF2* and *H19* genes in humans. These two genes are tightly linked on human chromosome 11p15.5 (Zemel *et al.*, 1992) and expressed from opposite parental chromosomes (Bartolomei *et al.*, 1991; DeChiara *et al.*, 1991); these findings have led to suggestions that the two genes may be coordinately regulated (Bartolomei *et al.*, 1993; Surani, 1993). The *H19* gene is driven by a single promoter and produces a single transcript, which seems to function at the RNA level (Brannan *et al.*, 1990; Pachnis *et al.*, 1988). The *IGF2* gene has four different promoters and can produce a family of different transcripts, although only one protein product has been found (Rotwein, 1991). Our examination of the expression of *H19* and the different transcripts of *IGF2* suggests that complex promoter-specific allele usage can occur. In addition, we find some evidence to suggest that an underlying counting mechanism may operate in parallel to the mechanism that can distinguish the parental origin of the chromosomes.

Results

Opposite allele usage of IGF2 *in human tumor cells: loss of imprinting?*

The loss of imprinting of *IGF2* in tumors has been speculated to lead to a growth advantage by allowing transcription from both alleles (Ogawa *et al.*, 1993; Rainier *et al.*, 1993). A problem inherent in these studies is that the extraction of RNA from whole pieces of tissue gives an averaging effect and so heterogeneity in expression across the tissue (due to, for instance, mosaicism in the allele usage) might be missed. To investigate possible *IGF2* tissue heterogeneity in cells of the trophoblast lineage, we have asked whether the allele usage in the tumor cell line Jeg-3, originating from the trophoblastic lineage, is identical in each cell and maintained cell-autonomously.

We first established a system for evaluating the allele usage of *IGF2* in normal tissues. To discriminate between the parental *IGF2* alleles we exploited the $(C-A)_n$ repeat polymorphism of exon nine, an exon common to all the known *IGF2* transcripts (except a 2.2 kb species) independent of the mode of regulation of expression (Fig. 12.1). The *IGF2* genotype was determined by analyzing such

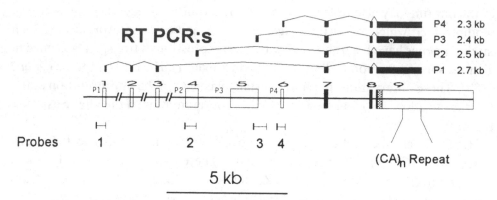

Fig. 12.1. A schematic view of the *IGF2* transcriptional unit with the four different promoters and polymorphic (C–A)$_n$ repeat indicated. The promoter-specific cDNA transcripts indicated in the figure were obtained by reverse transcribing total RNA primed at the 3' end of the (C–A)$_n$ repeat. Each promoter-specific cDNA was then singled out by PCR amplification using promoter-specific primers paired with a common primer at the 3' end of the (C–A)$_n$ repeat.

(C–A)$_n$ repeats by a polymerase chain reaction (PCR) amplification procedure followed by RNase protection analysis using ^{32}P-labeled RNA probes generated from either parental allele (schematically shown in Fig. 12.2) (Ohlsson *et al.*, 1993). In this assay, use of an RNA probe derived from the cDNA of one particular allele will fully protect only the corresponding identical mRNA: transcripts derived from other alleles will be clipped at mismatch sites, giving a banding pattern characteristic for each type of allele. Extensive screening has identified seven alleles assorting at the polymorphic (C–A)$_n$ repeat locus of *IGF2*. By PCR analysis of the DNA isolated from the same samples, the alleles present in the genome and the total cellular RNA can be directly compared. Figure 12.3 shows the allele usage pattern in a family in which the mother was heterozygous and the father was homozygous. When the DNA and RNA of the offspring were analyzed it was clear that only the paternally derived *IGF2* allele was expressed. This approach has been used to more extensively assay the allelic usage of *IGF2* during human pre- and postnatal development. *IGF2* was found to be functionally imprinted in all of the human prenatal and perinatal tissues examined except in the choroid plexus and leptomeninges of a perinatal patient (Ohlsson *et al.*, 1994). It is not known whether *IGF2* is expressed from the paternal chromosome only in the precursor cells from which the cells of the choroid plexus and leptomeninges are derived, in which case the imprint is ignored in their daughter cells, or whether these precursor cells fail to establish the imprint at all.

Primary cultures of fibroblasts have been shown to maintain a monoallelic

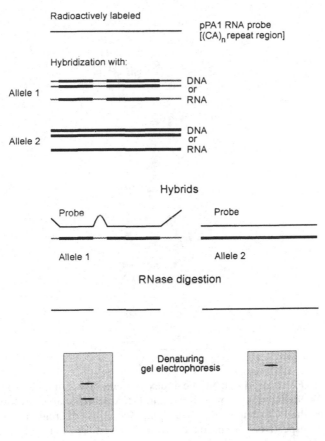

Fig. 12.2. The principle of RNase protection to assess *IGF2* allelic usage directly at the RNA level. The allele-specific fragmentation of the ^{32}P-labeled RNA probe (encompassing the polymorphic $(C-A)_n$ repeat within exon nine) is obtained when either total cellular RNA or PCR-amplified exon nine is analyzed. A comparison of the band patterns identifies the active allele. Reproduced from Nyström *et al.* (1994) with kind permission from the publisher.

expression pattern of *IGF2* (Eversole-Cire *et al.*, 1993). In Fig. 12.4 it is shown that an 'early' passage (passage 100) of the Jeg-3 cell line (obtained from ATCC) also appears to express *IGF2* monoallelically whereas a later passage (passage 150) appears to express both parental alleles. To establish whether the apparent biallelic expression of *IGF2* was due to the culture containing two subpopulations of cells, each expressing a different allele, we subcloned Jeg-3 cells by transfection with a psv2neo plasmid followed by neomycin selection. Individual clones (57 in all) were expanded and the *IGF2* allele usage analyzed. The surprising outcome was that three subclones expressed one allele type exclusively, three subclones expressed the other allele type exclusively and the rest

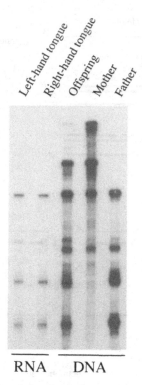

Fig. 12.3. *IGF2* is imprinted in the index patient of a familial form of the Beckwith–Wiedemann syndrome. RNA and DNA depict analysis of total cellular RNA and the PCR-amplified polymorphic $(C–A)_n$ repeat region within exon nine DNA, respectively. Reproduced from Nyström *et al.* (1994) with kind permission from the publisher.

expressed *IGF2* from both parental alleles. Because the Jeg-3 cell line has undergone serial cloning procedures prior to its availability at ATCC, there is the possibility of unusual *in vitro* artifacts occurring. If so, the mutability of the allele usage pattern in cultured cells suggests that the epigenetic modification pattern controlling a gene's expression is more susceptible to damage or to change than the DNA itself. If, on the other hand, these results are not due to *in vitro* artifacts or to epigenetic mutation, then an explanation for the allele usage in these cell lines would have to be found which could be fitted to what is already known about the imprinting of *IGF2* and other genes *in vivo*.

It is interesting in this context to consider the gene that seems to initiate X chromosome inactivation, *Xist* (Kay *et al.*, 1993). *Xist* is first expressed from the paternal allele only, then from about gastrulation onwards, from one randomly chosen parental allele exclusively in any given cell, a so-called chromosome counting mechanism. Here, the imprint on the gene may only serve to bias a

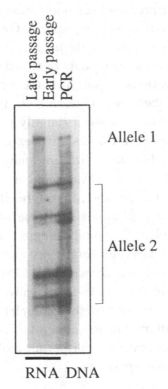

Fig. 12.4. *IGF2* allelic usage in an early and late passage of Jeg-3 choriocarcinoma cells. RNase protection analysis of total cellular RNA was performed, as outlined in Fig. 12.2.

basically random process under a certain developmental time period, after which the information as to parental origin represented by the imprint is ignored. It is interesting to speculate that this might be true of other imprinted genes, too. A certain leakiness in the bias might then be expected, so that the paternal allele, for instance, was shut down in 90% of the cells, but occasionally the wrong allele was chosen and the maternal allele became inactive. This might explain such results as the allele switching and biallelic expression seen in some tissues for *H19* (Zhang *et al.*, 1993) and the observation of monoallelic expression of *WT1* in only some placentas (Jinno *et al.*, 1994). Although the Jeg-3 cell clone was established by serial cloning, it is not possible to exclude an initial heterogeneity in the population as to *IGF2* allele usage. Even if only a tiny fraction of the cells initially expressed the maternal allele (or both alleles simultaneously) the serial cloning and selection could fix this allele usage in subsequent cell cultures. A relaxation of the monoallelic expression may also account for the transition from monoallelic to biallelic expression for the population of cells as a whole. It has been noted that the 'loss of imprinting' of *IGF2* seen in several tumor types might equally well reflect either a heterogeneity in the precursor cell population with respect to allele usage or a relaxation of a strict paternal allele expression (Ogawa *et al.*, 1993).

That a counting mechanism may underlie genetic imprinting of some loci derives more support from preliminary data obtained in dispermic hydatidiform moles. These preneoplastic tissues result from the fertilization of an empty egg by two sperm (Lawler & Fisher, 1993; Ohama *et al.*, 1981). Despite the fact that the *H19* gene is transcriptionally active primarily from the maternal allele in normal placenta, *H19* transcripts are abundant in extravillous trophoblasts of the complete moles. Southern blot hybridization analysis suggests that the two paternal *H19* alleles present in the dispermic complete moles appear to be differentially methylated. It is possible, therefore, that in the absence of differential marking of the two genomes the underlying counting mechanism ensures shut-down of one allele. The similarities in structure and function noted between the *H19* and *Xist* genes (Feinberg, 1993; Surani, 1993; Tilghman *et al.*, this volume) may well be more than coincidental. Chromosome counting to give random inactivation should be visible as clonally derived patches of cells expressing a single allele of *H19* in dispermic complete hydatidiform moles, if it occurs. We are currently attempting to address this issue by performing allele-specific *in situ* hybridization analysis on dispermic moles and associated tumors exhibiting aberrant allele usage patterns.

The loss of *IGF2* imprinting during human liver development reflects promoter-specific allele usage

Recent work suggests that a reversal to a paternal epigenotype on the maternal chromosome 11p15.5 in humans causes activation of the silent *IGF2* allele and repression of the active *H19* allele (Moulton *et al.*, 1994; Steenman *et al.*, 1994). Tumorigenesis in these tissues has therefore been speculated to be a consequence of the events leading to biallelic expression of *IGF2*. We have obtained data that suggest that the allelic usage of *IGF2* is temporally controlled during human liver development. Hence, although overall expression is monoallelic during embryonic, fetal and neonatal liver development, samples from later developmental time points show overall biallelic expression (Ekström *et al.*, 1995). These results might reflect a temporal relaxation of imprinting by the erasing or neutralization of parental imprints during human postnatal development. Alternatively, the allelic activity of the four promoters could have been modified so that one promoter is active from one parental allele while other promoters could be active from the other parental allele. To investigate this possibility we elaborated on a RT–PCR and RNase protection technique that we had previously developed. By combining a primer 3′ of the polymorphic $(C-A)_n$

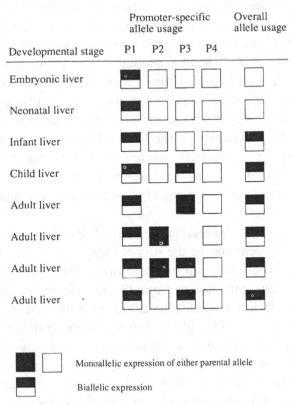

Developmental stage	Promoter-specific allele usage				Overall allele usage
	P1	P2	P3	P4	
Embryonic liver					
Neonatal liver					
Infant liver					
Child liver					
Adult liver					
Adult liver					
Adult liver					
Adult liver					

Monoallelic expression of either parental allele

Biallelic expression

Fig. 12.5. Schematic summary of promoter-specific *IGF2* allele usage during human liver development.

repeat in exon 9 with a 5′ primer for exon 1, 4, 5 or 6 (specific for promoters 1, 2, 3 and 4, respectively), each promoter-specific transcript can be amplified up from the total RNA (see Fig. 12.1). Subsequent analysis with RNase protection allowed us to specifically address the imprinting status for any of the promoters.

The results of our investigations are schematically summarized in Fig. 12.5, which shows that in all the informative liver specimens investigated (covering a range of developmental time points) the P1 promoter directed expression from both parental alleles. Because expression from the P1 promoter is very low prenatally, an examination of the pool of all the *IGF2* transcripts in the prenatal stages shows overwhelming predominance of paternal transcripts, explaining the apparent contradiction between the findings using promoter-specific and non-specific probes. The P4 promoter-derived transcripts were from one allele only in all liver cases examined. The picture becomes more complex with the P2 and P3 promoters. The P3 promoter-derived transcripts came from both parental alleles in three out of four adult specimens, as well as in the 18 months old liver sample.

Hence, the P3 promoter allelic usage can be relaxed during liver development. We also found that the parental allele transcribed via the P2 and P3 promoters was sometimes the opposite to the one used by the P4 promoter (Fig. 12.5). This could reflect mosaicism in allele usage among the population of cells in the liver. This issue was addressed by hybridizing ^{35}S-labeled antisense RNA probes of exons 4 and 6 (specific for P2- and P4-derived transcripts) to adjacent thin sections of one liver, which was expressing the P2 and P4 transcripts from opposite alleles. This revealed that the P2 and P4 promoters direct expression from opposite parental alleles in the same cell (R. Ohlsson et al., unpublished observations). It therefore seems that the parental chromosome from which transcription will occur can be specified for each promoter independently of the imprinted status of H19.

We conclude that the biallelic expression of IGF2 seen during postnatal human liver development may be the sum of many effects: (i) an increase in P1 promoter activity on both alleles during development; (ii) a frequent switch from monoallelic to biallelic transcription from P3; and (iii) the opposite allele usage seen for P2, P3 and P4 in some individuals. These results indicate that imprinting at the IGF2 locus is a complex phenomenon, involving different allele usage patterns for each promoter and variation of the pattern over developmental time. With such varied parental allele usage occurring at the different IGF2 promoters, it seems more reasonable to imagine that the imprint must be specified in a promoter-autonomous fashion than that there might be a single locus which specifies the imprinting pattern of both IGF2 and the neighboring H19 gene, as has been proposed (Bartolomei et al., 1993; Brandeis et al., 1993; Surani, 1993). It is possible to imagine, however, that the allele usage patterns of the IGF2 and H19 genes are initially synchronized, but that this coupling is unhitched in the later stages of development. The ability of the cell to grow and divide changes during development; it may be that the replication status of the cells can affect the ability to maintain the imprint. It has been shown that imprinted loci are replicated asynchronously on the two paternal chromosomes (Kitsberg et al., 1993), in contrast to the synchronous replication of the parental alleles at most loci. The liver specimens of older patients are likely to be dominated by non-replicating cells, which none the less express IGF2. It may be that it is harder for a cell to maintain the original imprint when it is not replicating, although this is, of course, very speculative.

Transcription and imprinting

The observation of distinct imprinting patterns for transcripts derived from the different promoters of IGF2 raises a number of potentially important issues.

Although this phenomenon has so far been referred to (and thought of) in terms of 'imprinted genes', the case of *IGF2* in the liver suggests that it may be prudent to think more in terms of 'imprinted gene regulatory elements'. Because imprinting involves the parental allele-specific *transcription* of genes, it would be expected that DNA sequences involved in transcriptional regulation (promoters, enhancers, silencers, locus control regions, etc.) would represent the targets for the imprinting mechanism. It may well be, therefore, that genes that are associated with several cell-type-specific or developmental-stage-specific promoters or enhancers will not exhibit the same imprinted status in all situations. Special care should, therefore, be taken in the evaluation of any potentially imprinted gene that may be driven by multiple promoters. This is particularly important with respect to the region of the mRNA targeted for RNase protection assays, where alternative choices of probe could result in very different conclusions, as seen here.

The plasticity of imprinting, as exhibited by *IGF2* in human liver, could be the result of either a change in the epigenetic imprint, or a change in the response of the transcriptional machinery to that imprint. Changes in the availability of the various components of the complex transcription apparatus (Buratowski, 1994), whether in a cell-type-specific, developmentally regulated or disease-related situation, could be envisaged to produce a new transcriptional response by 'imprinted' alleles. For example, if the 'imprint' is targeted to a particular protein-binding DNA sequence whose function becomes redundant in response to a new repertoire of available factors, then that cell could 'ignore' the original imprinting signal. This is all the more plausible in the light of the 'modular' nature of transcriptional control elements (Dynan, 1989), i.e. that promoters and enhancers are known to be made up of multiple modules that represent discrete protein binding sites, which can interact to produce a different overall effect of the element, depending on which of the potential element-binding factors are available (Tijan & Maniatis, 1994). It is possible that an imprint would be limited to one such key regulatory module within a promoter or enhancer and that plasticity in imprinting would not therefore be limited to genes that are regulated by multiple promoters and/or enhancers. The observation that the monoallelic expression patterns of imprinted genes can vary through time may not therefore be so surprising, given that the response to the imprint may change in concert with the variations in the transcription factor composition. Recent research has also indicated that some of the fundamental mechanisms involved in transcriptional regulation may change over developmental time; both the requirement for an enhancer to stimulate high-level transcription (Majumder *et al.*, 1993) and the requirement for a TATA box in activated transcription (Majumder & De Pamphilis, 1994) have been reported to be developmentally acquired in the mouse embryo. This may be of some relevance to the initially biallelic expression of the *Xist* gene during early mouse development.

Acknowledgements

This work was supported by funds from the Swedish Cancer Foundation, the Swedish Natural Science Council, the Wenner-Gren Foundation and the Swedish Medical Research Council.

References

Allen, N., Norris, M. & Surani, M. (1990). Epigenetic control of transgene expression and imprinting by genotype-specific modifiers. *Cell* **61**, 853–61.

Barlow, D., Stöger, R., Herrmann, B., Saito, K. & Schweifer, N. (1991). The mouse insulin-like growth factor type-2 receptor is imprinted and closely linked to the Tme locus. *Nature* **349**, 84–7.

Bartolomei, M. M., Webber, A. L., Brunkow, M. E. & Tilghman, S. M. (1993). Epigenetic mechanisms underlying the imprinting of the mouse *H19* gene. *Genes Devel.* **7**, 1663–73.

Bartolomei, M., Zemel, S. & Tilghman, S. (1991). Parental imprinting of the mouse *H19* gene. *Nature* **351**, 153–5.

Brandeis, M., Kafri, T., Ariel, M., Chaillet, J. R., McCarry, J., Razin, A. & Cedar, H. (1993). The ontogeny of allele-specific methylation associated with imprinted genes in the mouse. *EMBO J.* **12**, 3669–77.

Brannan, C., Dees, E., Ingram, R. & Tilghman, S. (1990). The product of the *H19* gene may function as an RNA. *Molec. Cell Biol.* **10**, 28–36.

Buratowski, S. (1994). The basics of basal transcription by RNA polymerase II. *Cell* **77**, 1–3.

DeChiara, T., Robertson, E. & Efstratiadis, A. (1991). Parental imprinting of the mouse insulin-like growth factor II gene. *Cell* **64**, 849–59.

Dynan, W. S. (1989). Modularity in promoters and enhancers. *Cell* **58**, 1–4.

Ekström, T. J., Cui, H., Li, X. & Ohlsson, R. (1995). Promoter-specific IGF2 imprinting status and its plasticity during human liver development. *Development* **121**, 309–16.

Engler, P., Haasch, D., Pinkert, C., Doglio, L., Glymour, M., Brinster, R. & Storb, U. (1991). A strain-specific modifier on mouse chromosome 4 controls the methylation of independent transgene loci. *Cell* **65**, 939–47.

Eversole-Cire, P., Ferguson-Smith, A. C., Sasaki, H., Brown, K. D., Cattanach, B. M., Gonzales, F. A., Surani, M. A. & Jones, P. A. (1993). Activation of an imprinted *Igf2* gene in mouse somatic cell cultures. *Molec. Cell Biol.* **13**, 4928–38.

Feinberg, A. J. (1993). Genomic imprinting and gene activation in cancer. *Nature Genet.* **4**, 110–13.

Forejt, J. & Gregorová, S. (1992). Genetic analysis of genomic imprinting: an *Imprintor-1* gene controls inactivation of the paternal copy of the mouse *Tme* locus. *Cell* **70**, 443–50.

Giddings, S. J., King, C. D., Harman, K. W., Flood, J. F. & Carnaghi, L. R. (1994). Allele specific inactivation of insulin 1 and 2, in the mouse yolk sac, indicates imprinting. *Nature Genet.* **6**, 310–13.

Jinno, Y., Yun, K., Nishiwaki, K., Kubota, T., Ogawa, O., Reeve, A. & Niikawa, N. (1994). Mosaic and polymorphic imprinting of the *WT-1* gene in humans. *Nature Genet.* **6**, 305–9.

Kay, G. F., Penny, G. D., Patel, D., Ashworth, A., Brockdorff, N. & Rastan, S. (1993). Expression of *Xist* during mouse development suggests a role in the initiation of X chromosome inactivation. *Cell* **72**, 171–82.

Kitsberg, D., Selig, S., Brandeis, M., I, S., Keshet, I., Driscoll, D. J., Nicholls, R. D. & Cedar H. (1993). Allele-specific replication timing of imprinted gene regions. *Nature* **364**, 459–63.

Lawler, S. D. & Fisher, R. A. (1993). The contribution of the paternal genome: hydatidiform mole and choriocarcinoma. In *The Human Placenta*, ed. C. W. G. Redman, I. L. Sargent & P. M. Starkey, pp. 82–112. Oxford: Blackwell Scientific Publications.

Majumder, S. & DePamphilis, M. L. (1994). TATA-dependent enhancer stimulation of promoter activity in mice is developmentally acquired. *Molec. cell Biol.* **14**, 4258–68.

Majumder, S., Miranda, M. & DePamphilis, M. L. (1993). Analysis of gene expression in mouse preimplantation embryos demonstrates that the primary role of enhancers is to relieve repression of promoters. *EMBO J.* **12**, 1131–40.

Moulton, T., Crenshaw, T., Hao, Y., Moosikasuwan, J., Lin, N., Dembitzer, F., Hensle, T., Weiss, L., McMorrow, L., Loew, T., Kraus, W., Gerald, W. & Tycko, B. (1994). Epigenetic lesions at the *H19* locus in Wilms' tumor patients. *Nature Genet.* **7**, 440–7.

Nyström, A., Hedborg, F. & Ohlsson, R. (1994). Insulin-like growth factor 2 cannot be linked to a familial form of Beckwith–Wiedemann syndrome. *Eur. J. Pediatr.* **153**, 574–80.

Ogawa, O., Eccles, M., Szeto, J., McNoe, L., Yun, K., Maw, M., Smith, P. & Reeve, A. (1993). Relaxation of insulin-like growth factor II gene imprinting implicated in Wilm's tumour. *Nature* **362**, 749–51.

Ohama, K., Kajii, T., Okamoto, E., Fukuda, Y., Imaizumi, K., Tsukahara, M., Kobayashi, K. & Hagiwara, K. (1981). Dispermic origin of XY hydatidiform moles. *Nature* **292**, 551–2.

Ohlsson, R., Hedborg, F., Holmgren, L., Walsh, C. & Ekström, T. J. (1994). Overlapping patterns of *IGF2* and *H19* expression during human development: biallelic *IGF2* expression correlates with a lack of *H19* expression. *Development* **120**, 361–8.

Ohlsson, R., Nyström, A., Pfeifer-Ohlsson, S., Töhönen, V., Hedborg, F., Schofield, P., Flam, F. & Ekström, T. J. (1993). *IGF2* is parentally imprinted during human embryogenesis and in the Beckwith–Wiedemann syndrome. *Nature Genet.* **4**, 94–7.

Pachnis, V., Brannan, C. & Tilghman, S. (1988). The structure and function of a novel gene activated in early mouse embryogenesis. *EMBO J.* **3**, 673–81.

Rainier, S., Johnson, L., Dobry, C., Ping, A., Grundy, P. & Feinberg, A. (1993). Relaxation of imprinted genes in human cancer. *Nature* **362**, 747–9.

Rotwein, P. (1991). Structure, evolution, expression and regulation of insulin-like growth factors I and II. *Growth Factors* **5**, 3–18.

Sapienza, C., Paquette, J., Tran, T. H. & Peterson, A. (1989). Epigenetic and genetic factors affect transgene methylation imprinting. *Development* **107**, 165–8.

Steenman, M. J., Rainier, S., Dobry, C. J., Grundy, P., Horon, I. L. & Feinberg, A. P. (1994). Loss of imprinting of *IGF2* is linked to reduced expression and abnormal methylation of *H19* in Wilms' tumour. *Nature Genet.* **7**, 433–9.

Surani, M. A. (1993). Silence of the genes. *Nature* **366**, 302–3.

Tijan, R. & Maniatis, T. (1994). Transcriptional activation: A complex puzzle with few easy pieces. *Cell* **77**, 5–8.

Xu, Y., Goodyer, C. G., Deal, C. & Polychronakos, C. (1993). Functional polymorphism in the parental imprinting of the human *IGF2R* gene. *Biochem. biophys. Res. Commun.* **197**, 747–54.

Zemel, S., Bartolomei, M. & Tilghman, S. (1992). Physical linkage of two mammalian imprinted genes, *H19* and insulin-like growth factor 2. *Nature Genet.* **2**, 61–5.

Zhang, Y., Shields, T., Crenshaw, T., Hao, Y., Moulton, T. & Tycko, B. (1993). Imprinting of human *H19*: allele-specific CpG methylation, loss of the active allele in Wilms' tumor and potential for somatic allele switching. *Am. J. Hum. Genet.* **53**, 113–24.

13

Regional regulation of allele-specific gene expression

ITAMAR SIMON AND HOWARD CEDAR

Most genes in the animal genome are expressed equally from both parental alleles, but there are a variety of exceptional gene sequences that undergo transcription in an allele-specific manner. The most striking example of this phenomenon is the random X chromosome inactivation in females. As a result of this event which takes place at the late blastula stage of development, each somatic cell expresses the genes from either the maternal or paternal X chromosome, but not both. Genomic imprinting represents another category of allele-specific gene expression; it is characterized by the gamete-directed inactivation of one particular parental allele in many cells of the embryo and adult organism. In the mouse, for instance, the genes *Igf2* and *Snrpn* are transcribed exclusively from the paternal allele, whereas *Igf2r* and *H19* are expressed from the maternal allele only (Efstratiadis, 1994).

Although the regulatory mechanisms involved in allele-specific gene expression are not yet understood, it is clear that unique molecular control processes must be employed. In general, molecular studies on the control of transcription have emphasized the role played by cellular *trans*-acting factors, which interact with gene-specific regulatory sequences and in this way modulate RNA synthesis. Although similar mechanisms may also take part in the expression of allele-specific genes, it is obvious that specialized *cis*-acting control elements must be recruited in order to distinguish between the two alleles.

In thinking about possible mechanisms for controlling allele-specific gene expression, one must take into account the critical observation that genes of this nature appear to be regulated in a regional manner. This phenomenon is seen both for X inactivation, which encompasses almost an entire chromosome, and for imprinted genes. By analyzing the phenotypes derived from uniparental disomies in mice, it was concluded that imprinted genes are restricted to a small number of fixed chromosomal regions (Cattanach & Kirk, 1985). This unique organization has been confirmed by molecular studies on individual genes. Thus,

Igf2 and *H19*, although reciprocally imprinted, are both located within 90 kb on mouse chromosome 7 (Zemel *et al.*, 1992); the nearby insulin gene is also expressed monoallelically in extraembryonic tissues during the early stages of development (Giddings *et al.*, 1994). In the Prader–Willi/Angelman syndrome (PWS/AS) region on human chromosome 15 at least two specific genes, *ZNF-127* and *SNRPN*, are expressed exclusively from the paternal allele, and genetic evidence suggests that there may be additional imprinted genes in this region (Nicholls, 1993). Although these observations only demonstrate a physical linkage between imprinted sequences, this genomic organization certainly suggests that the expression patterns themselves may be subject to domain-wide regulatory mechanisms. The immunoglobulin and T-cell receptor genes are also subject to allelic exclusion; in this case, too, allelic expression is governed by a region-specific mechanism involving a large cluster of individual genes.

DNA methylation represents a good potential candidate for differentially marking parental alleles. This mechanism is clearly utilized on the X chromosome, where housekeeping genes are exclusively modified on the inactive allele in all somatic tissues (Razin & Cedar, 1994). Because this modification is added to the DNA after the genes undergo transcriptional inactivation, the methyl moieties cannot possibly serve as a primary effector of inactivation (Lock *et al.*, 1987), but rather most likely play a key role in the maintenance of differential gene expression. Imprinted genes are also associated with small patches of differentially methylated DNA, but in this case, as well, it is unlikely that these methyl groups serve as a gamete-derived imprinting signal. For most of these genes, the gametic methylation patterns are erased in the early embryo and the allele-specific somatic pattern is only established after implantation (Fig. 13.1) (Brandeis *et al.*, 1993). Thus, this allele-specific modification is usually a secondary process, which must itself be directed by some other more stable molecular imprint. Many of the methyl moieties associated with these imprinted genes, although not directly derived from the gametes, probably play a role in the maintenance of allele-specific transcription. In embryos derived from DNA methyltransferase-deficient mice, for example, several imprinted gene sequences lack DNA modification on both alleles and this apparently causes a striking loss of imprinting (Li *et al.*, 1993).

In contrast to these somatically imprinted methylation patterns, unique sites in the *Igf2r* gene domain (Stöger *et al.*, 1993) and the RSVIgMyc imprinted transgene (Chaillet *et al.*, 1991) do undergo gamete-specific modification in the oocyte, but not in the sperm; this differential pattern is then maintained throughout early development. Although these loci may represent potential candidates for an imprinting signal, it should be noted that they are topographically limited to relatively small fragments of DNA. Thus, although

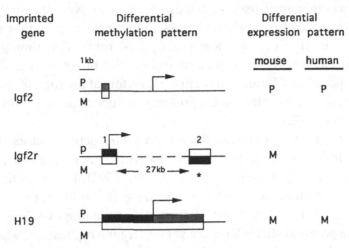

Fig. 13.1. Differential methylation and expression patterns of imprinted genes. Allele-specific methylation patterns are shown (see Razin & Cedar, 1994). The paternal (P) or maternal (M) allele can be fully methylated (closed boxes), partly methylated (hatched boxes) or unmethylated (open boxes). Each map is drawn to the same scale and indicated the start site for transcription. The region marked with an asterisk may represent a gamete-derived imprinting signal. These sites have all been shown to be methylated in the mature oocyte, to be unmethylated in sperm, and to maintain this allelic modification in the early preimplantation embryo. The other methylation patterns are established after implantation (Brandeis *et al.*, 1993). Each gene is transcribed exclusively from either the maternal or the paternal allele.

these signals may be intimately involved in the local regulation of individual imprinted genes, it is very likely that they themselves are under the control of a master imprinting box which regulates the entire domain.

Replication time zones represent a structural feature of the chromosome that is not only controlled in a regional manner, but may also serve to distinguish between parental alleles. During each cell cycle, the entire genome must undergo a single round of DNA replication; this is carried out as an ordered, programmed process in which each DNA region is duplicated at a specific time in S phase (Hand, 1978). This is best observed by growing cells in bromodeoxy-uridine (BrdU) for fixed time intervals and then mapping the location of this label in metaphase chromosomes. This analysis reveals that DNA synthesis takes place in a regional manner, generating a series of reproducible replication bands, which comap to structurally active and inactive domains on each chromosome (Kerem *et al.*, 1984). Molecular techniques have also been employed to measure the replication timing of individual gene sequences; these studies demonstrate that there is a straightforward relationship between DNA replication and gene expression (Holmquist, 1988). Housekeeping genes all replicate in the first half of S phase, whereas many tissue-specific genes have a developmentally regulated pattern characterized by early replication only in those cells that express the particular gene. It is not yet clear exactly how replication timing and RNA synthesis are causally related, but, as a result of this programming, each gene is probably exposed to different sets of protein factors at the time of its replication during S phase and this may have a profound influence on transcription (Fangman & Brewer, 1992).

In order to better understand the *cis-* and *trans-*acting factors that control replication timing, we have developed a new technique for the analysis of DNA synthesis at specific gene sequences (Selig *et al.*, 1992). In this method, fluorescence *in situ* hybridization is used to visualize genes in interphase nuclei. Two different patterns are then observed: in nuclei containing two single hybridization dots the parental alleles have not yet undergone replication, whereas those showing double dot hybridization signals represent cells in which this particular gene has already been replicated on both homologs (Plate 3). Thus, in a non-synchronous culture, a high percentage of cells with double dots indicates that this sequence replicates early in the cell cycle, whereas a predominance of singlets suggests that this gene replicates late.

By using this methodology it has been possible to map replication time zones at the molecular level. The cystic fibrosis gene (*CF*), for example, is located within a 1.5 Mb region on human chromosome 7, which has been completely cloned into phage and cosmid vectors. By using these DNA sequences as probes to carry out *in situ* hybridization, we have shown that the *CF* gene is positioned within a large, late-replicating domain in non-expressing cells. In tissues that transcribe the *CF* gene, however, a 500–700 kb region containing this sequence undergoes an alteration in its structure and becomes early-replicating (Fig. 13.2). The size of this time zone is consistent with the overall number of replication bands seen on highly resolved prometaphase chromosomes (Drouin *et al.*, 1990), suggesting that the entire genome is composed of approximately 2000 replication zones each about 1 Mb in length. It is likely that the timing of these units is regulated by means of long-range, domain-wide *cis-*acting sequences, but control sites of this nature have not been yet identified at the molecular level.

Replication timing analysis, using either the banding technique or *in situ* hybridization, has shown quite clearly that for most of the genome the two parental alleles replicate synchronously during the cell cycle. One striking exception to this rule is the X chromosome in female cells, where identical sequences on the two homologs replicate asynchronously, with the inactive chromosome undergoing DNA synthesis late in S phase. This shift in replication timing presumably reflects differences in overall chromatin structure between the active and inactive homologs (Kerem *et al.*, 1983). Assuming that this may

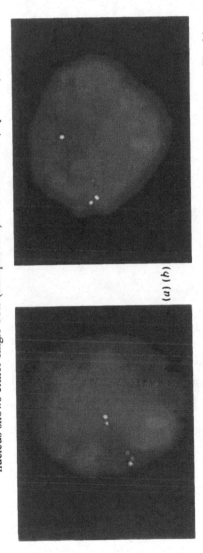

(a) (b)

Plate 3. *In situ* hybridization to interphase nuclei. Individual phage or cosmid clones labelled with biotin are hybridized to nuclei and these sequences are then detected with avidin-linked RITC (Selig *et al.*, 1992). Each nucleus shows either single dots (unreplicated) or double dots (replicated).

Plate 4. Olfactory receptor loci replicate without parental specificity. Nuclei from embryonic fibroblasts carrying a paternally derived deletion in the *Fah* region on chromosome 7 were hybridized with probes for *Fah* (red) and for the *I7* olfactory receptor (white). Double-label detection was performed as in Kitsberg *et al.* (1993). In some cells it is the paternal allele that is early-replicating (*a*), whereas in others it is the maternal copy (*b*).

These images are available in colour as a download from www.cambridge.org/9780521179997

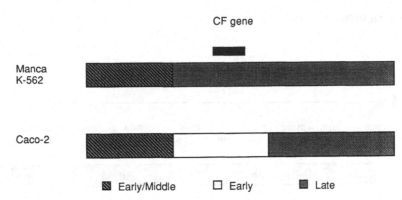

Fig. 13.2. Replication structure of the cystic fibrosis domain. *In situ* hybridization delineates three time zones in this region. The *CF* gene itself is located on a 500–700 kb domain, which is early-replicating in the expressing Caco-2 cell line or late replicating in lymphocytes (Manca) or erythroleukemia cells (K-562), which do not express this gene.

be a general property of allele-specific expression, we asked whether genomically imprinted genes might also be subject to a similar mechanism. To this end we carried out *in situ* hybridization using probes from the genomic regions harboring known imprinted genes (Kitsberg *et al.*, 1993). In this assay, asynchronous replication can be easily detected by the appearance of a high percentage of cells showing one single and one double hybridization dot. In these nuclei, it is possible to actually visualize the replicated (double) and unreplicated (single) alleles.

As shown in Fig. 13.3, imprinted genes appear to be embedded within large domains of asynchronously replicating DNA, which are bounded by normal synchronous regions and this has been confirmed by cytogenetic studies as well (Izumikawa *et al.*, 1991). In order to determine whether this pattern is also allele-specific, we examined replication timing in the *Igf2*, *Igf2r* and PWS/AS regions using cell lines which allow one to distinguish between the maternal and paternal chromosomal alleles. In many of these cases it is the paternal allele that replicates early, with all of the sequences in the domain undergoing DNA synthesis in a coordinate manner on each chromosome (Kitsberg *et al.*, 1993). The most striking example of this specificity is seen on the imprinted X chromosome in extraembryonic tissues where the inactive paternal allele is selectively early-replicating in almost every cell (Sugawara *et al.*, 1985).

It thus appears that imprinted genes are not only physically clustered in the genome, but are also organized into domains that have a unique, allele-specific chromosome structure. This differential configuration is not confined to the specific cell types that show the imprinted phenotype, but can be observed in a

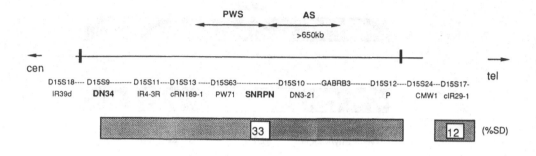

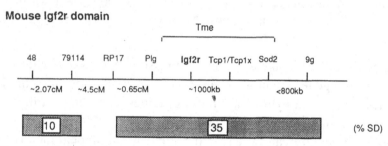

Fig. 13.3. Imprinted genes are in asynchronously replicating domains. *In situ* hybridization shows that large regions around the mouse *Igf2r* gene and the human PWS/AS locus are asynchronously replicating. This is indicated by a high percentage of nuclei with a single/double (SD) hybridization pattern in a variety of different cell types (Kitsberg *et al.*, 1993). The genes marked with bold lettering are known to be transcriptionally imprinted. *DN34* is the same as *ZNF-127*.

number of different cell lineages, suggesting that this is a basic genomic structure which is established early in development. In support of this, we have also found that these imprinted domains replicate asynchronously in the F9 embryonic carcinoma cell type, which serves as a model for the blastula stage of development. It is not known whether asynchronous replication plays a causative role in controlling allele-specific gene expression; it is likely that the relationship between replication and transcription is quite complex. In the imprinted region on the distal part of mouse chromosome 7, for example, both the active *Igf2* gene and the inactive *H19* gene are on the same early-replicating paternal allele. Furthermore, each imprinted domain includes many genes that do not have an imprinted phenotype (Barlow *et al.*, 1991; Kitsberg *et al.*, 1993) and this suggests that the regulation of imprinting must involve both regional and local effectors of expression.

Another form of allele-specific gene expression has been observed at the immunoglobulin and T-cell receptor gene loci. In these cases, single functional gene sequences are generated by a stochastic intramolecular rearrangement, and the resulting protein product evidently then acts to prevent further reorganization on the second allele (Alt *et al.*, 1984). This allelic exclusion process probably represents a critical step in the development of the B cell repertoire, since it insures that each cell only produces a single antibody type. Interestingly, at least in the heavy chain region in humans, this rearrangement brings about a striking change in the replication timing of the variable regions that are juxtaposed near the constant gene sequences, and this causes the two alleles to be asynchronously replicating (Calza *et al.*, 1984).

The olfactory receptor gene family may also be subject to a similar type of regulatory mechanism. Individual olfactory sensory neurons are functionally distinct; each neuron expresses only one or a small number of receptor genes out of a family containing at least 1000 distinct members (Vasser *et al.*, 1993). The signal elicited by the interaction of odorants with receptors is probably then decoded by the brain to determine which of the numerous receptors have been activated. As is the case for the immunoglobulin genes, the olfactory receptors are clustered within a number of chromosomal loci (authors' unpublished observations) and it is very likely that single genes are activated in a stochastic manner in each olfactory neuron. If this is the case, there must also be some mechanism for preventing gene expression from the second allele. Thus, one would expect that the receptor gene expressed in any particular neuron would only be transcribed from one of the parental alleles. In collaboration with A. Chess and R. Axel, we examined the expression pattern of *I7*, a specific member of the olfactory receptor gene family. Sequencing of this cDNA from *Mus spretus* and *M. musculus* indicated that these genes differ at several single polymorphic nucleotides within the mRNA. Thus, in F_1 hybrid mice from crosses between these two species, it is possible to distinguish between the maternal and paternal *I7* alleles. The strategy for analyzing the expression of *I7* RNA in single olfactory neurons is shown in Fig. 13.4. Following trypsinization of the sensory neurons from the nose, pools containing about 100–200 cells were prepared. Because only a small percentage of these pools showed *I7* expression by a sensitive PCR assay, we could be assured that all of the RNA from individual positive pools must have been derived from a single neuron. When these PCR products were then analyzed by hybridization to *I7* oligonucleotide probes specific to *M. musculus* or *M. spretus*, it was clearly seen that each cell expresses either the maternal or paternal *I7* allele, but not both, strongly suggesting that these genes are subject to allelic exclusion.

If, as these data strongly suggest, only one olfactory receptor allele is active at

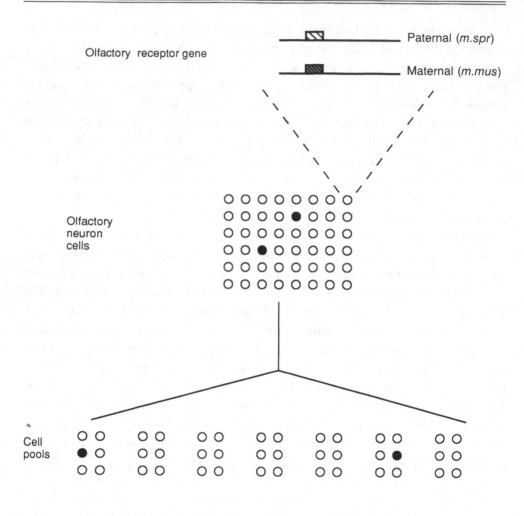

Fig. 13.4. Strategy for analysing allelic exclusion of olfactory receptor genes. Olfactory neurons were isolated from F_1 mice generated by crosses between a *Mus spretus* father and *M. musculus* mother. Following trypsinization, cells were divided into pools, which were then assayed for *I7* mRNA by PCR analysis (Chess *et al.*, 1994). PCR products from positive pools (●) were hybridized to *M. spretus* (*M. spr*) and *M. musculus* (*M. mus*) *I7* receptor-gene-specific oligonucleotide probes.

any given locus, these domains may have differential chromosomal structures, which replicate asynchronously. Indeed, an analysis of over 10 individual receptor gene probes by *in situ* hybridization showed them to undergo differential replication, with over 35% of all nuclei containing the single–double hybridization profile (Chess *et al.*, 1994). The genes, *I7* and *M50* are closely linked and map to mouse chromosome 7 at a position between the *Igf2* and *Snrpn* gene clusters. Using embryonic fibroblasts derived from mice carrying a small paternal deletion in the *Fah* domain on chromosome 7 (Kelsey *et al.*, 1992), it was possible to identify each individual parental homolog, and this enabled us to determine whether these olfactory receptor genes replicate in an allele-specific manner. As shown in Plate 4 (facing p. 198), the paternal allele is early-replicating in some cells and late-replicating in others. Different receptor genes in a given cluster, however, appear to replicate in a coordinated manner (Chess *et al.*, 1994), suggesting that asynchronous replication encompasses a large domain containing a number of individual genes.

When taken together, these results indicate that at each olfactory receptor gene locus the two parental alleles are structurally distinguishable, with one replicating early in S phase and the other replicating later in the cycle. We propose (Fig. 13.5) that only one of the alleles in each neuron is in an activatable configuration, while the genes on the other allele are in a repressed conformation that excludes transcription. Because the asynchronous replication pattern is observed in a number of different cell types and in F9 embryonic cells, it seems likely that this inactivation process occurs early in development and results in the random repression of one allele in every somatic cell. Although it takes place on autosomal domains, this process appears to be very similar to X inactivation.

Allelic inactivation also probably plays a role in the regulation of the red and green pigment genes that are expressed in retinal cones and make up the basis of color vision. Whereas the autosomal blue pigment gene is expressed in a fixed manner within a morphologically distinct subset of cones, the red and green pigment genes map to a single locus and are stochastically expressed in another subclass of retinal cones. It has been proposed that a locus control region (LCR) at this site serves as a common enhancer for both genes, but can only interact with a single pigment gene on any given allele (Winderickx *et al.*, 1992). Because these genes are present on the X chromosome, only one allele is active in any cone; the random inactivation of this chromosome in females thus serves to prevent the simultaneous transcription of a red and green pigment gene within a single cell.

In contrast to the expectations of simple Mendelian genetics, the genome appears to contain numerous sequences that are expressed from a single allele in each cell. This general process of allelic exclusion usually involves the stochastic

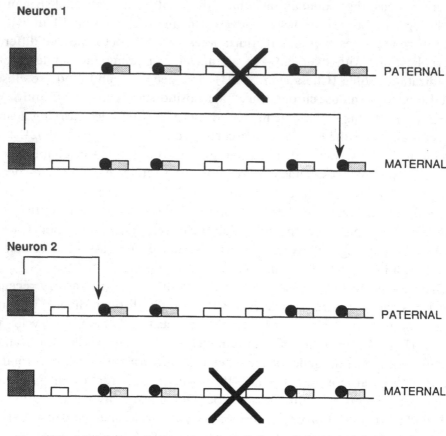

Fig. 13.5. Model for olfactory receptor allelic exclusion. A linked array of olfactory receptor genes are depicted in two neurons. The shaded boxes represent genes expressed in one topographic zone; the open boxes represent genes expressed in different zones of the nose. The black circles represent zone-specific transcription factors, which bind to a subset of the receptor genes within the array, affording these genes the potential to be activated in a given zone. The expression of these factors is likely to result from spatial information imparted in the epithelium, such that different genes can be expressed by virtue of transcriptional activation by a single *cis*-acting regulatory element (large gray box). This element may reflect a strong enhancer or a site of recombination, assuring the expression of only one receptor gene from the linked array. Only one allele is transcriptionally active since one allele is thought to be inactivated (large X) early in embryogenesis.

inactivation of a chromosomal locus, which takes place some time during normal development. Genomic imprinting represents a subset of this phenomenon, where the instructions for inactivation are engraved into the chromosome in the gametes of the previous generation, preserved in the early embryo and then used to generate a parent-specific monoallelic expression pattern. In all of these instances, the genes involved in allelic exclusion are organized into clusters embedded within chromosomal bands that replicate asynchronously during the cell cycle. These data thus suggest that the various manifestations of allele-specific expression observed in animal cells may all involve a common mechanism, which is based on chromosomal organization and regional regulation.

Acknowledgements

This research was supported by grants from the NIH, the Israel Cancer Research Fund and the Israel Academy of Sciences.

References

Alt, F. W., Yancopoulos, G. D., Blackwell, T. K., Wood, C., Thomas, E., Boss, M., Coffman, R., Rosenberg, N., Tonegawa, S. & Baltimore, D. (1984). Ordered rearrangement of immunoglobulin heavy chain variable region segments. *EMBO J.* **3**, 1209–19.

Barlow, D. P., Stöger, R., Herman, B. G., Saito, K. & Schweifer, N. (1991). The mouse insulin-like growth factor type 2 receptor is imprinted and closely linked to the Tme locus. *Nature* **349**, 84–7.

Brandeis, M., Kafri, T., Ariel, M., Chaillet, J. R., McCarrey, J., Razin, A. & Cedar, H. (1993). The ontogeny of allele-specific methylation associated with imprinted genes in the mouse. *EMBO J.* **12**, 3669–77.

Calza, R. E., Eckhardt, L. A., DelGiudice, T. & Schildkraut, C. L. (1984). Changes in gene position are accompanied by a change in the time of replication. *Cell* **26**, 689–96.

Cattanach, B. M. & Kirk, M. (1985). Differential activity of maternally and paternally derived chromosome regions in mice. *Nature* **315**, 496–8.

Chaillet, J. R., Voght, T. F., Beier, D. R. & Leder, P. (1991). Parental-specific methylation of an imprinted transgene is established during gametogenesis and progressively changes during embryogenesis. *Cell* **66**, 77–83.

Chess, A., Simon, I., Cedar, H. & Axel, R. (1994). Allelic inactivation regulates olfactory receptor gene expression. *Cell* **78**, 823–34.

Drouin, R., Lemieux, N. & Richer, C. L. (1990). Analysis of DNA replication during S phase by means of dynamic chromosome banding at high resolution. *Chromosoma* **99**, 273–80.

Efstratiadis, A. (1994). Parental imprinting of autosomal mammalian genes. *Curr. Opin. Genet. Devel.* **4**, 265–80.

Fangman, W. L. & Brewer, B. J. (1992). A question of time: replication origins of eukaryotic chromosomes. *Cell* **71**, 363–6.

Giddings, S. J., King, C. D., Harman, K. W., Flood, J. F. & Carnaghi, L. R. (1994). Allele specific inactivation of insulin 1 and 2, in the mouse yolk sac, indicates imprinting. *Nature Genet.* **6**, 310–17.

Hand, R. (1978). Eucaryotic DNA: organization of the genome for replication. *Cell* **15**, 317–25.

Holmquist, G. P. (1988). DNA sequences in G-bands and R-bands. In *Chromosomes and Chromatin*, ed. K. W. Adolphs, pp. 75–121. Boca Raton: CRC Press.

Izumikawa, Y., Naritomi, K. & Hirayama, K. (1991). Replication asynchrony between homologs 15q11.2: cytogenetic evidence for genomic imprinting. *Hum. Genet.* **87**, 1–5.

Kelsey, G., Schedl, A., Ruppert, S., Niswander, L., Magnuson, T., Klebig, M. L., Rinchik, E. M. & Schutz, G. (1992). Physical mapping of the albino-deletion complex in the mouse to localise alf/hsdr-1, a locus required for neonatal survival. *Genomics* **14**, 275–87.

Kerem, B., Goitein, R., Diamond, G., Cedar, H. & Marcus, M. (1984). Mapping of DNase-I sensitive regions on mitotic chromosomes. *Cell* **38**, 493–9.

Kerem, B. S., Goitein, R., Richler, C., Marcus, M. & Cedar, H. (1983). In situ nick-translation distinguishes between active and inactive X chromosomes. *Nature* **304**, 88–90.

Kitsberg, D., Selig, S., Brandeis, M., Keshet, I., Simon, I., Driscoll, D. J., Nicholls, R. D. & Cedar, H. (1993). Allele-specific replication timing of imprinted gene regions. *Nature* **364**, 459–63.

Li, E., Beard, C. & Jaenisch, R. (1993). The role of DNA methylation in genomic imprinting. *Nature* **366**, 362–5.

Lock, L. F., Takagi, N. & Martin, G. R. (1987). Methylation of the HPRT gene on the inactive X occurs after chromosome inactivation. *Cell* **48**, 39–46.

Nicholls, R. D. (1993). Genomic imprinting and candidate genes in the Prader-Willi and Angelman syndromes. *Curr. Opin. Genet. Devel.* **3**, 445–56.

Razin, A. & Cedar, H. (1994). DNA methylation and genomic imprinting. *Cell* **77**, 473–6.

Selig, S., Okumura, K., Ward, D. C. & Cedar, H. (1992). Delineation of DNA replication time zones by fluorescence in situ hybridization. *EMBO J.* **11**, 1217–25.

Stöger, R., Kubicka, P., Liu, C.-G., Kafri, T., Razin, A., Cedar, H. & Barlow, D. P. (1993). Maternal-specific methylation of the imprinted mouse *Igf2* locus identifies the expressed locus as carrying the imprinting signal. *Cell* **73**, 61–71.

Sugawara, O., Takagi, N. & Sasaki, M. (1985). Correlation between X-chromosome inactivation and cell differentiation in female preimplantation embryos. *Cytogenet. Cell Genet.* **39**, 210–19.

Vasser, R., Ngai, J. & Axel, R. (1993). Spatial segregation of odorant receptor expression in the mammalian olfactory epithelium. *Cell* **74**, 309–18.

Winderickx, J., Battisti, L., Motulsky, A. G. & Deeb, S. S. (1992). Selective expression on human X chromosome-linked green opsin genes. *Proc. Natl. Acad. Sci. USA* **89**, 9710–14.

Zemel, S., Bartolomei, S. M. & Tilghman, S. M. (1992). Physical linkage of two mammalian imprinted genes, H19 and insulin-like growth factor 2. *Nature Genet.* **2**, 61–5.

IV

Genomic imprinting in embryonal tumors and overgrowth disorders

14

Genomic imprinting in embryonal tumors and overgrowth disorders

ANTHONY E. REEVE

Introduction

Genomic imprinting is becoming increasingly recognized as playing an important role in a number of human diseases, including cancer. In 1988 Wilkins was the first to propose that imprinting could be involved in the onset of cancer when he reported that in Wilms' tumor the characteristic chromosome 11 loss of heterozygosity (LOH) consistently involved the maternal allele (Wilkins, 1988). The specific involvement of one parental allele in tumor-specific chromosome alterations has now been shown to occur in several embryonal tumors, which include neuroblastoma (Caron et al., 1993; Cheng et al., 1993) (1p LOH and N-myc amplification) and rhabdomyosarcoma (Scrable et al., 1989) (maternal 11p LOH). Imprinting mechanisms are not only restricted to embryonal tumors. For example, the 9;22 translocation in CML has been shown to involve the paternal chromosome 9 and maternal chromosome 22 (Haas et al., 1992) and defective IGF2 imprinting has recently been implicated in lung cancer (Suzuki et al., 1994). Wilms' tumor and other embryonal tumors have to date provided the most useful and practical experimental models for studying imprinting mechanisms in tumorigenesis. Several models that have been proposed to explain the role of genomic imprinting in the embryonal tumors are discussed in this chapter.

Wilkins model

In the mid-1980s the Knudson two-hit model was widely accepted as providing an explanation for the onset of Wilms' tumor and retinoblastoma (Knudson, 1971; Knudson & Strong, 1972). Translated into molecular terms, this model proposed the inactivation of both alleles of a gene on either chromosome 11 for Wilms' tumor (Koufos et al., 1984; Orkin et al., 1984; Reeve et al., 1984; Fearon et al., 1984) or chromosome 13 for retinoblastoma (Cavenee et al., 1983). A refinement

209

of this model later proposed by Comings (1973) suggested that the two hits or mutations sequentially inactivate each allele of a diploid pair of regulatory genes. The alleles of this regulatory gene would normally express a diffusible gene product, which would be capable of suppressing the transcription of both alleles of a transforming gene. In the event that the function of both alleles was lost, then this would lead to the expression of the transforming gene.

One of the assumptions of the Knudson and Comings models is that loss of heterozygosity (LOH) or allele inactivation should occur randomly. Schroeder *et al.* (1987) published the first data indicating that chromosome 11 LOH did not appear to be random in Wilms' tumor, with the maternal allele being lost in 5 out of 5 cases. Although these data were not explained, Wilkins pointed out that neither the frequency of germ cell mutations nor the epidemiological evidence could explain this bias towards maternal allele loss (Wilkins, 1988). To explain these data, Wilkins theorized that preferential maternal LOH was due to the differences in the imprinting of paternally and maternally inherited transforming genes (see Fig. 14.1).

The Wilkins model was based on a modified form of the Knudson two-hit model as proposed by Comings (1973). The model proposed that there are two genes on chromosome 11; the first gene consists of an allelic pair of negative regulatory genes (W_g), which are normally expressed in the embryo, and the second gene is a diploid pair of transforming genes (T_r), the maternal allele of which was proposed to be selectively inactivated by normal genomic imprinting involving selective methylation. It was suggested that the first mutational hit may occur randomly to either the maternal or paternal alleles of the W_g gene, while the second hit would most likely involve the loss of a whole chromosome 11. Tumors could only develop, however, if the maternal chromosome 11 was lost, thereby leaving the paternal T_r gene to express its gene product in the absence of the negative regulation by the W_g gene product. An important prediction from this model is that the T_r gene would be fully expressed only if the paternal chromosome 11 has been retained in a tumor, thus providing an explanation for the selective retention of paternal 11p alleles in Wilms' tumor. This was a foresighted model in view of recent studies on *IGF2* imprinting in Wilms' tumor.

Tumor suppressor gene model

A fundamentally different model has been proposed by Sapienza and colleagues to explain the preferential loss of maternal alleles in rhabdomyosarcoma and Wilms' tumor (Scrable *et al.*, 1989). This model is based on the two-hit scenario, which first involves the inactivation of the paternal allele of a tumor suppressor gene followed by the loss or inactivation of the remaining maternal allele. While

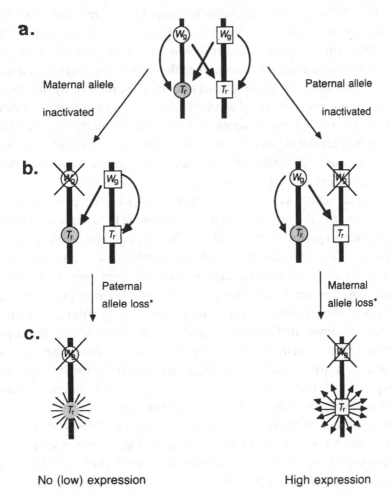

Fig. 14.1. Wilkins imprinting model for tumorigenesis. (a) In normal cells the two alleles of a transforming gene (T_r) are kept in a suppressed state by the diffusible product (arrowed) of the two Wilms' regulatory (W_g) alleles. (b) If one W_g allele is rendered inactive (through either somatic mutation in sporadic Wilms' or inheritance in familial Wilms'), suppression of T_r genes still continues irrespective of whether the paternal (unshaded square) of maternal (unshaded circle) alleles are involved. (c) When the second W_g is lost, the T_r genes are released from the suppressed state and are expressed at a high level (if unmethylated) or a low level or not at all (if methylated). In the model shown the maternal T_r allele is methylated (shaded circle). Reprinted from Wilkins (1988) with permission of the publisher.

it had been generally assumed that the first mutation in the two-hit model involved a change in the nucleotide sequence of a tumor suppressor gene on chromosome 11 (termed *Rd*), this model proposed that the first mutation is epigenetic and is due to the activity of an unlinked 'imprintase', which acts at the

Rd locus. Like Wilms' tumor, rhabdomyosarcoma also involves loss of hetero-zygosity on chromosome 11p; because both tumors are associated with the Beckwith–Wiedemann syndrome (see below) it is generally assumed that they both involve the same gene. The model therefore proposes that the first mutation would involve the inactivation of a locus on chromosome 11p by imprinting and that the imprinting may be viewed as a special form of dominance modification in which the activity of a gene is controlled by an unlinked modifier gene at another locus. However, unlike dominance modification, with genomic imprinting the modifier gene must act differently in males and females and thus have the properties of an imprintase (see Fig. 14.2).

A potential difficulty with this imprintase model is that because imprinting occurs in the gamete, the resulting tumors should have the characteristics of those occurring through a germline mutation, i.e. they should have an early age of onset and be bilateral. To explain the absence of unilateral tumors, somatic mosaicism is invoked as a result of an imprinting defect occurring some time after fertilization, thereby leading to an imprinting defect which would be present in only a limited range of tissues. The embryonal tumors are uncommon; in order to account for the low frequency of tumors in the population, the model proposes that the population frequency of the aberrant imprintase is low. Alternatively it is suggested that there could be genetic factors that affect the degree to which individuals could be mosaic for the imprinting defect; this could also explain the low frequency of tumors as well as the variable penetrance of the tumor phenotype.

Within the context of the tumor suppressor gene model it has been argued that tumors may arise by two classes of mutations affecting the tumor suppressor gene on chromosome 11, namely allele inactivation by nucleotide alteration or allele inactivation by imprinting (Scrable *et al.*, 1989). This argument led to the suggestion that familial forms of tumors may be linked either to the site of the nucleotide alteration on chromosome 11 or to another site at an unlinked locus. Support for the notion of an unlinked defective imprintase was therefore forthcoming from the observations that in rare Wilms' tumor pedigrees the disease predisposition locus was not on chromosome 11. Furthermore, in the tumor of one of the individuals in these pedigrees, the chromosone 11 that was lost was inherited from the affected mother; this event is inconsistent with the predisposing locus being on chromosome 11 (Grundy *et al.*, 1988; Huff *et al.*, 1988). While this observation is consistent with the unlinked imprintase hypo-thesis, another explanation is that 11p LOH in this Wilms' tumor patient simply represents a mitotic event associated with tumor progression. In an attempt to find the chromosomal location of the non-11 linked gene, a number of Wilms' tumors were examined for LOH throughout the autosomes. Only one major site on chromosome 16q was detected in addition to chromosome 11p (Maw *et al.*,

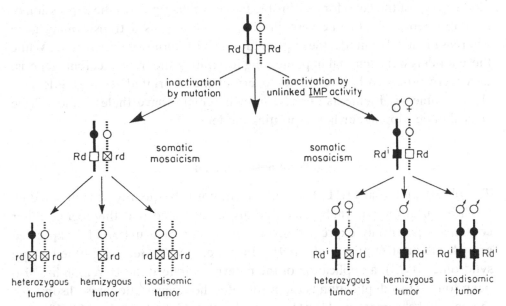

Fig. 14.2. Tumor suppressor gene model. This model involves inactivation of a tumor suppressor gene either by mutation and loss of heterozygosity, or by a mechanism invoking genomic imprinting as an alternative first step in the attainment of nullizygosity at the rhabdomyosarcoma locus (*Rd*). Open box, active locus; cross or filled box, inactive locus; *Rd*, wild type locus; *rd*, mutant locus. Part of this figure has been reprinted from Scrable *et al.* (1989) with permission of the publisher.

1992). A subsequent linkage analysis of the original Wilms' tumor pedigrees using probes on 16q indicated that this site was not linked to the phenotype (Huff *et al.*, 1992).

Reik & Surani (1989) have proposed a model for embryonal tumorigenesis which is similar to the model proposed by Sapienza and coworkers. The major difference in this model is the suggestion that within some cells in a developing tissue the maternal allele of a tumor suppressor gene may be *partly* repressed by imprinting while the paternal allele is lost by deletion or an LOH mechanism. Consequently, if the level of the tumor suppressor gene falls low enough due to repression, then this may lead to these cells gaining a proliferative preneoplastic advantage. This expanded population of cells then represents an increased target for the complete loss of the imprinted maternal allele, and this leads to neoplasia.

The Wilkins model and the tumor suppressor gene models differ fundamentally in that the first of these is proposed to involve the regulation of an imprinted transforming gene by a *trans*-acting factor. The second model involves the modulation of the activity of a tumor suppressor gene by an imprintase, although there is no requirement in this model for the imprintase to act in *trans*. Both models suggest the need for a diffusible factor which regulates the expression of an imprinted gene. In one case the imprinted gene is a transforming gene whereas in the other model the imprinted gene is a tumor suppressor gene. While these models were seminal in pioneering imprinting theories of carcinogenesis, they were proposed before the discovery of the imprinted *IGF2/H19* loci on chromosome 11. Elements of these models remain, nevertheless, and will be critical in developing further imprinting models.

Gene dosage model

The observation that 11p LOH in Wilms' tumor is frequently accompanied by duplication of the paternally inherited allele suggested that this region either contains a paternally expressed growth promoter or a maternally expressed growth inhibitor (Little *et al.*, 1991). In patients with Beckwith–Wiedemann syndrome (BWS), a duplication of the paternally inherited 11p region has also been found; this duplication is the result of either constitutional isodisomy for the paternal chromosome 11p (Henry *et al.*, 1991; Grundy *et al.*, 1991, 1994) or an unbalanced translocation resulting in an extra paternal chromosome 11p copy (Turleau & de Grouchy, 1985; Henry *et al.*, 1989). BWS is a complex syndrome which predisposes to the onset of several embryonal neoplasms including Wilms' tumor, and it is frequently characterized by somatic overgrowth (Wiedemann, 1964; Beckwith, 1969). Insulin-like growth factor 2 (*IGF2*) is a good candidate gene for the BWS because it is linked to the BWS phenotype in some BWS pedigrees (Koufos *et al.*, 1989; Ping *et al.*, 1989), is expressed at high levels in sporadic tumors associated with the syndrome (Reeve *et al.*, 1985; Scott *et al.*, 1985), and is expressed in the normal embryonal tissues from which the BWS tumors arise (Han *et al.*, 1987). Chimeric mouse embryos which contain a duplicated chromosomal segment syntenic with human chromosome 11p have been found to have overgrowth features similar to those of BWS (Ferguson-Smith *et al.*, 1991). It has been suggested that paternal 7p duplication in the chimeric mice and paternal 11p duplication in BWS individuals may lead to overgrowth because of a 'double dose' of an imprinted gene (Little *et al.*, 1991).

Support for the double dose hypothesis came from the discovery that the *Igf2* gene is imprinted in the mouse such that only the paternal allele is actively transcribed (DeChiara *et al.*, 1991). *IGF2* has recently been shown to be imprinted in humans also (Rainier *et al.*, 1993; Ogawa *et al.*, 1993b; Ohlsson *et al.*, 1993; Giannoukakis *et al.*, 1993). Accordingly, it is envisaged that in humans an overall increase in *IGF2* transcription may result from duplication or isodisomy of chromosome segments that encompass the paternally inherited 11p allele. It is possible that duplication of the active paternal *IGF2* allele may occur constitutionally and lead to the BWS, whereas mosaicism for the defect may lead to incomplete forms of the syndrome. Sporadic tumors may also arise as a consequence of the duplication of the paternal *IGF2* allele. It is intriguing to think that sporadic tumors may represent the end of a continuum of mosaicism beginning with mutations restricted to the somatic lineages such as the embryonal kidney and ending with constitutional mutations in the complete Beckwith–Wiedemann syndrome.

This concept of mosaicism is supported by the finding that chromosome 11p may be partly duplicated in the normal kidney tissue adjacent to some Wilms' tumors (Chao *et al.*, 1993). Within the developing embryonic kidney, mutations in the early development of this organ may lead to a clone of cells, which is then susceptible to further mutations. Although not proven, it is easy to envisage that gene duplications or other mechanisms affecting the imprinting of the *IGF2* locus (see below) could be involved in early clonal proliferation events within the developing kidney. A common feature of the neonatal kidney is the presence of nephrogenic rests, which contain persistent immature foci of undifferentiated mesenchyme (Beckwith *et al.*, 1990). Nephrogenic rests have recently been shown to contain mutations within the *WT1* gene and it will also be of interest to determine whether nephrogenic rests show LOH for 11p markers or imprinting changes at the *IGF2* locus.

A major unanswered question is whether there is a tumor suppressor gene (or genes) in 11p15. Loss of 11p15 heterozygosity suggests that a tumor suppressor gene may exist because this event is regarded as necessary to provide the second of two loss-of-function mutations (Scrable *et al.*, 1989; Koufos *et al.*, 1984; Orkin *et al.*, 1984; Fearon *et al.*, 1984; Reeve *et al.*, 1985; Solomon, 1984). Interpretation of the LOH data in Wilms' tumor is, however, not straightforward, because LOH usually leads to a duplication of 11p rather than a deletion (Little *et al.*, 1991; Henry *et al.*, 1989, 1991). The published data would therefore appear to support the gene duplication model. Another difficulty with interpreting the LOH data is that in some tumors reduction to homozygosity of 11p markers could reflect widespread 11p LOH, which includes the *WT1* tumor suppressor gene at 11p13 (Call *et al.*, 1990; Gessler *et al.*, 1990). Because of the physical linkage between the *WT1* tumor suppressor gene and the hypothetical 11p15 tumor suppressor gene, it is difficult to determine whether the 11p15 tumor suppressor gene is a reality. Before LOH data can be used to support the existence of a tumor suppressor gene, it will be necessary to show that LOH restricted to 11p15 involves hemizygous deletions as a frequent mechanism of allele loss. Alternatively, if the primary mechanism of 11p15 allele loss involves gene duplication, this would strengthen the argument that LOH simply leads to the doubling of the active paternal *IGF2* allele.

Although the LOH data do not yet provide a convincing case for the existence of an 11p15 tumor suppressor gene, other data have been proposed in support of this model. One candidate tumor suppressor gene is the *H19* gene, which is located within 90 kb of *IGF2* (Zemel *et al.*, 1992) in the mouse and is oppositely imprinted to *IGF2* (Bartolomei *et al.*, 1991) (maternally expressed). *H19* is abundantly transcribed in the mouse embryo and codes for an RNA molecule that might have a negative growth regulatory role; for example, its expression is low in undifferentiated cells but increases during early differentiation (Pachnis *et al.*, 1988; Brannan *et al.*, 1990). Tycko and colleagues have introduced an *H19* construct into G401 cells such that the stable cells lines were growth-retarded, less clonogenic in soft agar, and non-tumorigenic in nude mice (Hao *et al.*, 1993). This is a particularly interesting experiment, although it is difficult to compare the levels of *H19* in cultured cells with the situation *in vivo* because only a minority of cells in an expressing tissue (e.g. fetal kidney) expresses the gene whereas each cell in a transfected cell culture will express the gene. This approach therefore has the inherent problem that the level of the expressed gene in cultured cells might be considerably higher than *in vivo* and consequently lead to non-specific cytotoxic effects. The answer as to whether *H19* is a tumor suppressor gene will ultimately have to come from the detection of genetic or epigenetic mutations within the gene.

Another approach used to gain evidence for 11p15 tumor suppressor genes involved introducing fragments of chromosome 11 into the G401 cell line and then measuring tumorigenicity in nude mice (Weissman *et al.*, 1987; Dowdy *et al.*, 1991). Fragments containing the 11p13 region had no effect, whereas chromosome fragments encompassing 11p15 suppressed tumorigenicity (Dowdy *et al.*, 1991). The conclusion of these experiments is that there is a gene in the 11p15 region which is capable of altering the tumorigenic phenotype of G401 cells in the nude mouse assay. This finding is of considerable interest, although whether this is relevant to the Wilms' tumor model is not clear since it has subsequently been shown that the G401 cell line was derived from a kidney tumor of a different histology (Garvin *et al.*, 1993). Other groups have shown by complementation methods that regions within 11p15 can cause growth suppression in a rhabdomyosarcoma cell line, although tumorigenicity was not examined (Koi *et al.*, 1993; Loh *et al.*, 1992). These findings demonstrating growth suppression could be relevant to the embryonal tumor two-hit model, although caution is needed when extrapolating from the findings from these *in vivo* systems to the solid embryonal tumors.

Imprinting switch model

IGF2 is considered as a candidate for the BWS and for the development of embryonal tumors, for reasons discussed in the previous section. One reason supporting the role of *IGF2* in tumorigenesis is that LOH and the concomitant duplication of 11p would lead to an increased dosage of the actively transcribed paternal allele *IGF2* (Little *et al.*, 1991). The difficulty with this argument is that only 30–40% of Wilms' tumors involve 11p LOH (Koufos *et al.*, 1984; Orkin *et al.*, 1984; Reeve *et al.*, 1984; Fearon *et al.*, 1984; Junien & van Heyningen, 1991), suggesting that either the majority of Wilms' tumors arise by a mechanism not involving chromosome 11p, or that there are other changes at the *IGF2* locus which would not be detectable by conventional LOH analyses. The latter possibility led two groups of researchers to investigate whether the imprinting of the *IGF2* gene was altered in Wilms' tumors (Rainier *et al.*, 1993; Ogawa *et al.*, 1993b). Whereas *IGF2* is expressed monoallelically from the paternal allele under normal circumstances in the mouse and humans (with the exception of the choroid plexus, leptomeninges and liver (DeChiara *et al.*, 1991)), it was found in approximately 70% of informative Wilms' tumors that *IGF2* was also transcribed from the maternal allele (Rainier *et al.*, 1993; Ogawa *et al.*, 1993b). The finding of defective *IGF2* imprinting in a large proportion of Wilms' tumors led to the concept of 'relaxation of imprinting', a term that arose from the notion of an imprint being a positive process involving chromatin condensation and gene silencing. Consequently, if *IGF2* was inappropriately expressed from the maternal allele this process could be conceived as resulting from the 'relaxation' of the condensed chromatin structure. Although the process of chromatin condensation is partly understood for X inactivation, the connection between chromatin condensation and *IGF2* imprinting is not well understood. At this stage a more appropriate expression for the inappropriate activation of an imprinted gene may therefore be loss of imprinting (LOI).

Biallelic *IGF2* transcription detected in Wilms' tumors could have its origins as a somatic event occurring in one cell in the developing kidney; alternatively, tumors could arise from within a minor population of cells in the fetal kidney that normally express *IGF2* biallelically. It is conceivable that a small population of cells could express *IGF2* biallelically during the early stages of differentiation of the fetal kidney; however, very low levels of biallelic transcription would not have been detectable with the techniques previously used (Rainier *et al.*, 1993; Ogawa *et al.*, 1993b). *IGF2* is transcribed at high levels in nephrogenic rests, which are believed to be a precursor to Wilms' tumor, and have been found at a high frequency in juvenile kidneys (Yun *et al.*, 1993). Loss of *IGF2* imprinting is possibly an early event which leads to the production of these rests.

The notion that sporadic Wilms' tumors could arise from a population of cells within the fetal kidney which express *IGF2* biallelically is relevant to the current thinking of the role that genetic mosaicism plays in the onset of the embryonal tumors. *IGF2* is a strong candidate gene for the BWS in which paternal isodisomy may sometimes occur (Henry *et al.*, 1993; Grundy *et al.*, 1991, 1994) and consequently lead to a doubling of the active paternal *IGF2* allele. The loss of *IGF2* imprinting, either in a limited way and restricted to individual organs, or in its entirety throughout the body, may account for a spectrum of pathology ranging from unilateral to bilateral tumors to the complete BWS with all its overgrowth manifestations. Which pathologic manifestations of this spectrum of overgrowth and neoplasia will be observed may depend on the embryonic stage at which the imprint becomes defective. For example, the variable nature of overgrowth patterns in the BWS suggests that the event(s) leading to the constitutional loss of *IGF2* imprinting can occur during the postfertilization phase, as has been previously suggested for the events that lead to paternal 11p isodisomy and somatic mosaicism for the BWS (Henry *et al.*, 1993).

Compelling evidence has recently been obtained for the role of a defective *IGF2* imprinting mechanism in tumorigenesis and somatic overgrowth. In one study, 4 out of 6 fibroblast cultures from individuals with BWS were found to have biallelic *IGF2* expression (Weksberg *et al.*, 1993). In another report, constitutional biallelic expression was demonstrated in an individual with gigantism and who had previously had a Wilms' tumor in which *IGF2* was transcribed biallelically (Ogawa *et al.*, 1993a). Unlike the BWS cases, the individual with gigantism had only a few manifestations of BWS (Wilms' tumor and generalized somatic overgrowth), suggesting that a simple defect in *IGF2* imprinting might not provide the whole answer for predisposition to BWS.

Another relevant locus on chromosome 11p15 is the *H19* gene, which is actively transcribed in the embryo into an RNA of unknown function (see above, gene dosage model). The close proximity of the *H19* and *IGF2* genes and their opposite patterns of imprinting have suggested that these genes might be coordinately regulated, or alternatively that *H19* might control *IGF2* expression (Tilghman, 1993). In one study it was shown that the imprinting of *IGF2* and *H19* could both be disrupted in Wilms' tumors; however, the biological relevance of this finding is uncertain because it is unclear whether *H19* was actively transcribed in these tumors (Rainier *et al.*, 1993). We have recently examined the relationship between *H19* and *IGF2* transcription in Wilms' tumors in order to investigate the nature of the *IGF2/H19* imprinting mechanism (T. Taniguchi *et al.*, in preparation). *H19* was transcribed in only approximately 20% of Wilms' tumors, in marked contrast to *IGF2*, which was transcribed in all tumors examined. Furthermore, in all tumors that had undergone 11p15 LOH, the *H19*

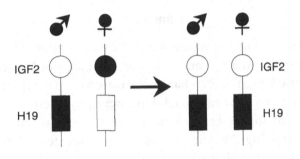

Fig. 14.3. Imprinting switch model in Wilms' tumor. *IGF2* and *H19* are normally expressed monoallelically from the maternal and paternal alleles respectively. In some Wilms' tumors, loss of imprinting occurs such that the maternal *IGF2* allele becomes active (open circles) resulting in biallelic *IGF2* expression. At the same time transcription from the maternal *H19* allele is suppressed (filled boxes).

RNA was either non-detectable or transcribed at very low levels, consistent with the *H19* maternal expression pattern and maternal 11p15 LOH.

Furthermore, in all tumors that expressed *H19* monoallelically and retained heterozygosity at the *H19* locus, *H19* was abundantly transcribed, as would be expected for a tissue of this embryonal nature. This finding was in marked contrast to the finding that in those tumors that expressed *IGF2* biallelically, *H19* transcription was absent. These data therefore indicate that the activation of the maternal *IGF2* allele in Wilms' tumor is associated with the concomitant inactivation of the maternal *H19* allele. This observation provides strong evidence for an imprinting switch mechanism which is involved in controlling the parental specificity of *IGF2* and *H19* transcription (see Fig. 14.3).

Figure 14.3 indicates that in Wilms' tumors the activation of the maternal *IGF2* allele leads to biallelic *IGF2* expression and is associated with the silencing of the maternal *H19* allele. It is possible that in Wilms' tumors one of the primary genetic lesions lies within the *H19/IGF2* switch mechanism. There are many questions that remain to be answered. For example, is the *H19/IGF2* switch mechanism related to a change in methylation patterns within this locus? Can mutations occur within nucleotide sequences which form part of a hypothetical imprinting box which coordinates *H19/IGF2* imprinting? Is it possible that *H19* controls *IGF2* directly, such that mutations that inactivate *H19* lead to *IGF2* activation? Can the *H19/IGF2* switch mechanism be altered by the inappropriate action of an unlinked imprintase? Answers to these questions will provide an important basis for comprehending the mechanism of embryonal tumor onset and the Beckwith–Wiedemann syndrome.

Summary

The potential role of genomic imprinting in the onset of tumors was first invoked to explain the preferential retention of paternal alleles in Wilms' tumor. Since that time, parent-of-origin effects have been observed in a number of embryonal and some adult tumors. Several models have been proposed to explain the loss of maternal alleles in the embryonal tumors, but most recently attention has focused on determining the role of critical genes located within chromosome 11p15. Among these, the *H19* gene may serve as a tumor suppressor gene, while *IGF2* may act as a growth enhancer, either as a result of duplication of the paternal allele or by increased transcription resulting from defective imprinting of the maternal allele. In addition, constitutionally defective imprinting of the maternal *IGF2* allele provides a conceptual basis for rationalizing the mechanism of growth disorders associated with the embryonal tumors.

Acknowledgements

A.E.R. thanks Ian Morison, Takanobu Taniguchi, Kankatsu Yun and Michael Eccles for valuable comments on the manuscript. This work was supported by the Cancer Society of NZ and the NZ Lottery Board.

References

Bartolomei, M. S., Zemel, S. & Tilghman, S. M. (1991). Parental imprinting of the mouse *H19* gene. *Nature* **351**, 153–5.

Beckwith, J. B. (1969). Macroglossia, omphalocele, adrenal cytomegaly, gigantism and hyperplastic visceromegaly. *Birth Defects* **5**, 188–90.

Beckwith, J. B., Kiviat, N. B. & Bonadio, J. F. (1990). Nephrogenic rests, nephroblastomatosis, and the pathogenesis of Wilms' tumor. *Pediat. Pathol.* **1990**, 1–35.

Brannan, C. I., Dees, E. C., Ingram, R. S. & Tilghman, S. M. (1990). The product of the *H19* gene may function as an RNA. *Molec. Cell Biol.* **10**, 28–36.

Call, K. M. *et al.*, (1990). Isolation and characterization of a zinc finger polypeptide gene at the human chromosome 11 Wilms' tumor locus. *Cell* **60**, 509–20.

Caron, H. *et al.* (1990). Allelic loss of chromosome 1p36 in neuroblastoma is of preferential maternal origin and correlates with N-*myc* amplification. *Nature Genet.* **4**, 187–90.

Cavenee, W. K. *et al.* (1983). Expression of recessive allele by chromosomal mechanisms in retinoblastoma. *Nature* **305**, 779–84.

Chao, L.-Y. *et al.* (1993). Genetic mosaicism in normal tissues of Wilms' tumour patients. *Nature Genet.* **3**, 127–31.

Cheng, J. M. *et al.* (1993). Preferential amplification of the paternal allele of the N-*myc* gene in human neuroblastomas. *Nature Genet.* **4**, 191–4.

Comings, D. E. (1973). A general theory of carcinogenesis. *Proc. Natn. Acad. Sci. U.S.A.* **70**, 3324–8.

DeChiara, M., Robertson, E. J. & Efstratiadis, A. (1991). Parental imprinting of the mouse insulin-like growth factor II gene. *Cell* **64**, 849–59.

Dowdy, S. F. *et al.* (1991). Suppression of tumorigenicity in Wilms tumor by the p15.5–p14 region of chromosome 11. *Science* **254**, 293–5.

Fearon, E. R., Vogelstein, B. & Feinberg, A. P. (1984). Somatic deletion and duplication of genes in chromosome 11 in Wilms' tumours. *Nature* **309**, 176–8.

Ferguson-Smith, A. C., Cattanach, B. M., Barton, S. C., Beechey, C. V. & Surani, M. A. (1991). Embryological and molecular investigations of parental imprinting on mouse chromosome 7. *Nature* **351**, 667–70.

Garvin, A. J., Re, G. G., Tarnowski, B. I., Hazen-Martin, D. J. & Sens, D. A. (1993). The G401 cell line, utilized for studies of chromosomal changes in Wilms' tumor, is derived from a rhabdoid tumor of the kidney. *Am. J. Path.* **142**(2), 375–80.

Gessler, M. *et al.* (1990). Homozygous deletion in Wilms' tumours of a zinc-finger gene identified by chromosome jumping. *Nature* **343**, 774–7.

Giannoukakis, N., Deal, C., Paquette, J., Goodyer, C. G. & Polychronakos, C. (1993). Parental genomic imprinting of the human *IGF2* gene. *Nature Genet.* **4**, 98–101.

Grundy, P. *et al.* (1991). Chromosome 11 uniparental isodisomy predisposing to embryonal neoplasms. *Lancet* **338**, 1079–80.

Grundy, P. *et al.* (1988). Familial predisposition to Wilms' tumour does not map to the short arm of chromosome 11. *Nature* **336**, 374–6.

Grundy, P., Wilson, B., Telzerow, P., Zhou, W. & Paterson, M. C. (1994). Uniparental disomy occurs infrequently in Wilms tumor patients. *Am. J. Hum. Genet.* **54**, 282–9.

Haas, O. A., Argyriou-Tirita, A. & Lion, T. (1992). Parental origin of chromosomes involved in the translocation t(9;22). *Nature* **359**, 414–16.

Han, V. K. M. *et al.* (1987). Identification of somatomedin/insulin-like growth factor immunoreactive cells in the human fetus. *Pediat. Res.* **22**, 245–9.

Hao, Y., Crenshaw, T., Moutlon, T., Newcomb, E. & Tycko, B. (1993). Tumour-suppressor activity of *H19* RNA. *Nature* **365**, 764–7.

Henry, I. *et al.* (1989). Molecular definition of the 11p15.5 region involved in Beckwith–Wiedemann syndrome and probably in predisposition to adrenocortical carcinoma. *Hum. Genet.* **81**, 273–7.

Henry, I., Bonaiti-Pellie, C., Chehensse, V., Beldjord, C., Schwartz, C., Utermann, G. & Junien, C. (1991). Uniparental paternal disomy in a genetic cancer-predisposing syndrome. *Nature* **351**, 665–7.

Henry, I., Puech, A., Riesewijk, A., Ahnine, L., Manners, M., Beldjord, C., Bitoun, P., Tournade, M., Landrieu, P. & Junien, C. (1993). Somatic mosaicism for partial paternal isodisomy in Wiedemann–Beckwith syndrome: a post-fertilisation event. *Eur. J. Hum. Genet.* **1**, 19–29.

Huff, V. *et al.* (1988). Lack of linkage of familial Wilms' tumour to chromosomal band 11p13. *Nature* **336**, 377–8.

Huff, V. *et al.* (1992). Nonlinkage of 16q markers to familial predisposition to Wilms tumor. *Cancer Res.* **52**, 6117–20.

Junien, C. & van Heyningen, V. (1991). Report of the committee on the genetic constitution of chromosome 11. *Cytogenet. Cell Genet.* **58**, 459–554.

Knudson, A. G. (1971). Mutation and cancer: statistical study of retinoblastoma. *Proc. Natn. Acad. Sci. U.S.A.* **68**, 820–3.

Knudson, A. G. & Strong, L. C. (1972). Mutation and cancer: a model for Wilms' tumor of the kidney. *J. Nat. Cancer Inst.* **48**, 313–24.

Koi, M., Johnson, L. A., Kalikin, L. M., Little, P. F. R., Nakamura, Y. & Feinberg, A. P. (1993). Tumor cell growth arrest caused by subchromosomal transferable DNA fragments from chromosome 11. *Science* **260**, 361–4.

Koufos, A., Grundy, P., Morgan, K., Aleck, K., Hadro, T., Lampkin, B., Kalbakji, A. & Cavenee, W. (1989). Familial Wiedemann–Beckwith syndrome and a second Wilms' tumor locus both map to 11p15.5. *Am. J. Hum. Genet.* **44**, 711–19.

Koufos, A. *et al.* (1984). Loss of alleles at loci on human chromosome 11 during genesis of Wilms' tumour. *Nature* **309**, 170–4.

Little, M., van Heyningen, V. & Hastie, N. (1991). Dads and disomy and disease. *Nature* **351**, 609–10.

Loh, W. E. *et al.* (1992). Human chromosome 11 contains two different growth suppressor genes for embryonal rhabdomyosarcoma. *Proc. Natn. Acad. Sci. U.S.A.* **89**, 1755–9.

Maw, M. A. *et al.* (1992). A third Wilms' tumor locus on chromosome 16q. *Cancer Res.* **52** 3094–8.

Ogawa, O., Becroft, D. M., Morrison, I. M., Eccles, M. R., Skeen, J. E., Mauger, D. C. & Reeve, A. E. (1993a). Constitutional relaxation of insulin-like growth factor 2 gene imprinting associated with Wilms tumour and gigantism. *Nature Genet.* **5**, 408–12.

Ogawa, O., Eccles, M. R., Szeto, J., McNoe, L. A., Yun, K., Maw, M. A., Smith, P. J. & Reeve, A. E. (1993b). Relaxation of insulin-like growth factor gene imprinting implicated in Wilms' tumour. *Nature* **362**, 749–51.

Ohlsson, R., Nyström, A., Pfeifer-Ohlsson, S., Töhönen, V., Hedborg, F., Schofield, P., Flam, F. & Ekström, T. J. (1993). *IGF2* is parentally imprinted during human embryogenesis and in the Beckwith–Wiedemann syndrome. *Nature Genet.* **4**, 94–7.

Orkin, S. T., Goldman, D. S. & Sallan, S. E. (1984). Development of homozygisty of chromosome 11p markers in Wilms tumor. *Nature* **309**, 172–4.

Pachnis, V., Brannan, C. I. & Tilghman, S. M. (1988). The structure and expression of a novel gene activated in early mouse embryogenesis. *EMBO J.* **7**, 673–81.

Ping, A. J., Reeve, A., Law, D., Young, M., Boehnke, M. & Feinberg, A. (1989). Genetic linkage of Beckwith–Wiedemann syndrome to 11p15. *Am. J. Hum. Genet.* **44**, 720–3.

Rainier, S., Johnson, L. A., Dobry, C. J., Ping, A. J., Grundy, P. E. & Feinberg, A. P. (1993). Relaxation of imprinted genes in human cancer. *Nature* **362**, 747–9.

Reeve, A. E. *et al.* (1985). Expression of insulin-like growth factor-II transcripts in Wilms' tumour. *Nature* **317**, 258–60.

Reeve, A. E. *et al.* (1984). Loss of a Harvey *ras* allele in sporadic Wilms' tumour. *Nature* **309**, 174–6.

Reik, W. & Surani, M. A. (1989). Genomic imprinting and embryonal tumours. *Nature* **338**, 112–13.

Schroeder, W. T., Chao, L.-Y., Dao, D. T., Strong, L. C., Pathak, S., Riccardi, V. M., Lewis, W. K. & Saunders, G. F. (1987). Nonrandom loss of maternal chromosome 11 alleles in Wilms tumors. *Am. J. Hum. Genet.* **40**, 413–20.

Scott, J., Cowell, J. & Robertson, M. E. (1985). Insulin-like growth factor-II gene expression in Wilms' tumour and embryonic tissues. *Nature* **317**, 261–2.

Scrable, H. *et al.* (1989). A model for embryonal rhabdomyosarcoma tumorigenesis that involves genome imprinting. *Proc. Natn. Acad. Sci. U.S.A.* **86**, 7480–4.

Solomon, E. (1984). Recessive mutation in aetiology of Wilms tumour. *Nature* **309**, 111–12.

Suzuki, H., Ueda, R., Takahashi, T. & Takahashi, T. (1994). Altered imprinting in lung cancer. *Nature Genet.* **6**(4), 332–3.

Tilghman, S. M. (1993). Parental imprinting in the mouse. *The Harvey Lectures,* Series **87**, pp. 69–84.

Turleau, C. & de Grouchy, J. (1985). Beckwith–Wiedemann syndrome – clinical comparison between patients with and without 11p15 trisomy. *Ann. Genet. 1985*, pp. 93–6.

Weissman, B. E. *et al.* (1987). Introduction of a normal human chromosome 11 into a Wilms' tumor cell line controls its tumorigenic expression. *Science* **236**, 175–236.

Weksberg, R., Shen, D. R., Fei, Y. L., Song, Q. L. & Squire, J. (1993). Disruption of insulin-like growth factor 2 imprinting in Beckwith–Wiedemann syndrome. *Nature Genet.* **5**, 143–9.

Wiedemann, H.-R. (1964). Complexe malformatif familial avec hernie ombilicale et macroglossie – un syndrome nouveau. *J. Genet. Hum.* **13**(2/3), 223–32.

Wilkins, R. J. (1988). Genomic imprinting and carcinogenesis. *Lancet* **i**, 329–31.

Yun, K. *et al.* (1993). Insulin-like growth factor II messenger ribonucleic acid expression in Wilms tumor, nephrogenic rest, and kidney. *Lab. Invest.* **69**(5), 603–15.

Zemel, S., Bartolomei, M. S. & Tilghman, S. M. (1992). Physical linkage of two mammalian imprinted genes, *H19* and insulin-like growth factor 2. *Nature Genet.* **2**, 61–5.

15

Tracking imprinting: the Beckwith–Wiedemann syndrome

MARCEL MANNENS

Introduction

The Beckwith–Wiedemann syndrome (BWS) was first described independently by Beckwith (1963) and Wiedemann (1964) and is therefore also cited as the Wiedemann–Beckwith syndrome, often depending on the nationality of those who refer to this syndrome. It occurs with an incidence of 1:13 700 births and is characterized by numerous growth abnormalities, especially the Exomphalos (umbilical hernia), Macroglossia (enlarged tongue) and Gigantism triad, explaining the EMG acronym used for this syndrome. These features are variably present and can be found in association with multiple abnormalities including neonatal hypoglycemia (low blood glucose levels), typical ear creases and pits, and a unilateral growth abnormality of parts of the body called hemihypertrophy.

There is a striking increase of 7.5% in the incidence of different types of tumors found in BWS patients, including the following childhood tumors: Wilms' tumor (59% of all tumors found in this disorder), adrenocortical carcinoma (15%), and a few instances of hepatoblastoma and rhabdomyosarcoma (Wiedemann, 1983).

The clinical findings in BWS tend to become less distinctive with age, and therefore the syndrome can be underdiagnosed in adults (Niikawa et al., 1986). In 30% of BWS patients, hypoglycemia has been diagnosed, which might be caused by the overproduction of insulin (INS) or insulin-like growth factor 2 (IGF2) genes (Engström et al., 1988). Children with BWS and children born to mothers with diabetes share certain clinical features (Gardner, 1973). Infants of diabetic mothers also develop high insulin levels to cope with their mother's high blood glucose levels, and sometimes have gigantism and craniofacial and cardiac defects, as do children with BWS. Low blood glucose levels have been described in non-BWS patients with mesenchymal tumors, including the BWS-associated tumors (reviewed by Macaulay, 1992). In this respect, the assignment of BWS to chromosome region 11p15 by linkage analysis, near the *INS* and immediately adjacent *IGF2* gene, is interesting (Ping *et al.*, 1989; Koufos *et al.*, 1989). Indeed, in some cases of BWS, overproduction of these genes has been noted (Mannens *et al.*, 1994 and references therein). Increased expression of *IGF2* has also been found in Wilms' tumors and many other tumors, including all those associated with BWS (Rechler & Nissley, 1990).

Chromosome 11, the imprinting chromosome

The localization of BWS to chromosome region 11p15 was hardly surprising, since BWS cases with chromosomal abnormalities involving this region had been described as early as 1983 (Mannens *et al.*, 1994 and references therein). In addition, genetic changes found in the BWS-associated childhood kidney tumor, Wilms' tumor, were found to be often limited to this same region (Mannens *et al.*, 1988). Other investigators showed that loss of heterozygosity limited to this same region could be found in all BWS-associated tumors, suggesting a common pathogenetic mechanism (Fig. 15.1). Surprisingly, we found that the lost allele in Wilms' tumor was always of maternal origin. Again, the same could be demonstrated for the other BWS-associated tumors. This phenomenon was first described by Schroeder *et al.* (1987), who suggested that increased mutation rates in male germ cells might explain their finding. The high numbers of maternal losses that we and others noticed made this explanation highly unlikely and enabled us to suggest a role for genomic imprinting in the etiology of Wilms' tumor.

Imprinting is a gamete-of-origin-dependent allele-inactivation process. An imprinted gene is therefore differentially expressed depending on whether this gene was inherited from father or mother. One of the two alleles of an imprinted gene is thus totally or partly 'silenced'. Genomic, or parental, imprinting was found to play a role in all BWS-associated tumors but also in other tumors, such as neuroblastoma, osteosarcoma, glomus tumors and leukemia (CML). The same holds for a number of genetic disorders such as the Prader–Willi/Angelman syndromes, atopy and, last but not least, the Beckwith–Wiedemann syndrome. Of these, the BWS-associated tumors, glomus tumors, atopy and BWS all map to chromosome 11. In addition, of the few cloned autosomal genes that are known to have monoallelic expression in humans or mice, four map to 11p (*WT1*, *INS*, *IGF2* and *H19*). One might therefore refer to this chromosome as the 'imprinting chromosome'.

For the Beckwith–Wiedemann syndrome, it became overwhelmingly clear that imprinting played a major role in this syndrome. Apart from the preferential maternal loss of alleles seen in BWS-associated tumors, the syndrome itself is often only transmitted through females. This parental bias in familial

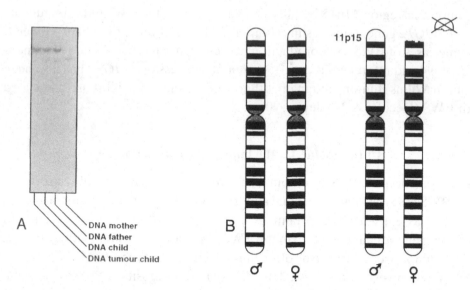

Fig. 15.1. Maternal LOH in BWS-associated tumors. (A) Example of loss of heterozygosity in a Wilms' tumor. A chromosome 11p15 marker with a 2-allelic restriction fragment length polymorphism (RFLP) has been used. The mother is homozygous for the smaller band. Father and child are heterozygous. In the tumor, the maternal allele is lost. (B) Comparison of the genetic situation in normal and tumor tissue. In normal tissue there is an equal contribution of the maternal and paternal chromosomes 11. In the tumor, there is no contribution of the maternal 11p15 region.

transmission points to imprinting. Of even more importance, however, is the fact that in all cases with chromosomal abnormalities, the origin of the abnormality is always paternal if the chromosomal abnormality is a duplication of 11p15, or maternal if the chromosomal abnormality is a balanced chromosomal rearrangement (Mannens *et al.*, 1994 and references therein) (Fig. 15.2). Apart from trisomy 11p or balanced chromosomal abnormalities involving 11p15, uniparental disomy of the region containing *IGF2* has been reported (Henry *et al.*, 1991, 1993). All the parental effects observed in the etiology of BWS and associated childhood tumors are apparently contradictory under a single-locus hypothesis. Therefore we proposed a model in which, apart from a growth-promoting gene such as *IGF2*, one or more suppressor genes are involved in the etiology of BWS and tumorigenesis (Fig. 15.3). The growth-promoting and growth-suppressing genes obviously have to show opposite parental imprinting to explain the parental effects discussed above. As will be outlined below, detailed analysis of BWS-associated chromosomal breakpoints suggest that multiple suppressor genes are involved.

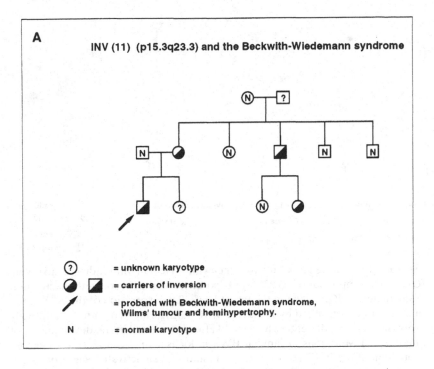

A   INV (11) (p15.3q23.3) and the Beckwith-Wiedemann syndrome

(?) = unknown karyotype

= carriers of inversion

= proband with Beckwith-Wiedemann syndrome, Wilms' tumour and hemihypertrophy.

N = normal karyotype

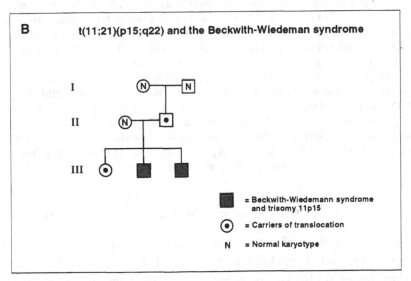

B   t(11;21)(p15;q22) and the Beckwith-Wiedeman syndrome

I

II

III

= Beckwith-Wiedemann syndrome and trisomy 11p15

= Carriers of translocation

N = Normal karyotype

Fig. 15.2. (A) Expression of the BWS phenotype, including hemihypertrophy and Wilms' tumor after maternal transmission of an INV(11) (p15.3q23.3). Note that carriers of the inversion are not affected after paternal transmission (Mannens *et al.*, 1994). (B) Expression of the BWS phenotype after paternal transmission of a t(11;21)(p15;q22) resulting in a trisomy 11p15. Note that paternal transmission of the balanced rearrangement (not leading to a trisomy 11p15) does not result in the BWS phenotype (pedigree courtesy Dr M. Nordenskjöld).

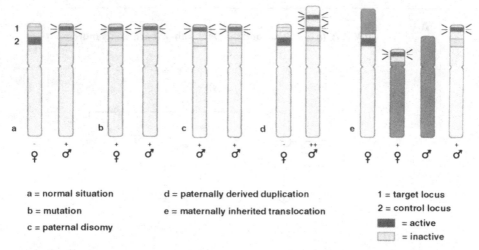

a = normal situation

b = mutation

c = paternal disomy

d = paternally derived duplication

e = maternally inherited translocation

1 = target locus

2 = control locus

■■■ = active

☐ = inactive

Fig. 15.3. Imprinting model for the Beckwith–Wiedemann syndrome involving *IGF2* and a suppressor of *IGF2*. (a) Proposed normal situation with inactivation of the maternal *IGF2* gene in the target locus. The expression of the *IGF2* gene (marked +) is controlled by locus 2 (BWSCR1/2), which contains a maternally expressed suppressor gene (which could also be involved in the development of tumors). (b) Mutations in familial BWS in locus 1 or 2 can lead to increased expression of the IGF2 gene. Maternal mutations can activate locus 1 or inactivate locus 2 or both (as shown). (c) Paternal disomy with two paternal and no maternal copies of locus 1 and 2 (as shown) or only two paternal copies of either locus. (d) Paternally derived duplication with two active copies of *IGF2*. (e) Maternally inherited translocations involving 11p15 and another chromosome, leading to loss of the existing maternal imprint and consequently two active *IGF2* alleles (as shown). The translocation chromosomes are shown to the left, the normal chromosomes to the right. The translocation breakpoint might also fall within locus 2 and thus disrupt the suppressor. A breakpoint proximal to locus 2 might also have an effect on the imprinting status of both loci. Maternal loss of the suppressor might lead to an increased tumor risk (alleles lost in tumors are always maternal); indeed, BWS patients with paternal disomy 11p15 have a much higher chance of developing a tumor.

Cloning of BWS-associated chromosomal breakpoints

Our cytogenetic analysis of the balanced chromosomal rearrangements found in BWS patients revealed breakpoints in the distal region of 11p15. Most of them seemed to cluster in 11p15.5; a few breakpoints were mapped more proximal at 11p15.3. In order to investigate these breakpoints in more detail at the molecular level, a physical map of this region had to be constructed. Using a combination of pulsed field gradient electrophoresis (PFGE) and fluorescent *in situ* hybridization (FISH) techniques, we were able to construct a contiguous map of 10 Mb. Several hundred markers were positioned on to this map and their position

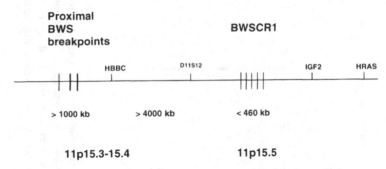

Fig. 15.4. Physical localization of the BWS-associated balanced chromosomal breakpoints. Chromosome bands, reference markers and physical distances (in kb) are given. Vertical lines indicate the location of the breakpoints. The two bold vertical lines represent the patients with hemihypertrophy.

relative to the BWS breakpoints was established (Mannens *et al.*, 1994; Redeker *et al.*, 1994, 1995). In this way we could position the breakpoints on the map and demonstrate clustering of these breakpoints in two distinct regions (Fig. 15.4).

Markers that were localized close to these breakpoints were then used to isolate yeast artificial chromosomes (YACs). These YACs were subcloned into cosmids. This strategy of chromosome walking and positional cloning enabled us to find cosmids that overlapped 7 out of 8 BWS breakpoints studied. Only for the most proximal breakpoint has no overlapping cosmid or YAC yet been found.

Five breakpoints clustered in band 11p15.5 near, but clearly distinct from, the imprinted genes *IGF2* and *H19* in a DNA fragment of less than 460 kb (Fig. 15.5). In this BWSCR1 cluster (Beckwith–Wiedemann syndrome chromosome region 1), all breakpoints were identified by overlapping cosmids.

Three additional breakpoints were mapped 4000 kb more proximal of BWSCR1. Two of these breakpoints (B05 and B14) could be mapped within the range of a single cosmid (Fig. 15.6). The third breakpoint, however, was found to be 2000 kb more proximal. This region was provisionally called BWSCR2, although the most proximal breakpoint might even suggest a third BWS locus.

Long-range position effect or gene disruption?

The finding that BWSCR1 was mapped less than 400 kb from the *INS*, *IGF2* and *H19* genes is highly suggestive of a long-range position effect. Indeed, altered expression of these genes has been found in BWS patients and associated tumors, as discussed before. In addition, loss of imprinting for these genes has been noted in BWS patients (Weksberg *et al.*, 1993) or associated tumors

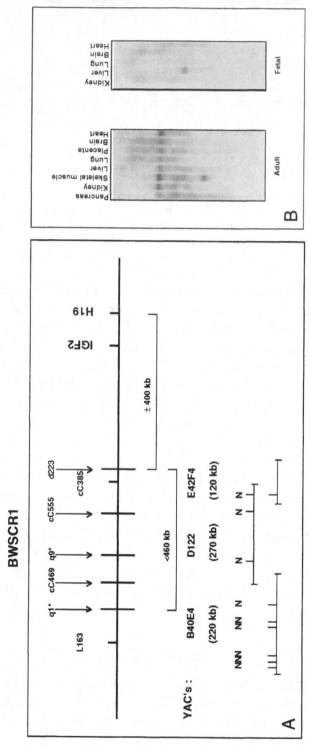

Fig. 15.5. (A) Schematic representation of BWSCR1. The DNA markers used are shown. The five BWS breakpoints are indicated with arrows and the cosmids overlapping the breakpoints are listed above. *Not*I sites within the YACs used are shown. Cosmids q1 and q9 were subcloned; CpG islands from these cosmids were evolutionarily conserved and used as probes on Northern blots. (B) Northern blot analysis of single copy probes from q1 and q9 (not shown). Both probes recognize a major 6.7 kb transcript in various adult tissues (especially skeletal muscle and heart) and less abundantly in fetal tissues.

BWSCR2

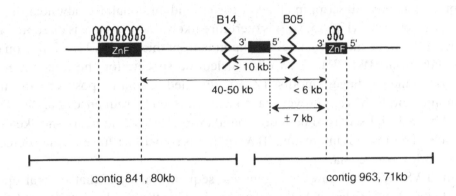

u280-u2001-ZnFP83-e4983-q29-q43-u3369-q27   u581-q25-q24-q26

Fig. 15.6. Schematic representation of the location of the hemihypertrophy and BWS-associated breakpoints (B05 and B14) within BWSCR2. B05 is also associated with the development of Wilms' tumor. Open reading frames (ORFs) are shown in gray boxes. The ZnF motifs are listed. Estimated distances and the order of cosmids within the cosmid contigs is given.

(Rainier *et al.*, 1993). Such relaxation of imprinting for *IGF2* and/or *H19*, however, was also found in non-BWS-associated tumors, such as lung cancer (Suzuki *et al.*, 1994) or testicular germ cell tumors (L. Looijenga, personal communication). Methylation is often used to monitor the imprinting status of a gene. In our experiments, hypomethylation of the *INS/IGF2* region was found in all EBV-transformed lymphoblastoid cell lines, in placenta and in Wilms' tumors. In addition, the same genes were hypomethylated in lymphocytes from a BWS patient described here, carrying the most proximal chromosome 11p15.3 breakpoint. Since this breakpoint is more than 4000 kb from the *INS/H19* genes, a 'very long range position effect' has to be assumed. Relaxation of the *IGF2/H19* imprint is obviously a very general phenomenon in cancer cells or in an overgrowth syndrome such as BWS.

Although we cannot rule out the possibility of such a long-range position effect, caused by balanced chromosomal translocation in 11p15, there is of course another obvious explanation. These breakpoints might identify genes that are involved in the etiology of BWS. At present, we believe that this is the case. Preliminary data from our laboratory suggest that, in both BWS regions, genes are present that are disrupted by multiple BWS breakpoints.

In BWSCR1 we cloned a number of CpG islands (CG-rich sequences, often involved in gene regulation). CpG islands cloned from cosmids q1 and q9 (Fig. 15.5, indicated with an asterisk) were found to be evolutionarily highly conserved (to yeast). Both probes identified the same 6.7 kb mRNA on Northern blots as a major transcript in all adult tissues and, although less abundantly, in fetal tissues tested (Fig. 15.5). It is therefore likely that this gene is disrupted by at least the three most proximal breakpoints from this cluster. Hybridization of cosmids from BWSCR1 to an oligonucleotide specific for the linker region of zinc-binding finger motifs (ZnF) revealed cosmids positive for the oligonucleotide. This, however, has to be confirmed by sequence analysis. The 6.7 kb transcript seems to be more abundantly expressed in heart and skeletal muscle. This result is interesting: BWS patients sometimes have cardiac defects or rhabdomyosarcoma.

In BWSCR2, we know from genomic sequence analysis that several open reading frames (ORFs) of 200–1000 bp are flanking the breakpoints of two BWS patients (Fig. 15.6). Two ORFs coded for 8 and 2 ZnF motifs, respectively. Although no expression was found on a multiple tissue Northern blot in both adult and fetal tissues, we were able to analyze a 600 bp mRNA fragment with RT–PCR using primers from the ORFs flanking the B05 breakpoint (Fig. 15.6). We therefore believe that the B05 breakpoint disrupts a gene that contains ZnF motifs.

Overgrowth syndromes and childhood tumor development: the same genetic background?

Because there are at least two chromosome 11p15 regions associated with BWS, one might ask whether there is genetic heterogeneity in this syndrome and whether both regions are associated with the same spectrum of clinical features. In our series of BWS patients there are some remarkable clinical findings. Two out of eight patients have only minor symptoms of BWS (patients B05 and B14) such as ear pits in patient B05 and increased birth weight and hypoglycemia in patient B14. Both patients, however, have a pronounced hemihypertrophy; patient B05 developed a Wilms' tumor. None of the other patients had hemihypertrophy or tumors. It is therefore highly suggestive that the ZnF gene in BWSCR2 is responsible for the hemihypertrophy and Wilms' tumor. Indeed, hemihypertrophy is frequently present in BWS patients with Wilms' tumor (40% in cases with Wilms' tumor compared with 12.5% in BWS patients without Wilms' tumor (Wiedemann, 1983)). This probably means that the ZnF gene plays an important role in early embryonic development and maybe in lateralization of the body. It also means that the gene is involved in malignant growth of kidney cells or, alternatively, in embryonic growth of kidney cells, since Wilms'

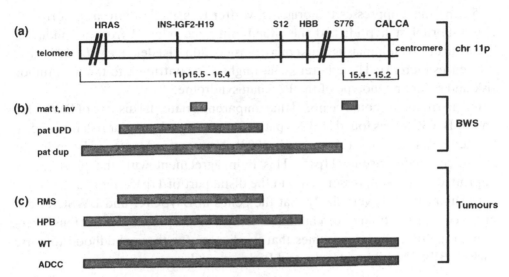

Fig. 15.7. Summary of the 11p15 regions involved in the etiology of BWS (maternal translocations or inversions; paternal uniparental disomy; paternal duplications) and associated childhood tumors (rhabdomyosarcoma; hepatoblastoma; Wilms' tumor; adrenocortical carcinoma). Reference markers are listed. Note that for Wilms' tumor, two chromosome regions were identified that coincide with BWSCR1 and BWSCR2 (adapted from Junien, 1992).

tumors are thought to develop from remnants of immature kidney tissue. In addition, genetic changes (loss of heterozygosity) limited to BWSCR2 have been described in Wilms' tumors (Fig. 15.7) (Junien, 1992). The increased birth weight, hypoglycemia and ear pits found in these patients, however, suggest some common genetic pathway in the etiology of BWS in patients with chromosomal abnormalities in BWSCR1 and BWSCR2. Both regions also seem to be associated with tumor development, as shown by LOH studies (Fig. 15.7). In addition, Newsham *et al.* (1994) placed a balanced translocation found in a rhabdoid tumor near or in BWSCR1.

There are other overgrowth malformation syndromes that have a highly increased risk of the development of Wilms' tumor. One of them is the Perlman syndrome (renal hamartomas, nephroblastomatosis and fetal gigantism) with a 100% chance of developing Wilms' tumor. Recently, a deletion of both BWSCR1 and BWSCR2 was found in 2 out of 2 Perlman patients studied (R. Grundy, personal communication). The concurrent loss of two tumor suppressor genes might explain the high Wilms' tumor risk. In addition, we mapped other candidate tumor suppressor genes to BWSCR2 that are not disrupted by the BWS breakpoints. These genes are: the *WEE1* gene, a human homolog of *Schizosaccharomyces pombe wee1* that functions as an inhibitor of mitosis: the

ST5 gene that suppresses tumorigenicity after transfection into a tumorigenic HeLa–fibroblast hybrid; and the rhombotin gene, cloned from a childhood T-cell acute lymphoblastic leukemia translocation (Redeker *et al.*, 1995 and references therein). These latter genes might also contribute to the high tumor risk and severe phenotype of the Perlman syndrome.

Furthermore, it should be noted that uniparental paternal disomy of BWSCR2 and/or BWSCR1, as found in BWS patients, increases the tumor risk from 7.5% to over 50% (Fig. 15.7) (Henry *et al.*, 1993). No increased tumor risk was found in patients with trisomy 11p15. This is in agreement with the presence of imprinted tumor suppressor genes in the distal part of 11p15 (Fig. 15.3).

In summary: it is very likely that the genes in BWSCR1 and BWSCR2 are involved in the etiology of childhood tumor development and various over-growth malformation syndromes that predispose for these childhood tumors, such as BWS, hemihypertrophy and Perlman syndrome.

Experiments to be done

Although we have identified two genes that are probably involved in the etiology of the above-mentioned disorders, many experiments have to be done to prove this assumption. Although these genes seem to be disrupted by BWS break-points and one of these breakpoints is associated with the development of a Wilms' tumor, the data collected so far are far from complete. First of all, we only have partial sequences of these genes. The complete sequence will enable us to look for point mutations in patients with BWS, hemihypertrophy and/or child-hood tumors. The existence of such point mutations will exclude the possibility of a long-range effect of the BWS breakpoints on other genes such as *IGF2* and *H19*. Furthermore, the gene's DNA sequence might partly reveal its function. As discussed, we already know that ZnF motifs are present. These ZnF motifs are found in the DNA binding proteins that are often associated with transcription regulation of genes. Such a gene function is, of course, compatible with a tumor suppressor function or, more generally, a growth-promoter function. On the other hand, DNA binding might have a more general effect associated with imprinting. One might postulate that such DNA binding proteins are modifier genes that are able to establish and maintain the imprint of a gene (possibly through methylation). The BWSCR1 and BWSCR2 genes might be involved in the loss of imprinting of *IGF2* and *H19*. Therefore, one experiment that should be done is of course to determine the DNA target of the ZnF genes. Mouse models might also be used to study the function of these ZnF proteins. The gene in BWSCR1 is highly conserved and a mouse homolog is likely to be found. This is not the case for the gene in BWSCR2. Monoallelic expression of these genes is to be expected, given the bias in parental transmission of the BWS phenotype. This, however, has to be proven, including possible aberrant imprinting in patients. Finally, tumor suppressor (or any other growth-promoting) activity has to be studied with transfection assays of these genes into tumorigenic cells. Given the broad spectrum of fascinating clinical features seen in the patients described above, we expect that the study of these genes will contribute significantly to our understanding of imprinting, tumor development and embryonic development or aberrant growth in general.

References

Beckwith, J. (1963). *Extreme cytomegaly of the adrenal fetal cortex, omphalocele hyperplasia of kidneys and pancreas, and Leydig-cell hyperplasia: Another syndrome?* Los Angeles: Western Society of Pediatric Research.

Engström, W., Lindham, S. & Schofield, P. (1988). Wiedemann–Beckwith syndrome. *Eur. J. Pediatr.* **147**, 450–7.

Gardner, L. (1973). Pseudo-Beckwith–Wiedemann syndrome: Interaction with maternal diabetes. *Lancet* ii, 911–12.

Henry, I., Bonaiti-Pellie, C., Chehensse, V., Beldjord, C., Schwartz, C., Utermann, G. & Junien, C. (1991). Uniparental paternal disomy in a genetic cancer predisposing syndrome. *Nature* **351**, 665–7.

Henry, I., Puech, A., Riesewijk, A., Ahnine, L., Mannens, M., Beldjord, C., Bitoun, P., Tournade, M., Landrieu, P. & Junien, C. (1993). Somatic mosaicism for partial paternal isodisomy in Wiedemann–Beckwith syndrome; a postfertilization event. *Eur. J. Hum. Genet.* **1**, 19–29.

Junien, C. (1992). Beckwith–Wiedemann syndrome, tumorigenesis and imprinting. *Curr. Opin. Genet. Devel.* **2**, 431–8.

Koufos, A., Grundy, P., Morgan, K., Aleck, K., Hadro, T., Lampkin, B., Kalbakji, A. & Cavenee, W. (1989). Familial Wiedemann–Beckwith syndrome and a second Wilms' tumor locus both map to 11p15.5. *Am. J. Hum. Genet.* **44**, 711–19.

Macaulay, V. (1992). Insulin-like growth factors and cancer. *Br. J. Cancer* **65**, 311–20.

Mannens, M., Hoovers, J., Redeker, E. *et al.* (1994). Parental imprinting of human chromosome region 11p15.3-pter involved in the Beckwith–Wiedemann syndrome and various human neoplasias. *Eur. J. Hum. Genet.* **2**, 3–23.

Mannens, M., Slater, R. M., Heyting, C., Bliek, J., de Kraker, J., Coad, N., de Pagter-Holthuizen, P. & Pearson, P. (1988). Molecular nature of genetic changes resulting in loss of heterozygosity of chromosome 11 in Wilms' tumours. *Hum. Genet.* **81**, 41–8.

Newsham, I., Daub, D., Besnard-Guerin, C. & Cavenee, W. (1994). Molecular sublocalization and characterization of the 11;22 translocation breakpoint in a malignant rhabdoid tumour. *Genomics* **19**, 433–40.

Niikawa, N., Ishikiriyama, S., Takahashi, S., Inagawa, A., Tonoki, H., Ohta, Y., Hase, N., Kamei, T. & Kajii, T. (1986). The Wiedemann–Beckwith syndrome: Pedigree studies on five families with evidence for autosomal dominant inheritance with variable expressivity. *Am. J. med. Genet.* **24**, 41–55.

Ping, A., Reeve, A., Law, D., Young, M., Boehnke, M. & Feinberg, A. (1989). Genetic linkage of Beckwith–Wiedemann syndrome to 11p15. *Am. J. Hum. Genet.* **44**, 720–3.

Rainier, S., Johnson, L. A., Dobry, C., Ping, A., Grundy, P. & Feinberg, A. (1993). Relaxation of imprinted genes in human cancer. *Nature* **362**, 747–9.

Rechler, M. & Nissley, S. (1990). Insulin-like growth factors. In *Handbook of Experimental Pharmacology*, vol. 95, pp. 263–367. Heidelberg: Springer-Verlag.

Redeker, E., Hoovers, J., Alders, M., van Moorsel, C., Ivens, A., Gregory, S., Kalikin, L., Bliek, J., de Galan, L., van den Bogaard, R., Visser, J., van der Voort, R., Feinberg, A., Little, P., Westerveld, A. & Mannens, M. (1994). An integrated physical map of 210 markers assigned to the short arm of human chromosome 11. *Genomics* **21**, 538–50.

Redeker, E., Alders, M., Hoovers, J., Richard, C. III, Westerveld, A. & Mannens, M. (1995). Physical mapping of 3 candidate tumour suppressor genes relatives to BWS associated chromosomal breakpoints at 11p15.3. *Cytogenet. Cell Genet.* **68**, 222–5.

Schroeder, W., Chao, L., Dao, D., Strong, L., Pathak, S., Riccardi, V., Lewis, W. & Saunders, G. (1987). Nonrandom loss of maternal chromosome 11 alleles in Wilms' tumours. *Am. J. Hum. Genet.* **40**, 413–20.

Suzuki, H., Ueda, R., Takahashi, T. & Takahashi, T. (1994). Altered imprinting in lung cancer. *Nature Genet.* **6**, 332–3.

Weksberg, R., Shen, D., Fei, Y., Song, Q. & Squire J. (1993). Disruption of insulin-like growth factor 2 imprinting in Beckwith–Wiedemann syndrome. *Nature Genet.* **5**, 143–50.

Wiedemann, H. (1964). Complexe malformatif familial avec hernie ombilicale et macroglossie – un syndrome nouveau? *J. Genet. Hum.* **13**, 223–32.

Wiedemann, H. (1983). Tumours and hemihypertrophy associated with Wiedemann–Beckwith syndrome. *Eur. J. Pediatr.* **141**, 129.

16

Genomic imprinting in Beckwith–Wiedemann syndrome

ROSANNA WEKSBERG AND JEREMY SQUIRE

Introduction

Beckwith–Wiedemann syndrome (BWS) is a human syndrome characterized by generalized and regional overgrowth and a predisposition to the development of specific embryonal tumors, most commonly Wilms' tumor (WT) (Pettenati *et al.*, 1986; Wiedemann, 1983). Although most cases of BWS are karyotypically normal and sporadic, there are patients with chromosome 11 duplications (Waziri *et al.*, 1983) or translocations (Pueschel & Padre-Mendoza, 1984), as well as families exhibiting autosomal dominant transmission with linkage to chromosome 11p15 (Ping *et al.*, 1989; Koufos *et al.*, 1989). Evidence that the gene(s) for BWS is likely to be imprinted comes from the finding of specific parent-of-origin effects for the karyotypic abnormalities seen in this condition (Mannens *et al.*, 1994; Weksberg *et al.*, 1993b) and from the increased maternal transmission pattern in autosomal dominant pedigrees. Moreover, patients with sporadic BWS have been found to exhibit paternal uniparental disomy (UPD), most commonly involving the genes for insulin and insulin-like growth factor 2 (*IGF2*) on 11p15.5 (Henry *et al.*, 1991). In addition, the clinical features of this syndrome, i.e. somatic overgrowth and tumor development, also suggest the involvement of a dysfunctional growth factor.

A number of hypotheses have been advanced to explain the etiology of BWS. The involvement of more than one locus is suggested by several independent observations. The 11p15.5 translocations associated with BWS map to two distinct translocation clusters, one proximal to β-hemoglobin and the second between *D11S12* and *IGF2* (Weksberg *et al.*, 1993b; Mannens *et al.*, 1994). Junien (1992) also proposed more than one locus based on the clinical features of BWS, autosomal dominant pedigrees and tumor development. Recently Cohen (1994) proposed the existence of two BWS loci based on the differences in clinical presentation in autosomal dominant versus sporadic cases. Ramesar *et* al. (1993) proposed a second locus on 11p15 to explain the preferential maternal transmission of BWS in autosomal dominant pedigrees (Moutou et al., 1992), which they designate 'paternal imprinting'. Furthermore, they suggest that this second locus on 11p15.5 could be *H19*, which is imprinted in the opposite direction to *IGF2*. Current linkage analysis would not distinguish between these two genes, because they are within 100 kb of each other (Zemel et al., 1992). In summary, models to explain BWS usually include more than one gene, imprinting, and aberrations of imprinted domains involving multiple genes, among them *H19* and *IGF2*. Such a model has been used to explain mutations leading to disease phenotypes in other imprinted regions, e.g. Prader–Willi syndrome (PWS) and Angelman syndrome (AS) on 15q11 (Nicholls, 1994; Francke et al., this volume).

Studies of the various BWS patient subgroups are likely to identify a variety of mutational events in one or more loci which can explain this condition and its associated tumors. Altered *IGF2* expression might account for a number of the genetically heterogeneous subgroups of BWS or at least partial BWS features in some of these groups. *IGF2* functions as a fetal growth factor (Humbel, 1990) and has been shown to be imprinted in both mice and humans; its expression in a variety of tissues is allele-specific and derived from the paternally inherited chromosome (DeChiara et al., 1991; Giannoukakis et al., 1993; Ohlsson et al., 1993). The 11p15 duplications associated with BWS almost always carry a paternally derived 11p15 segment. Since *IGF2* has, so far, been included in all of the duplicated segments, some of the BWS features may result from transcription of both of the paternally derived *IGF2* genes. In cases of BWS with uniparental disomy, all the disomic regions have been paternally derived; although most do not involve a whole chromosome 11, the disomic regions always include *IGF2*. Therefore, at least part of the BWS phenotype might be explained by the transcription of *IGF2* from both the paternally derived genes, and *IGF2* overexpression could occur in BWS patients with duplications or UPD of 11p15. This mechanism would also explain the preferential loss of maternal 11p15 alleles in WT, in that a transcriptionally inactive *IGF2* maternal allele could be replaced with a second transcriptionally active paternal allele by mechanisms such as somatic recombination.

Studies on a number of BWS patient subgroups are presented below to determine whether uniparental disomy involving *IGF2*, or aberrations in *IGF2* expression, might account for the phenotypic features of BWS. In addition, our experiments have been extended to include *H19*, a second imprinted gene on 11p15. Because *IGF2* and *H19* are linked and exhibit reciprocal expression (Ferguson-Smith et al., 1993), they are likely to constitute part of an imprinted domain, which might share some common regulatory elements.

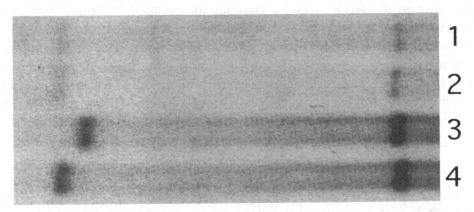

Fig. 16.1. Inheritance of insulin alleles in monozygotic twins discordant for BWS. Southern blot analysis of DNA from skin fibroblasts digested with *Pvu*II and probed with insulin 310. The affected twin is shown in lane 1, the unaffected twin in lane 2, father in lane 3, and mother in lane 4. The same contribution from each parent is seen for both the affected and the unaffected twins.

Studies on monozygotic twins discordant for BWS

A significant number of female monozygotic (MZ) twins discordant for BWS have been reported (Franceschini *et al.*, 1993; Olney *et al.*, 1988). Recently, we have identified one twin pair that is male and discordant for BWS. In addition, the affected twin of this pair developed a hepatoblastoma, the first reported case of a tumor in MZ twins with BWS.

Several explanations are possible for the apparent excess of MZ twins discordant for BWS, especially in females (only one female and one male pair are concordant). Because mosaicism for paternal UPD is seen in 20% of sporadic BWS, we examined the twin pairs for differences in paternal UPD that might have arisen after the twins had separated. Because MZ twin pairs can share their fetal circulation, we carried out the experiments on skin-derived fibroblasts from three MZ twin pairs (two female, one male) discordant for BWS. In all three cases, no evidence for UPD was found in either twin using probes for *INS* and *IGF2* (Fig. 16.1). In particular, on graded exposures of Southern blots, no evidence of differential intensity of bands was seen, suggesting equivalent contributions of 11p15 from the parents.

Alternative explanations for the discordance of the BWS phenotype in female MZ twins are possible. For example, a gene on the X chromosome might be involved in the imprinting of autosomal loci. In this way, different patterns of X inactivation may have a secondary effect on imprinting of loci on 11p (Lubinsky & Hall, 1991). Alternatively, the phenotypic differences among these twins may relate not to the BWS locus on 11p, but to a related syndrome on the X chromosome called Simpson–Golabi–Behmel syndrome (Simpson *et al.*, 1975; Behmel *et al.*, 1984; Golabi & Rosen, 1984; Hughes-Benzie *et al.*, 1992). Studies of X inactivation are therefore highly relevant to determine whether the twin pairs exhibit skewed patterns of X inactivation. Such skewed patterns have been documented for MZ twins who are discordant for X-linked disorders (Richards *et al.*, 1990).

Expression of *IGF2* in human control tissues and cell lines

To further evaluate the role of *IGF2* in BWS, we decided to study the expression of *IGF2* in various tissues and cell lines from normal individuals and from sporadic BWS patients with normal karyotypes and biparental chromosome 11 contributions. A reverse transcriptase polymerase chain reaction (RT–PCR) assay using an *Apa*I polymorphism in *IGF2* (Tadokoro *et al.*, 1991) was used to examine *IGF2* expression in five heterozygous control fibroblast cell strains, two placentas, and a control tongue. In all five strains where parental origin was informative, expression was from the paternally derived allele (Fig. 16.2). *IGF2* expression in control tongue tissue was largely, but not exclusively, from one allele. In summary, these data, taken together with other studies in humans and mice, suggest that transcriptional activity of the paternal *IGF2* allele represents the normal pattern of expression for most tissues (Giannoukakis *et al.*, 1993; Ohlsson *et al.*, 1993). In contrast to other normal cell types and tissues, biallelic expression of *IGF2* was observed for adult human liver by using the RT–PCR assay and the transcription assays discussed below.

Direct analysis of normal *IGF2* transcription

To validate the RT–PCR studies, primer extension analyses of the same region of *IGF2* were undertaken. An antisense oligonucleotide primer four base pairs 3' of the *Apa*I polymorphism was synthesized and used in extension analyses of RNA (Fig. 16.3). Primer extension analysis of control template RNA (Fig. 16.3, lanes 3, 4, and 13) and of total RNA obtained from snap-frozen heterozygous human tissue was performed. For two placentas, paternal-allele-specific expression of *IGF2* was detected, confirming earlier results of allele-specific expression in normal tissue determined by PCR-based assays. Surprisingly, RNA from all three normal livers exhibited biallelic expression of *IGF2* by primer extension analysis (Fig. 16.3, lanes 8, 9 and 10), indicating significant expression from both paternal and maternal alleles and relaxation of allele-specific *IGF2* expression in mature human liver (cf. Davies, 1994; Ekström *et al.*, 1995).

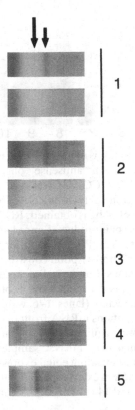

Fig. 16.2. Expression of *IGF2* in normal tissue. Expression of *IGF2* RNA by RT–PCR in three control fibroblast strains (panels 1–3) and two term placentas (panels 4 and 5), showing monoallelic expression. RNA was extracted and subjected to RT–PCR analysis as previously described (Wcksberg *et al.*, 1993a). Panels 1–4 only express allele 1; panel 5 expresses allele 2. Allele 1 and the larger fragment of allele 2 are identified by the shorter and longer arrows, respectively.

The observed constant ratio of the *IGF2* alleles seen in three independent live samples is consistent with uniform biallelic promoter 1 (P1) transcription. The maintenance of constant allelic proportions makes it less likely that biallelic *IGF2* transcription is a result of relaxed imprinting of one or more of the fetal P2–P4 promoters (Fig. 16.4), which have very low activity in adult liver. Hence, the biallelic *IGF2* expression that we have observed probably corresponds to transcription from the P1 promoter. Our data are consistent with promoter-specific imprinting of the *IGF2* gene as a mechanism for controlling developmental expression of *IGF2*.

Normal adult human liver expresses both paternal and maternal transcripts in approximately equal amounts demonstrating that, unlike most mature tissues, adult liver is not imprinted. This finding contrasts with observations in human

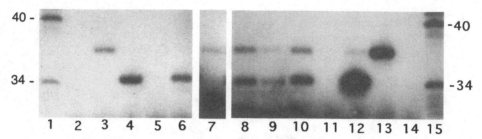

Fig. 16.3. Primer extension analysis of mRNA from liver and placental tissue and exon 9 antisense controls. An antisense oligonucleotide primer (TCT-TTAGTGTCCACCCGTGCAGCGAGCATG) 4 bp 3' of the *Apa*I polymorphism was used in the extension analyses of RNA. For detection of allele 1 RNA, a shorter extension product of 34 bp is obtained. RNA from allele 2 RNA extends further, resulting in a 37 base pair product. Lanes 1 and 15 are sequencing ladders used as molecular mass standards. Primer extension analysis of control template RNA generated from allele 2 transcription constructs is shown in lanes 3 and 13 and allele 1 constructs in lanes 4 and 12. For both placentas, paternal allele-specific expression of *IGF2* was detected. Lane 6 contains mRNA from placenta 2; only allele 1 can be detected (lanes 1–6 were developed after 24 hours autoradiography). Lane 7 contains mRNA from placenta 1; only allele 2 can be detected (a 5 day exposure was required for detection of extension products in this sample). In all three normal liver mRNA samples (lanes 8, 9 and 10) both extension products are seen, indicating equal expression from both paternal and maternal alleles. (Lanes 8–15 were developed after 48 hours exposure.) Lanes 2, 5, 11 and 14 contain tRNA controls.

and rodent fetal liver, where monoallelic *IGF2* expression is seen (DeChiara *et al.*, 1991; Rainier *et al.*, 1993; Sasaki *et al.*, 1992). Furthermore, transcriptional inactivity of the maternal *IGF2* allele is the normal pattern for most tissues in humans (Weksberg *et al.*, 1993a; Ogawa *et al.*, 1993; Rainier *et al.*, 1993; Giannoukakis *et al.*, 1993; Ohlsson *et al.*, 1993) and mice (DeChiara *et al.*, 1991; Sasaki *et al.*, 1992). Because *IGF2* is normally transcribed from distinct fetal and adult promoters in human liver (Van Dijk *et al.*, 1991; Schneid *et al.*, 1993), these observations not only indicate that *IGF2* imprinting is stage-specific, but further suggest that *IGF2* imprinting may be restricted to specific promoters.

Expression of *IGF2* in sporadic cases of BWS

We identified a group of karyotypically normal BWS patients who did not have any detectable UPD. Six of these patients were heterozygous for the *Apa*I polymorphism and had fibroblasts and/or tissue samples available for study. We then used RT–PCR to examine the expression of the fibroblast strains. Two of the six patients maintained monoallelic expression of *IGF2*. For the other four

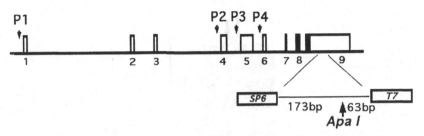

Fig. 16.4. Schematic diagram of *IGF2* gene based on published maps (de Pagter-Holthuizen *et al.*, 1985) to indicate the position of the four known *IGF2* promoters, the exon structure (boxes) and coding region (solid boxes). The non-coding part of exon 9 contains the *Apa*I RFLP used in these studies.

patients, however, biallelic expression of *IGF2* was evident in fibroblasts as well as in tongue tissue. The expression patterns are shown in Fig. 16.5.

Biallelic expression of *IGF2* in heterozygous individuals could be caused either by aberrant expression of the maternally inherited allele or by paternal heterodisomy. We excluded the possibility of paternal heterodisomy by studying a series of restriction fragment length polymorphisms (RFLPs) in the *IGF2* region (see example, Table 16.1). Using RFLPs for tyrosine hydroxylase, insulin, and *IGF2* genes, it was possible to demonstrate a maternal contribution of 11p15 in each case. Furthermore, mosaicism for paternal heterodisomy could be excluded in most cases, since a proportion of the fathers in these families were homozygous for the *Apa*I RFLP. These data strongly suggest that the one common defect in these patients is a disruption of the normal repression of the maternally derived *IGF2* allele.

IGF2 and *H19*: is reciprocal expression maintained in BWS?

We went on to enquire whether biallele *IGF2* expression occurs in BWS as an isolated imprinting defect in 11p15, e.g. as a result of mutation in *IGF2* or in a critical *cis*-acting regulator. Alternatively, biallelic expression of *IGF2* in these patients may be just one manifestation of a general disruption of an imprinted domain or region. To address the issue, we began a study of *H19* expression in BWS patients.

The *H19* gene encodes an RNA for which no protein product has been identified (Brannan *et al.*, 1990). Although the function of *H19* is unclear, a number of roles have been suggested including a tumor suppressor function (Hao *et al.*, 1993) and a regulatory function for the RNA itself, analogous to the *Xist* gene on the X chromosome (Bartolomei *et al.*, 1993; Brockdorff *et al.*, 1992; Tilghman *et al.*, this volume). That stringent regulation of *H19* is required is

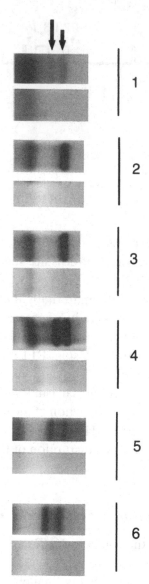

Fig. 16.5. Expression of *IGF2* (Weksberg *et al.*, 1993a) fibroblasts from six BWS patients. Panels 2 and 3 from two BWS patients show monoallelic expression of *IGF2* (allele 1). Panels 1 and 4–6 clearly show biallelic expression.

suggested by several observations: in particular, that transgenic embryos over-expressing *H19* die *in utero* (Brunkow & Tilghman, 1991). In addition, *H19* produces an abundant developmentally regulated transcript in a variety of fetal tissues, but in the adult its expression is confined to a small number of tissues, including skeletal and cardiac muscle (Zhang & Tycko, 1992).

Table 16.1. *Insulin, IGF2 and tyrosine hydroxylase RFLPs*

IGF2 *and* INS *RFLPs are two-allele systems whereas the tyrosine hydroxylase RFLP is a six-allele system (Weksberg* et al., *1993a). For each gene tested, this patient is informative and paternal heterodisomy can be excluded.*

	Tyrosine hydroxylase	Insulin	IGF2/ApaI
BWS patient	1,6	1,2	1,2
Father	5,6	1,1	2,2
Mother	1,2	1,2	1,1

Of special interest is the reciprocal expression pattern of *H19* and *IGF2* (Bartolomei *et al.*, 1993). In most tissues, monoallelic expression of *IGF2* arises almost exclusively from the paternal allele (Giannoukakis *et al.*, 1993; Ohlsson *et al.*, 1993; DeChiara *et al.*, 1991), whereas the opposite is true for *H19* (Zhang & Tycko, 1992). In human choroid plexus and leptomeninges, however, *IGF2* expression is biallelic whereas expression of *H19* is repressed (Ohlsson *et al.*, 1994). These observations have led to the idea that there may be coordinate regulation of these two loci; or that *H19* may actually regulate *IGF2* expression (Bartolomei *et al.*, 1993; Bird, 1993). Thus, if BWS involved aberrations of the whole imprinted domain, abnormalities in *H19* expression might be expected, at least for a subset of patients.

H19 expression in controls and sporadic BWS

In order to evaluate *H19* expression for individuals with BWS, we first tested human skin fibroblasts from controls to assess whether *H19* expression could be studied in these cells. Using an *Rsa*I polymorphism in *H19* (Zhang & Tycko, 1992), we found that of five human skin fibroblast strains tested, all of them expressed *H19*, and that this expression was monoallelic from the maternally derived allele (Fig. 16.6). We then went on to study *H19* expression in fibroblasts from BWS patients. In all six cases studied, *H19* expression was maintained, even in the one patient in whom biallelic *IGF2* expression was documented (Fig. 16.6). Further studies will be needed to support our preliminary data that the usual inverse relationship between *H19* and *IGF2* expression is not maintained in at least some BWS patients. This may mean that when biallelic *IGF2* expression occurs in BWS, there is escape from the normal coordinate regulation of *IGF2* and *H19*; for example, *IGF2* may become unresponsive to *H19* or other *cis*-

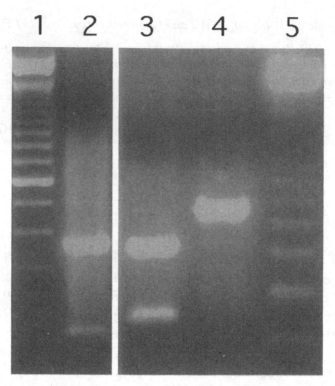

Fig. 16.6. Allele-specific expression of *H19* in controls and BWS patients. Expression of a transcribed *RsaI* polymorphism in *H19* was used to determine allele-specific expression by RT–PCR (Zhang & Tycko, 1992). Allele 1 lacks the *RsaI* site, whereas allele 2 carries the site and is cut. Lane 1 shows a 100 bp ladder and lane 5 a 123 bp ladder. Monoallelic expression of *H19* is shown in two fibroblast control strains (lanes 3 and 4) expressing alleles 2 and 1, respectively, and in one BWS fibroblast strain (lane 2) expressing allele 2.

acting elements. Of interest is the fact that for many WTs (Tycko, this volume) biallelic expression of *IGF2* is accompanied by a reduction in *H19* expression (Tycko, this volume). Although these data suggest that the altered expression profiles of *IGF2* and *H19* in BWS and WT may be etiologically different, a more detailed analysis of *H19* expression, especially for BWS, is needed.

Studies in BWS autosomal dominant pedigrees

The basis for BWS in autosomal dominant (AD) pedigrees remains unclear. The observation of increased transmission through female carriers was labeled paternal imprinting and led to the proposal of a second BWS locus (Ramesar *et al.*, 1993). This is based on the assumption that the BWS phenotype is caused by a loss-of-function mutation. This may be true, but an alternative and simpler model would account for the autosomal dominant pedigrees by using only one locus, e.g. *IGF2*, and a gain-of-function mutation. In this model, females in BWS pedigrees may carry a genetic alteration which does not allow normal suppression of their *IGF2* gene, i.e. a gain-of-function mutation. This mechanism does not involve paternal imprinting, but rather an abnormality in maternal imprinting. In fact, if one looks at the subgroup of BWS patients carrying cytogenetic translocations and inversions through 11p15, they present the same transmission patterns seen in most of the autosomal dominant pedigrees, i.e. the BWS phenotype is expressed only when the translocation or inversion is transmitted by the mother (Mannens *et al.*, 1994; Weksberg *et al.*, 1993b). Paternal transmission of the cytogenetic alteration is not associated with the BWS phenotype (Tommerup *et al.*, 1993). Thus, the translocations might disrupt normal repression of *IGF2* or other imprinted genes in the region. Supporting data for this view comes from the PWS/AS region, where genomic alterations generate *cis*-acting effects over 1 Mb (Horsthemke, this volume; Nicholls, 1994); there is at least one *cis*-acting regulatory element that acts over very long distances. In autosomal dominant pedigrees, however, a disruption of imprinted gene expression could occur via other more subtle DNA alterations, e.g. a critical methylation change or another *cis*-acting regulatory unit which has a more limited target in the imprinted domain.

We recently studied one placenta informative for both *H19* and *IGF2* from an autosomal dominant BWS pedigree. The BWS phenotype in this family has been shown to be linked to chromosome 11p15. In the informative placenta, both *H19* and *IGF2* expression were clearly monoallelic when studied by using standard PCR assays. Thus, a gross change in *IGF2* and *H19* allele-specific expression is not the basis of BWS in at least one autosomal dominant pedigree showing 11p15.5 linkage. This means that the biallelic expression of *IGF2* in sporadic cases is caused either by genetic heterogeneity or by aberrant regulation of an imprinted domain. That is, *IGF2* still remains a candidate gene for direct involvement in the etiology of BWS, analogous to the involvement of imprinted genes in the PWS/AS region where hierarchical regulatory mechanisms and chromosomal domain events can be invoked to explain the experimental findings. In fact, for the PWS/AS region, coordinate regulation of imprinted gene expression is probably driven by at least two *cis*-acting 'imprinting control elements' (Nicholls, 1994).

Models for BWS

Numerous models have already been proposed for BWS. It has become clear that a true understanding of this disease and its related tumors will depend on defining the critical imprinted domains on 11p15 and identifying the genes involved. In order to achieve this, a thorough investigation of the various patient subgroups is required with respect to expression of imprinted genes in the region, DNA methylation, replication timing, and *cis*-acting regulators. Furthermore, biological pathways encoded by genes on other chromosomes may be critical to the imprinting process on 11p15.5. Specifically, genes on the X chromosome may be involved in the phenotypic overlap between SGB, BWS and the excess of MZ female twins discordant for features of BWS.

A second issue in building models for diseases involving imprinted genes is our current terminology. There is mounting evidence that imprinting is not simply the transcriptional silencing of one paternal allele in gametogenesis. Rather, parental alleles are selectively marked during gametogenesis so that, after subsequent interactions with the cellular transcriptional machinery in early development, there is differential expression of the two parental alleles. These interactions, at critical periods in development or in specific tissues, might have differential expression via a number of mechanisms. Different cell types each producing specific regulatory molecules to recognize the imprint could lead to modulation of transcription, translation, message stability, etc. The ability of an individual cell to interpret imprints in particular genes is supported by a number of recent observations in mice and humans. For example, the insulin gene shows differential expression of maternal and paternal alleles limited to specific tissues and/or stages in development (Giddings *et al.*, 1994). For the *IGF2* gene, expression in cells from the choroid plexus and adult liver is typically biparental (DeChiara, *et al.*, 1991; Ohlsson *et al.*, 1994; Rainier *et al.*, 1993). The *H19* gene in humans appears susceptible to tissue-specific modulation in somatic development (Zhang *et al.*, 1993). Such observations on imprinting will necessitate a review of our current models for the imprinting process and a novel approach to our models for BWS.

References

Bartolomei, M. S., Webber, A. L., Brunkow, M. E. & Tilghman, S. M. (1993). Epigenetic mechanisms underlying the imprinting of the mouse *H19* gene. *Genes Devel.* **7**, 1663–73.

Behmel, A., Plöchl, E. & Rosenkranz, W. (1984). A new X-linked dysplasia gigantism syndrome: Identical with Simpson dysplasia syndrome? *Hum. Genet.* **67**, 409–13.

Bird, A. P. (1993). Imprints in islands. *Curr. Biol.* **3**, 275–7.

Brannan, C. I., Dees, E. C., Ingram, R. S. & Tilghman, S. M. (1990). The product of the *H19* gene may function as an RNA. *Molec. Cell Biol.* **10**, 28–36.

Brockdorff, N., Ashworth, A., Kay, G. F., McCabe, V. M., Norms, D. P., Cooper, P. J., Swift, S. & Rastan, S. (1992). The product of the mouse *Xist* gene is a 15 kb inactive Z-specific transcript containing no conserved ORF and located in the nucleus. *Cell* **71**, 515–26.

Brunkow, M. E. & Tilghman, S. M. (1991). Ectopic expression of the *H19* gene in mice causes parental lethality. *Genes Devel.* **5**, 1092–101.

Cohen, M. M. Jr. (1994). Beckwith–Wiedemann Syndrome. Imprinting, *IGF2* and *H19*: Implications for hemihyperplasia, associated neoplasms and overgrowth. *Am. J. med. Genet.* **52**, 233–4.

Davies, S. M. (1994). Developmental regulation of genomic imprinting of the *IGF2* gene in human liver. *Cancer Res.* **54**, 2560–2.

DeChiara, T. M., Robertson, E. J. & Efstratiadis, A. (1991). Parental imprinting of the mouse insulin-like growth factor II gene. *Cell* **64**, 849–59.

Ekström, T. Cui, H., Li, X. & Ohlsson, R. (1995). Promoter-specific *IGF2* imprinting status and its plasticity during human liver development. *Development* **121**, 309–16.

Ferguson-Smith, A. C., Sasaki, H., Cattanach, B. M. & Surani, M. A. (1993). Parental-origin-specific epigenetic modifications of the mouse *H19* gene. *Nature* **362**, 751–5.

Franceschini, P., Guala, A., Vardeu, M. P. & Franceschini, D. (1993). Monozygotic twinning and Wiedemann–Beckwith syndrome. *Am. J. med. Genet.* **46**, 353–4.

Giannoukakis, N., Deal, C., Paquette, J., Goodyer, C. & Polychronakos, C. (1993). Parental genomic imprinting of the human *IGF2* gene. *Nature Genet.* **4**, 98–101.

Giddings, S. J., King, C. D., Harman, I. W., Flood, J. F. & Carnaghi, L. R. (1994). Allele specific inactivation of insulin 1 and 2, in the mouse yolk sac, indicates imprinting. *Nature Genet.* **6**, 310–13.

Golabi, M. & Rosen, L. (1984). A new X-linked mental retardation-overgrowth syndrome. *Am. J. med. Genet.* **17**, 345–58.

Hao, Y., Crenshaw, T., Moulton, T., Newcomb, E. & Tycko, B. (1993). Tumour-suppressor activity of *H19* RNA. *Nature* **365**, 764–7.

Henry, I., Bonaiti-Pellié, C., Chehensee, V., Beldjord, C., Schwartz, C., Utermann, G. & Junien, C. (1991). Uniparental paternal disomy in a genetic cancer-predisposing syndrome. *Nature* **351**, 665–7.

Hughes-Benzie, R., Allanson, J., Hunter, A. & Cole, T. (1992). The importance of differentiating Simpson–Golabi–Behmel and Beckwith–Wiedemann syndromes. [Letter.] *J. med. Genet.* **29**, 928.

Humbel, R. (1990). Insulin-like growth factors I and II. *Eur. J. Biochem.* **190**, 445–62.

Junien, C. (1992). Beckwith–Wiedemann syndrome, tumorigenesis and imprinting. *Curr. Opin. Genet. Devel.* **2**, 431–8.

Koufos, A., Grundy, P., Morgan, K., Aleck, K. A., Hadro, T., Lampkin, B. C., Kalbakji, A. & Cavenee, W. K. (1989). Familial Wiedemann–Beckwith syndrome and a second Wilms tumor locus both map to 11p15.5. *Am. J. Hum. Genet.* **44**, 711–19.

Ledbetter, D. (1994). Presentation at FISH Conference, Lake Tahoe, California.

Lubinsky, M. S. & Hall, J. G. (1991). Genomic imprinting, monozygous twinning, and X inactivation. *Lancet* **337**, 1288.

Mannens, M., Hoovers, J. M. N., Redeker, E., Verjaal, M., Feinberg, A. P., Little, P., Boavida, M., Coad, N., Steenman, M., Bilek, J., Niikawa, N., Tonoki, H., Nakamura, Y., de Boer, E. G., Slater, R. M., John, R., Cowell, J. K., Junien, C., Henry, I., Tommerup, N., Weksberg, R., Peuschel, S. M., Leschot, N. J. & Westerveld, A. (1994). Parental imprinting of human chromosome region 11p15.3-pter involved in the Beckwith–Wiedemann syndrome and various human neoplasia. *Eur. J. Hum. Genet.* **2**, 3–23.

Moutou, C., Junien, C., Henry, I. & Bonaiti-Pellie, C. (1992). Beckwith–Wiedemann syndrome: A demonstration of the mechanisms responsible for the excess of transmitting females. *J. med. Genet.* **29**, 217–20.

Nicholls, R. D. (1994). New insights reveal complex mechanisms involved in genomic imprinting. *Am. J. Hum. Genet.* **54**, 733–40.

Ogawa, O., Eccles, M. R., Szeto, J., McNoe, L. A., Yun, K., Maw, M. A., Smith, P. J. & Reeve, A. E. (1993). Relaxation of insulin-like growth factor II gene imprinting implicated in Wilms tumor. *Nature* **362**, 749–51.

Ohlsson, R., Hedborg, F., Holmgren, L., Walsh, C. & Ekström, T. J. (1994). Overlapping patterns of *IGF2* and *H19* expression during human development: biallelic *IGF2* expression correlates with a lack of H19 expression. *Development* **120**, 361–8.

Ohlsson, R., Nyström, A., Pfeifer-Ohlsson, S., Töhönen, V., Hedborg, F., Schofield, P., Flam, F. & Ekström, T. J. (1993). *IGF2* is parentally imprinted during human embryogenesis and in the Beckwith–Wiedemann syndrome. *Nature Genet.* **4**, 94–7.

Olney, A. H., Buehler, B. A. & Waziri, M. (1988). Wiedemann–Beckwith syndrome in apparently discordant monozygotic twins. *Am. J. med. Genet.* **29**, 491–9.

de Pagter-Holthuizen, P., Hoppener, J. W., Jansen, M., Geurts van Kessel, A. H., van Ommen, G. J. & Sussenbach, J. S. (1985). Chromosomal localization and preliminary characterization of the human gene encoding insulin-like growth factor II. *Hum. Genet.* **69**, 170.

Pettenati, M. J., Haines, J. L., Higgins, R. R., Wappner, R. S., Palmer, C. G. & Weaver, D. D. (1986). Wiedemann–Beckwith syndrome: Presentation of clinical and cytogenetic data on 22 new cases and review of the literature. *Hum. Genet.* **74**, 143–54.

Ping, A. J., Reeve, A. E., Law, D. J., Young, M. R., Boehnke, M. & Feinberg, A. P. (1989). Genetic linkage of Beckwith–Wiedemann syndrome to 11p15. *Am. J. Hum. Genet.* **44**, 720–3.

Pueschel, S. M. & Padre-Mendoza, T. (1984). Chromosome 11 and Beckwith–Wiedemann syndrome. *J. Pediatr.* **104**, 484–5.

Rainier, S., Johnson, L. A., Dobry, C. J., Ping, A. J., Grundy, P. E. & Feinberg, A. P. (1993). Relaxation of imprinted genes in human cancer. *Nature* **362**, 747–9.

Ramesar, R., Babaya, M. & Viljoen, D. (1993). Molecular investigation of familial Beckwith–Wiedemann syndrome: A model for paternal imprinting. *Eur. J. Hum. Genet.* **1**, 109–13.

Richards, C. S., Watkins, S. C., Hoffman, E. P., Schneider, N. R., Milsark, I. W., Katz, K. S., Cook, J. D., Kunkel, L. M. & Cortada, J. M. (1990). Skewed X inactivation in a female MZ twin results in Duchenne muscular dystrophy. *Am. J. Hum. Genet.* **46**, 672–81.

Sasaki, H., Jones, P. A., Chaillet, J. R., Ferguson-Smith, A. C., Barton, S. C., Riek, W. & Surani, M. A. (1992). Parental imprinting: potentially active chromatin of the repressed maternal allele of the mouse insulin-like growth factor II (*Igf2*) gene. *Genes Devel.* **6**, 1843–56.

Schneid, H., Seurin, D., Vazquez, M.-P., Gourmelen, M., Cabrol, S. & Bouc, Y. L. (1993). Parental allele specific methylation of the human insulin-like growth factor II gene and Beckwith–Wiedemann syndrome. *J. Med. Genet.* **30**, 353–62.

Simpson, J. L., Landey, S., New, M. & German, J. (1975). A previously unrecognized X-linked syndrome of dysmorphia. In *Malformation Syndromes* (Birth Defects:

Original Article series XI(2)), ed. D. Bergsma, pp. 18–24. White Plains, New York: The National Foundation.

Tadokoro, K., Fujii, H., Inoue, T. & Yamada, M. (1991). Polymerase chain reaction (PCR) for detection of Apa1 polymorphism at the insulin-like growth factor II gene (*IGF2*). *Nucleic Acids Res.* **19**, 6967.

Tommerup, N., Brandt, C. A., Pedersen, S., Bolund, L. & Kamper, J. (1993). Sex dependent transmission of Beckwith—Wiedemann syndrome associated with a reciprocal translocation t(9;11)(p11.2; p15.5). *J. med. Genet.* **30**, 958–61.

Van Dijk, M. A., van Schaik, F. M. A., Bootsma, H. J., Holthuizen, P. & Sussenbach, J. S. (1991). Initial characterization of the four promoters of the human IGF-II gene. *Molec. Cell Endocrinol.* **81**, 81–94.

Waziri, M., Patil, S. R., Hanson, J. W. & Bartley, J. A. (1983). Abnormality of chromosome 11 in patients with features of Beckwith–Wiedemann syndrome. *J. Paediatr.* **102**, 873–6.

Weksberg, R., Shen, D. R., Fei, Y.-L., Song, Q. L. & Squire, J. (1993a). Disruption of insulin like growth factor 2 imprinting in Beckwith–Wiedemann syndrome. *Nature Genet.* **5**, 143–50.

Weksberg, R., Teshima, I., Williams, B. R. G., Greenberg, C. R., Peuschel, S. M., Chernos, J. E., Fowlow, S. B., Hoyme, E., Anderson, I. J., Whiteman, D. A. H., Fisher, N. & Squire, J. (1993b). Molecular characterization of cytogenetic alterations associated with the Beckwith–Wiedemann syndrome (BWS) phenotype refines the localization and suggests the gene for BWS is imprinted. *Hum. molec. Genet.* **2**, 549–56.

Wiedemann, H. R. (1983). Tumours and hemihypertrophy associated with Wiedemann–Beckwith syndrome. *Eur. J. Pediatr.* **141**, 129.

Zemel, S., Bartolomei, M. S. & Tilghman, S. M. (1992). Physical linkage of two mammalian imprinted genes, *H19* and insulin-like growth factor 2. *Nature Genet.* **2**, 61–5.

Zhang, Y., Shields, T., Crenshaw, T., Hao, Y., Moulton, T. & Tycko, B. (1993). Imprinting of human *H19*: Allele-specific CpG methylation, loss of the active allele in Wilms tumor, and potential for somatic allele switching. *Am. J. Hum. Genet.* **53**, 113–24.

Zhang, Y. & Tycko, B. (1992). Monoallelic expression of the human *H19* gene. *Nature Genet.* **1**, 40–4.

17

Mitotic crossing over and the disruption of genomic imprinting

GILBERT B. CÔTÉ

Abstract

Mitotic crossing over does occur in humans and is expected to cause a *cis–trans* disruption of differential parental imprinting and X inactivation. A model is presented, and ten predictions are made, often at odds with classical views, but supported by available data. The model is applied to Wilms' tumor as an example.

Introduction

Although the occurrence of mitotic crossing over is well documented in men and women, human geneticists have generally relegated it to the unimportant albeit entertaining category of historical curiosities. This state of affairs was based until recently on the superficial thought that mitotic crossing over cannot be of any great significance, because it only occurs in one out of several thousand cell divisions. More serious reasons were the absence of known mechanisms that could link it to relevant clinical conditions, and the naïve belief that if not present at birth, mosaicism can generally be ruled out for life. However, DNA analysis of the human genome has gradually unveiled the frequent occurrence of a mosaic loss of heterozygosity (LOH) in tumors and other conditions, and the importance and intricacies of the *cis* effects of imprints, promoters and enhancers on syntenic DNA sequences.

This new outlook must prompt us to re-examine the implications of the forgotten mitotic crossing over, the occurrence of which precisely leads to a *cis–trans* change of configuration every time it takes place, and to LOH in half of cases. Under this new light, its effects are bound to suddenly appear significant. And if one recalls that, unlike meiotic products, all daughter cells are kept together after mitosis, one quickly realizes that the apparently modest rate of occurrence of mitotic crossing over is not negligible at all in organisms that have billions upon billions of dividing cells.

Theoretical genetics

The precise mechanisms and timing of both imprinting and crossing over are presently unknown. We do not know which one precedes the other, or whether they can overlap. Both are likely to involve complex processes: imprinting certainly comprises more than sheer methylation, while the relationship of mitotic crossing over with DNA repair indicates that it must be more than just a useless random event. Mitotic crossing over – also called somatic crossing over – is often *assumed* to take place during mitosis but can theoretically occur anytime after DNA replication. Indeed, there is no known zygotene stage at mitosis for homologs to pair, while *trans*-sensing mechanisms and the FISH (fluorescence *in situ* hybridization) technique clearly show that homologs or parts thereof occasionally pair during interphase. Pairing may be limited to only some portions of homologous chromosomes; it may occur only when precipitating factors are at play; we may not know exactly how, when and why; but we do know that it *does* happen. In the text that follows, I have chosen to depict the completion of the imprinting process after that of crossing over because this order is simpler to draw and seems to offer more possibilities. However, the reverse may also be true; time and research will tell.

Figure 17.1 shows an anonymous pair of chromosomes within a cell. The stripes on the chromosomes correspond to the parental origin: horizontal for one parent, and oblique for the other. In order to keep the model general, we purposely do not specify which parent is which, with the understanding that imprinting may differ according to parental origin, tissue type, developmental stage and metabolic circumstances. Shading shows the completed imprint.

Interaction

When DNA duplication takes place, the newly synthesized DNA strands are not imprinted instantaneously, and a copying mechanism must reproduce the old imprint from the four parental (shaded) strands to the four newly synthesized (not shaded) ones. Whatever the exact mechanism, the copying process must be repeated on each chromosome separately, for differential imprinting to be maintained. Obviously, introducing crossing over at this stage, and shuffling the chromatids about, *must* disrupt the maintenance of differential imprinting, as special enzymes and other molecules busy themselves along each chromatid and keep on copying a particular parental imprint from strand to strand, only to

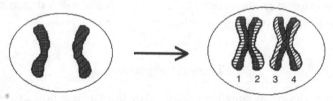

Fig. 17.1. Imprinting of a homologous pair of chromosomes. The horizontal and slanted stripes correspond to the parental origin. The original (shaded) imprint has to be reproduced onto the unshaded area after DNA replication. (The stripes, shading and numbering of chromatids from 1 to 4 also apply to Figs. 17.2, 17.3 and 17.4.)

suddenly find out that parts of some chromatids have been switched and the imprint from the other parent must now be copied! The disruption can be imagined to be akin to the variable and inappropriately maintained spreading of the X chromosome inactivation into an X-translocated autosome (Schanz & Steinbach, 1989). Clearly, the cellular consequences of a *cis–trans* exchange will be serious, and even disastrous on occasion, especially when the disruption occurs *within* an imprint.

Crossing over does not occur absolutely randomly at any chromosomal site but at preferred DNA sequences. If we consider an imprint as any series of contiguous genes, the expression of which depends on their parental origin, some imprints will involve very long DNA stretches and contain enough crossing-over-prone sequences to allow such internal disruption. Functional disruption in subsequent cell generations can then be expected whether crossing over occurs before or after the imprint is copied.

Uniparental partial isodisomy

The four different ways in which crossing over can involve two chromatids at a time are shown on the left of Fig. 17.2. The chromatids are numbered from 1 to 4 (as in Fig. 17.1) and the four types of exchange designated (1,3), (1,4), (2,3) and (2,4) according to the chromatids involved. After each exchange, random segregation of the four chromatids (two crossed and two uncrossed) offers two possibilities: (a) chromatids 1 + 3 can head towards one pole and chromatids 2 + 4 to the other, or (b) chromatids 1 + 4 to one pole and 2 + 3 to the other.

Whichever two chromatids are involved in crossing over, one of the two segregation patterns leads to uniparental partial isodisomy in the daughter cells, but the other does not. This partial isodisomy therefore happens half of the time, in two out of four possible daughter cells, and is detectable as LOH whenever constitutional heterozygosity existed in the parental cells.

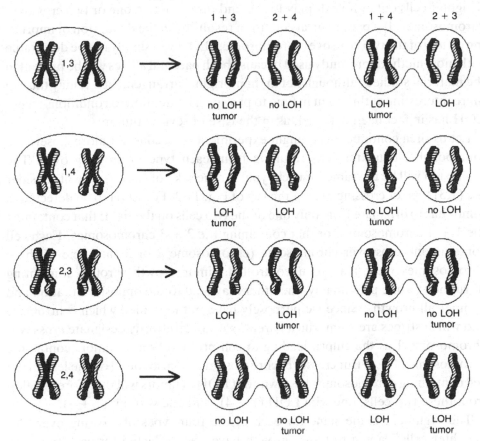

Fig. 17.2. Relationship between a single mitotic crossing over, imprinting and uniparental partial isodisomy. The chromatids are numbered as in Fig. 17.1, and the four types of exchanges designated (1,3), (1,4), (2,3) and (2,4) according to the chromatids involved. For each type, random segregation offers two possibilities, only one of which leads to partial isodisomy. See text for discussion.

Loss of heterozygosity

In the absence of imprinting, LOH alone can lead to the unexpected expression of recessive diseases or the reduced expressivity of dominant ones. Although LOH consequent to mitotic crossing over will only explain a very small minority of cases with truly Mendelian conditions, the outlook is very different for disorders of disputed etiology or irregular inheritance, because of the non-Mendelian interaction with imprinting, and a rate of occurrence compatible with that of such disorders. A crossing over etiology is especially compatible with reports of mosaic and partial isodisomy in individuals or their tumors.

Figure 17.2 shows that, after any of the four types of crossing over, two daughter cells out of four display LOH, and three contain one or two crossover chromosomes. If a pathological condition results from the disruption of imprinting on *any* of the two crossover chromosomes, LOH will simply not be detectable with most methods presently used because both parental alleles will be present in the material studied (although not in their original arrangement). It may thus be more interesting at this point in time to pay special attention to conditions where LOH has in fact been detected, as in the case of several tumors.

Let us then continue this thought experiment, and consider more closely the four possible daughter cells resulting from each type of crossing over. The discussion will be the same for each type; for the sake of clarity, we will consider the (1,3) type of crossing over at the top of Fig. 17.2. For LOH to be detected, a tumor has to originate from only one of the two cells on the right: that containing the 1 + 4 chromosomes, or that containing the 2 + 3 chromosomes. Each cell contains one crossover chromosome (chromosome 1 or 3) and one of these chromosomes must lead to uncontrolled tumor growth through imprinting disruption (while presumably, the other may lead to the opposite situation and hamper all growth). Since we purposely have not identified which centromere and which stripes are from which parent, we can arbitrarily designate crossover chromosome 1 as the culprit leading to cell proliferation in tumors containing chromosomes 1 + 4. But crossover chromosome 1 is also found on the left, in the cell containing chromosomes 1 + 3 without LOH. Tumors will therefore develop from these two cells, one with LOH (1 + 4), and one without (1 + 3).

The argument is the same for each of the four types of crossing over. All daughter cells leading to tumor growth have been selected for each type and redrawn in Fig. 17.3, where it is obvious that half of them display LOH.

Intrachromosomal switch over

If we abstract a bit further and isolate the culprit chromosomes in Fig. 17.4 (those found at the left of each cell in Fig. 17.3), we can see a further difference between them: all have a *cis–trans* exchange of parental imprinting pattern, but in half of them (those on the right, originating from crossing over types (1,4) and (2,3)) there is an additional interstrand switch within the chromosome. These are only possible if copying the imprinting pattern is completed after crossing over, and it is suggested that the disruption resulting from this further switch would be worse than it is without, and that the resulting tumors could then be differentiated not only by the presence or absence of LOH, but by an additional property also found in half of cases (half of those with LOH, and half of those without).

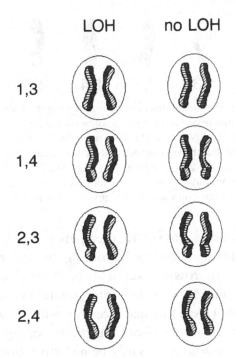

Fig. 17.3. Daughter cells from Fig. 17.2 leading to tumor growth. Half show LOH, half do not. In each cell, the chromosome on the left is the one causing the tumor.

Further complexity

Multiple crossing over between the same two chromatids will lead to interstitial LOH and leave intact the heterozygosity of more distal genes. Multiple exchanges involving three or four chromatids will result in more complex combinations, all showing LOH, but of different regions. However complex or simple the crossing over, all exchanges within an imprint will lead to a disruption of its original pattern.

Triggering factors

As a last theoretical reminder, it is worth noting that inherited chromosomal defects such as microdeletions and fragile sites are expected to sharply increase the probability of molecular attempts at DNA repair and thus be associated with mitotic crossing over. Such Mendelian defects, here called *A*, are thus expected to be associated with crossing over and the ensuing disruption of imprinting that will affect more distant regions, here called *Z*. Classical analyses based on strict Mendelian principles would definitely be mistaken in such situations, and would reach the strange conclusion that a particular gene *A* causes condition *Z* 'often

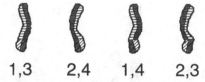

1,3   2,4   1,4   2,3

Fig. 17.4. The four chromosomes causing tumor growth, found on the left of all cells in Fig. 17.3, and originating from crossing over types (1,3), (1,4), (2,3) and (2,4) shown in Fig. 17.2. All four chromosomes display a *cis–trans* disruption of parental imprinting, but the two on the right have an additional interstrand switch of imprinting within the chromosome. It is suggested the consequences of this additional disruption may be worse than that experienced by the two chromosomes on the left. See text for discussion.

but not always' (the classical case of 'reduced penetrance'), whereas in fact gene A would cause condition A, and an imprinting disruption of region Z would cause condition Z (after crossing over at A, or B, or C, or at any intervening sequence between A and Z). Such a misinterpretation would be especially easy to believe if condition A were rare and recessive, while Z were a more common and serious disorder. A, B and C can thus be important (although optional) precipitating factors without necessarily being active elements in disorder Z. Similar arguments also apply to any triggering candidate (genetic or environmental) capable of increasing the probability of mitotic crossing over within a particular chromosomal region.

Assumptions and expectations

The paragraph above gives us a glimpse of the difficulties encountered in genetic analyses if assumptions are not clearly defined, and if mutually exclusive ones are not all considered. The wrong choice of assumptions can easily predetermine outcome and lure us into studies of doubtful value, false surprises or misleading conclusions. This is certainly not a new idea; after all, it explains why imprinting took so long to be discovered, despite what we now see as flagrant evidence in favor of its existence.

By definition, conditions where imprinting is involved will show a non-Mendelian mode of inheritance in at least some instances, and sometimes in all cases. Genetic analyses and linkage studies based on strict Mendelism and the underlying assumption that phenotype is determined once and for all by constitutional genotype are bound to lead to erroneous conclusions when applied to somatically disrupted imprinting. This is especially evident for meiotic linkage studies with phase (*cis–trans*) unknown, whether or not assisted by computer chips and impressive software.

In addition, *any* model involving the somatic disruption of differential parental imprinting will expect an organism to show local differences unheard of in strict Mendelism, at both the phenotypic and DNA levels. Under such models, bilateral tumors, discordant monozygotic (MZ) twins and the two sides of asymmetric individuals are *not* expected to have identical DNA and imprinting; it follows from this that the several studies assuming that DNA analyses of only *one* tumor, of *one* twin, or of *blood* are respectively sufficient and representative of both tumors, both twins and both sides, are unquestionably incomplete and exclude a proper explanation based on the disruption of imprinting before they even start.

The predictions based specifically on a mitotic crossing over etiology are at odds with classical views on mutation rates, penetrance, expressivity, asymmetry and twinning (Côté, 1989b; Côté & Gyftodimou, 1991) and incompatible with *strict* Mendelism. Fortunately, the assumptions adopted with a mitotic crossing over model are much less numerous and restrictive than those of strict Mendelism, and are specifically confined to a disruption of autosomal imprinting and X chromosome inactivation after a *cis–trans* change of configuration, with the occasional addition of a sex difference in the rate of mitotic crossing over (similar to that seen in its meiotic counterpart).

Predictions

Useful theoretical models must include specific predictions that can be compared with the data at hand; the better they fit, the more relative support they deserve. Model-specific predictions are especially useful since they lead to a scientific ordering of rival hypotheses.

In brief, one can list ten predictions of the mitotic crossing over model.

1. By definition, mosaicism will be frequent.
2. Uniparental *partial* isodisomy is expected, whether terminal or interstitial. On the contrary, uniparental heterodisomy is ruled out.
3. Because differential imprinting is involved, LOH should usually demonstrate retention of the same parental allele.
4. Affected tissues will show LOH in less than half of cases (less, because other causes are always possible). The proportion of cases due to mitotic crossing over will be at least twice the proportion of LOH (at least, because LOH detection is often an underestimate).
5. Frequent imprinting differences and LOH discrepancies are expected between the two sides of patients with asymmetric conditions, between bilateral tumors, and between discordant MZ twins. An association is expected between asymmetric disorders and MZ twinning.

6. MZ twin discordance is expected to be *high*. Concordance may be even less than the recurrence rate in non-twin sibs. For some diseases, discordance should be the rule.
7. LOH is expected more often in unilateral than in bilateral conditions.
8. DNA defects and imprinting anomalies will affect distant regions in *cis*. The DNA anomalies detected will not always correspond to the pathologically active or inactive regions causing the disorder under consideration.
9. Other characteristics may be expected to occur with a 0.5 probability in tissues with and without LOH.
10. Inherited disorders of DNA repair will show a higher incidence of diseases caused by the disruption of imprinting.

The implications of these predictions are certainly at odds with classical views, and even with some interpretations offered to explain imprinting problems.

Sorting out the differences is not an easy task, as one tries to brush off the old assumptions in the sudden blinding light brought about by the unexpected discovery of genomic imprinting. Finding and collecting appropriate new data is especially demanding, as much remains untouched, unreported, or not even discussed in several instances, because the old assumptions die hard.

Certainly, there will be many causes for imprinting anomalies, and several have already been found. Unbiased data are rare, but an attempt at applying the present model to a candidate disease may help uncover new paths to discovery.

Applied genetics

Wilms' tumor is of particular interest in this context, not only because imprinting is certainly involved in its pathogenesis, but because mitotic recombination has been specifically and repeatedly claimed *not* to play a major role in its etiology.

The largest and most detailed molecular study on Wilms' tumor is probably that of Coppes *et al.* (1992). In sharp contrast to articles speckled with 'data not shown' and 'unpublished observations', this international outstanding effort presents a meticulous two-page long table that enables one to make comparisons beyond what was covered in the article's too short discussion.

The authors' results and those they gathered from the literature show that 26 out of 60 investigated cases of Wilms' tumor displayed partial isodisomy of some genes on the short arm of chromosome 11 (11p), a percentage of 43.3%. According to our model, this means that at least $2 \times 43.3 = 86.6\%$ of all these cases underwent mitotic crossing over, an indication of the importance of this phenomenon in the development of this tumor. Heterodisomy was not encountered, and has more recently been excluded by Grundy *et al*. (1994), as expected.

In addition, 52 out of 53 tumors demonstrated preferential retention of the same parental allele (paternal in this case), as expected.

Approximately half of the tumors showed decreased WT1 and WIT1 mRNA levels (as defined and measured by Coppes *et al*., 1992). The tumors were also histopathologically classified as homotypic or heterotypic, and half were found to be heterotypic: 8/14 of those with 11p LOH, and 12/24 of those without. The correlation between histopathology and mRNA levels was strong but not absolute. Could any of these findings result from the intrachromosomal switch over described above? Whatever the reason, this 0.5 probability is unlikely to be due to chance!

Coppes *et al*. (1992) also found that 6/32 of the tumors had an additional LOH for genes on the long arm of chromosome 16 (16q): 3 of those with 11p LOH, and 3 of those without. This means that at least $2 \times (6/32) = 37.5\%$ have undergone an additional mitotic crossing over on 16q. This is between ⅓ and ½, too low to be a major cause of the disease, too high to be a rare inherited cause, but certainly high enough to be part of a cascade of chromosomal anomalies, as found in most cancers, once started. Because only two genes were tested for LOH on 16q, the result is certainly an underestimate. Again, the true incidence is probably very close to 50%, and certainly not due to chance.

Incidentally, under the assumptions of the crossing over model, there is as yet no convincing evidence for the existence of a third WT gene not linked to 11p.

Mutations of the WT1 zinc finger gene on 11p13 seem to impair binding to the consensus EGR-1 sequences of promoters of the insulin-like growth factor II (*Igf2*) gene on more distal 11p15, and thus suppress the transcriptional regulation of *Igf2* mRNA synthesis (Drummond *et al*., 1992; Yun *et al*., 1993). If all that DNA length on 11p is involved in renal biochemistry (and other things), it is not surprising that a *cis–trans* disruption of its imprinting pattern anywhere along it may end up in tumor induction: it does not really matter whether *H19*, *Igf2* and *Hras1* on 11p15 are all overproduced because of a specific DNA mutation in a regulatory gene, or through an impossibility for the normal paternal genes to proceed to inactivation; the result is chaotic all the same. Less than 13.4% of cases could then be due to the direct pathological effects of *de novo* and inherited mutations of structural genes, their suppressors, promoters, or enhancers, and more than 86.6% to the disruptive influence of crossing over, with or without mutations. It is therefore not surprising that LOH at 11p13 or 11p15 usually does not involve mutations of the WT1 gene (Cowell *et al*., 1993). Mutations of any innocent gene that simply happens to be linked to the critical region can lead to the same tumor association; such seems indeed to be the case for the aniridia gene of WAGR fame.

To continue with our list of fulfilled expectations, 11p LOH is less frequent in bilateral than in unilateral Wilms' tumors (Little *et al.*, 1992), and it has been found in one but not the other tumor of a bilateral case (Little *et al.*, 1992). Wilms' tumor is associated with the Beckwith–Wiedemann syndrome (BWS), itself characterized by a high rate of hemihypertrophy (asymmetry, as expected) and discordant female MZ twins (also as expected) (Côté, 1989a, b; Côté & Gyftodimou, 1991).

Finally, the discovery in a Wilms' tumor of telomeric fusions (Fett-Conte *et al.*, 1993), a rare abnormality found in patients with DNA repair defects and an increased propensity to cancer, is certainly not fortuitous. DNA repair syndromes all have a very increased rate of various cancers; Bloom syndrome in particular is very well known for its increased rate of symmetrical quadriradials, a sure demonstration of mitotic crossing over.

Conclusion

In conclusion, all predictions of the model are fulfilled in this supposedly difficult case. The model has the additional advantage of offering an explanation not only for the existence of LOH, but also for its particular frequency. It also advances a simpler, more normal alternative to the postzygotic mitotic non-disjunction suggested by Schinzel (1993) as a cause of mosaic uniparental disomy possibly leading to asymmetric growth, and seems to deserve its good share of relative support.

Caution is none the less indicated, as imprinting surprises are still looming on the horizon. The model is necessarily still incomplete and may very well be wrong, but it should at least prove useful by helping the reassessment of old and new assumptions mandated by the discovery of genomic imprinting. An additional and important point in its favor is that its consequences are far-ranging and seem to offer a solution to a wide variety of long-standing genetic problems, from mutation rates and penetrance to twinning and cancer, and their interaction with imprinting.

Acknowledgements

The expert bibliographic assistance of Mr D. Hawryliuk is gratefully acknowledged. The contribution of my better half, Alexandra, was also significant; this paper would not have been written, had we not crossed over.

References

Coppes, M. J., Bonetta, L., Huang, A., Hoban, P., Chilton-MacNeill, S., Campbell, C. E., Weksberg, R., Yeger, H., Reeve, A. E. & Williams, B. R. G. (1992). Loss of heterozygosity mapping in Wilms tumor indicates the involvement of three distinct regions and a limited role for nondisjunction or mitotic recombination. *Genes, Chromosomes Cancer* **5**, 326–34.

Côté, G. B. (1989a). Wilms tumour and related syndromes. A unifying theory. *Ann. Génét.* **32**, 69–72.

Côté, G. B. (1989b). The cis-trans effects of crossing-over on the penetrance and expressivity of dominantly inherited disorders. *Ann. Génét.* **32**, 132–5.

Côté, G. B. & Gyftodimou, J. (1991). Twinning and mitotic crossing-over: some possibilities and their implications. *Am. J. Hum. Genet.* **49**, 120–30.

Cowell, J. K., Groves, N. & Baird, P. (1993). Loss of heterozygosity at 11p13 in Wilms' tumours does not necessarily involve mutations in the WT1 gene. *Br. J. Cancer* **67**, 1259–61.

Drummond, I. A., Madden, S. L., Rohwer-Nutter, P., Bell, G. I., Sukhatme, V. P. & Rauscher, F. J. (1992). Repression of the insulin-like growth factor II gene by the Wilms tumor suppressor WT1. *Science* **257**, 674–8.

Fett-Conte, A. C., Liedtke, II., Chaves, H., Thomé, J. A. & Tajara, E. H. (1993). Telomeric fusions in a Wilms' tumor. *Cancer Genet. Cytogenet.* **69**, 141–5.

Grundy, P., Wilson, B., Telzerow, P., Zhou, W. & Paterson, M. C. (1994). Uniparental disomy occurs infrequently in Wilms tumor patients. *Am. J. Hum. Genet.* **54**, 282–9.

Little, M. H., Clarke, J., Byrne, J., Dunn, R. & Smith, P. J. (1992). Allelic loss on chromosome 11p is a less frequent event in bilateral than in unilateral Wilms' tumours. *Eur. J. Cancer* **28A**, 1876–80.

Schanz, S. & Steinbach, P. (1989). Investigation of the 'variable spreading' of X inactivation into a translocated autosome. *Hum. Genet.* **82**, 244–8.

Schinzel, A. (1993). Genomic imprinting: consequences of uniparental disomy for human disease. *Am. J. med. Genet.* **46**, 683–4.

Yun, K., Fidler, A. E., Eccles, M. R. & Reeve, A. E. (1993). Insulin-like growth factor II and WT1 transcript localization in human fetal kidney and Wilms' tumor. *Cancer Res.* **53**, 5166–71.

18

Evaluating H19 *as an imprinted tumor suppressor gene*

BENJAMIN TYCKO

Abstract

According to a simple model, the selective loss of maternal chromosome 11p15.5 alleles in Wilms' tumors (WTs) predicts the existence of a paternally imprinted 11p15.5 tumor suppressor gene. Human *H19* maps to chromosome 11p15.5 and is paternally imprinted. *H19* RNA can exert growth-inhibitory and/or tumor suppressor activity in certain tumor cell lines; 'one-hit' inactivation of *H19* expression, either through deletion of the active maternal allele or through an epigenetic pathway resulting in hypermethylation of this allele, occurs in a majority of primary WTs. In addition, *H19* DNA is biallelically hypermethylated in the non-neoplastic kidney parenchyma of some WT patients. Although they do not constitute proof, these observations are consistent with a role for *H19* as a tumor suppressor gene in WTs. The epigenetic lesions at the *H19* locus in WT patients could also be a component of a more global switch to a paternal epigenotype. Long-range mapping of alterations in functional imprinting and DNA methylation on chromosome 11p15.5 in non-neoplastic and tumor tissues of these patients may be useful for further testing these possibilities.

Introduction

As an evolutionarily conserved genetic phenomenon, parental imprinting is likely to confer some selective advantage to the species, but it is also interesting to consider whether aberrations in this form of gene regulation could have adverse consequences for rare individuals in the population. We have been interested in the possibility that there might exist imprinted genes with tumor suppressor activity which, because of their monoallelic expression and consequent susceptibility to 'one-hit' functional inactivation, could represent weak links in the chain of genetic safeguards against tumorigenesis (Tycko, 1994). To begin to examine this experimentally we have focused on the human *H19* gene. This gene produces a spliced and polyadenylated RNA which is highly expressed in a variety of murine and human fetal tissues, including differentiating blastemal cells of the fetal kidney, the precursor cells of WTs (Pachnis *et al.*, 1988; Wiles, 1988; Davis *et al.*, 1987; Poirier *et al.*, 1992; Rachmilewitz *et al.*, 1992a; Han & Liau, 1992; Goshen *et al.*, 1993; Ohlsson *et al.*, 1994). Expression is markedly down-regulated in most adult tissues, but remains detectable in several adult human organs, including the kidney (Hao *et al.*, 1993; Moulton *et al.*, 1994). As reviewed by Tilghman *et al.* (this volume) the *H19* gene is unusual in that, although its transcription is highly regulated and *H19* RNA levels (molecules per cell) can equal or exceed those of β-actin RNA in expressing tissues, the RNA appears to lack long or evolutionarily conserved protein-coding reading frames (Brannan *et al.*, 1990).

H19 was among the first defined genes shown to be subject to imprinting: RNase protection experiments using tissues from interspecific mouse hybrids demonstrated selective expression of the maternal allele (Bartolomei *et al.*, 1991) and reverse PCR with analysis of exonic restriction fragment polymorphisms showed that *H19* was expressed monoallelically in human fetal and adult organs (Zhang & Tycko, 1992). In both species, the active allele is maternal (Rachmilewitz *et al.*, 1992b; Rainier *et al.*, 1993; Zhang *et al.*, 1993; Moulton *et al.*, 1994). Significantly for the discussion that follows, it was also found that the inactive paternal *H19* allele in both mice and humans was fully methylated at numerous cytosines within CpG dinucleotides in the body of the gene and in the promoter region, with the active maternal allele unmethylated at all or most of these sites (Zhang *et al.*, 1993; Bartolomei *et al.*, 1993; Ferguson-Smith *et al.*, 1993). This situation is consistent with the possibility that allele-specific DNA methylation may play a role in establishing and/or maintaining monoallelic expression at this locus. Also consistent with this, *in vitro* methylation of the *H19* mimimal promoter region renders it inactive (Zhang *et al.*, 1993) and demethylation of the silent *H19* allele by treatment of cells in culture with 5-azacytidine leads to its transcriptional activation (T. Moulton & B.T., unpublished observations). Further, deletion of a DNA methyltransferase gene in the germline of mice resulted in relaxation of *H19* imprinting (Li *et al.*, 1993).

Human *H19* maps to chromosome 11p15.5 (Glaser *et al.*, 1989; Richard *et al.*, 1993), a region that is subject to loss of heterozygosity (LOH), presumably *via* mitotic recombination, in about 45% of WTs, with a striking and nearly complete bias towards the loss of maternal alleles (Schroeder *et al.*, 1987; Williams *et al.*, 1989; Pal *et al.*, 1990; Mannens *et al.*, 1990). It would be predicted that the transcriptionally active (maternal) *H19* allele would be deleted from these tumors; this prediction is born out of direct analysis (Zhang *et al.*, 1993;

Moulton *et al.*, 1994). Also, although rare cases may show relaxation of *H19* imprinting when examined by a PCR assay (Rainier *et al.*, 1993), in general the silence of the paternal *H19* allele is maintained in WTs that have lost the maternal allele, and these tumors are therefore null for *H19* expression (Moulton *et al.*, 1994).

The first suggestion of functional activity of *H19* RNA came from experiments in which the inappropriate expression of an *H19* transgene in mice caused fetal mortality (Brunkow & Tilghman, 1991). Motivated by this observation and by the provocative concordance of chromosomal localization and direction of parental imprinting of *H19* with the putative 11p15.5 WT suppressor gene, we decided to test whether *H19* RNA could affect the phenotype of human tumor cells in culture. The introduction of a human *H19* expression construct into two human embryonal tumor lines had growth-inhibitory (RD cells) or anti-clonogenic and anti-tumorigenic effects (G401 cells) (Hao *et al.*, 1993). How this effect is exerted biochemically remains to be determined, but if *H19* in fact functions directly at the level of its RNA then the mechanism is likely to be novel.

Although the transfection experiments indicated the ability of *H19* RNA to suppress certain parameters of cellular transformation when the RNA was introduced into a previously non-expressing tumor cell background, a proof that *H19* functions as a *bona fide* tumor suppressor gene in the natural evolution of WTs or other human tumors will require data from analysis of the primary tumors. In particular, if *H19* is in fact a WT suppressor gene, then it would be predicted to be inactivated not only in those WTs that show gross 11p15.5 LOH (and which have therefore lost maternal alleles of a large number of 11p15.5 genes in addition to *H19*) but also in at least some of the tumors that retain 11p15.5 heterozygosity. We have tested this by analyzing *H19* expression and CpG methylation in a series of primary WTs and correlating these data with 11p15.5 allelic status (Moulton *et al.*, 1994). In our series of 25 WTs, Northern analysis showed very low (at least 20-fold reduced from the levels in fetal kidneys by densitometry) or undetectable *H19* RNA in 18 cases (72%). Of the remaining cases, three showed detectable *H19* expression at a level about 10-fold reduced from fetal kidney and four showed expression at a level comparable to that of fetal kidney. The cases that showed low but detectable expression may reflect low expression in the neoplastic cells or, alternatively, contributions from non-neoplastic cells, such as newly formed vascular elements, which are known to express *H19* (Han & Liau, 1992). The presence or absence of *H19* RNA in the tumors did not correlate with any obvious differences in the proportion of blastemal, epithelial and stromal components, suggesting that the loss of *H19* expression could not be trivially explained as a function of cellular differentiation phenotype.

To assess the presence or absence of 11p15.5 LOH, we typed each WT for a series of DNA polymorphisms at *TH/IGF2*, *H19* and *HRAS* loci. Consistent with a generally stable paternal *H19* imprint, most of the tumors that showed gross 11p15.5 LOH did not express *H19* RNA and the two tumors that showed LOH but did express *H19* RNA were not entirely devoid of the active *H19* allele, since they showed only partial loss of one allelic band for each marker examined (these cases might therefore be examples of progressive loss of *H19* expression during tumor progression). Of more importance for testing the tumor suppressor hypothesis were the findings in the tumors that retained 11p15.5 heterozygosity. Among these cases, only 4/16 showed *H19* expression at a level comparable to that of fetal kidney; two showed trace expression and ten cases (63%) showed very low or undetectable expression. Among the four cases that were scored as retaining 11p15.5 alleles and which expressed significant amounts of *H19*, one showed a small but reproducible reduction in one allelic band on Southern analysis of the *H19* RsaI polymorphism, suggesting that this tumor contained a subclone of cells which had lost the active allele.

These data suggested that abrogation of *H19* expression in WTs could occur either by gross loss of 11p15.5 heterozygosity or, in the cases that retained heterozygosity, by an alternative mechanism, possibly epigenetic. Because CpG methylation of *H19* DNA shows a perfect correlation with inactivation of expression at the imprinted allele in normal tissues, one possibility was that the maternal *H19* allele in the non-expressing retention cases had become hyper-methylated and thereby inactivated. When we tested this by using a simple Southern blotting method, which we had previously applied in an extensive analysis of *H19* allelic methylation patterns in normal human fetal and adult tissues (Zhang *et al.*, 1993), we found that all but one of the non-expressing WTs showed either complete or partial biallelic hypermethylation of *H19* DNA (Moulton *et al.*, 1994). Figure 18.1 summarizes our observations on the fate of the *H19* gene in WTs: about 25% of cases continue to express the gene at levels comparable to those in fetal kidney, about 45% of cases lose expression via the 'genetic pathway', i.e. mitotic recombination, and the remaining 30% of cases lose expression via the 'epigenetic pathway'. In a separate study Feinberg and co-workers have made similar findings (Steenman *et al.*, 1994).

In the course of our analysis we also found that the non-neoplastic kidney parenchyma from two patients whose WTs had retained 11p15.5 alleles (as indicated by *TH/IGF2* and *HRAS* heterozygosity), but which did not express *H19*, showed biallelic hypermethylation throughout the *H19* gene, an abnormality not seen in any of six fetal, six juvenile and fifteen adult control kidneys. The abnormal methylation was widespread within the kidney (found in two separate samples of non-neoplastic renal cortex in the one case in which multiple samples were available) and, based on densitometry of the Southern blot

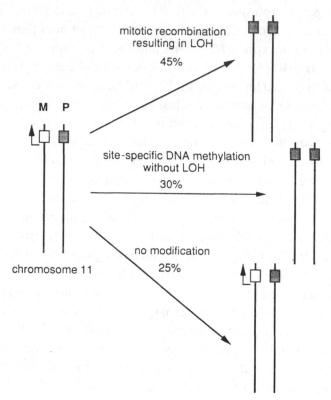

Fig. 18.1. Pathways for inactivation of the *H19* gene in Wilms' tumors.

autoradiograms, affected at least 80% of the non-neoplastic kidney cells in both cases. As would be predicted from the correlation of hypermethylation with transcriptional silencing, when compared with an age-matched control kidney, both WT kidneys showed a significant reduction in *H19* RNA. The finding that the large majority of cells in the non-neoplastic kidney parenchyma contained abnormally methylated *H19* DNA suggested that these WT patients had undergone a specific epigenetic alteration at the *H19* locus early in their somatic development.

We next asked whether the *H19* hypermethylation in these two cases reflected a local or a regional abnormality at the level of the chromosomal DNA. To map the region of abnormal methylation along the DNA we hybridized Southern blots containing the WT and non-neoplastic kidney DNAs with a series of probes from a cosmid and phage contig spanning a 100 kb region centered around the 3.5 kb *H19* gene. In contrast to the results obtained with probes within the body of the gene and its promoter, band patterns with each of four probes for 5′ or 3′ flanking DNA gave no indication of abnormal CpG methylation in the non-neoplastic kidney cells. Thus, within the limits of this initial intermediate-range mapping, the region of abnormal methylation in the two cases appeared to be confined to the *H19* gene.

It is interesting to ask how this biallelic *H19* hypermethylation might have come about. Although alterations of DNA methylation are well recognized in cancer cells, the abnormal hypermethylation in the non-neoplastic kidney cells in our two cases seems much less likely to reflect a global derangement in DNA methylation. Although we cannot yet answer this mechanistic question, we have noticed a large excess of *H19* homozygotes among the WT patients who grossly retain 11p15.5 heterozygosity and whose tumors do not express *H19*. The excess homozygosity among this subgroup of WT patients was statistically significant when compared with three different control cohorts of individuals with non-neoplastic diseases (random autopsies) or unrelated malignant tumors (Moulton *et al.*, 1994). We can therefore speculate that *H19* homozygosity might weakly but significantly predispose to transfer of the paternal 'methylation imprint' to the maternal allele, perhaps via a transvection or *trans*-sensing mechanism (Tartof & Henikoff, 1991; Fidler *et al.*, 1992).

Alternative mechanisms that could account for the observed biallelic hyper-methylation would be stochastic aberrations in the regulation of methylation in early development not dependent on allelic cross-talk or a genetic rather than epigenetic pathway, i.e. localized 11p15.5 mitotic recombination with crossover points closely flanking *H19*, resulting in physical replacement of the maternal *H19* allele by the inactive paternal allele. A different and very interesting possibility has been suggested, predicated on regional disruption of imprinting by mitotic recombination followed by segregation of sister chromatids, in which a single recombination crossover event could underlie the observed altered *H19* methylation state even in WT patients whose tumors retain 11p15.5 hetero-zygosity (Côté, this volume). According to this model, the 'epigenetic pathway' for *H19* inactivation in WT patients would not differ fundamentally from the 'genetic pathway'. Significantly, this model also predicts a regional switch in 'epigenotype' at multiple 11p15.5 loci in the critical category of patients with retention of heterozygosity and inactivation of *H19* (see below).

The *IGF2* gene, located within 200 kb of *H19*, has been proposed as a candidate dominant growth-promoting gene in the pathogenesis of Beckwith–Wiedemann syndrome (BWS) and WT (Giannoukakis *et al.*, 1993; Ogawa *et al.*, 1993; Ohlsson *et al.*, 1993; Rainier *et al.*, 1993; Weksberg *et al.*, 1993). As reviewed by Weksberg & Squire (this volume) and Tilghman *et al.* (this volume) there may be competition between the *IGF2* and *H19* promoters for the *H19* enhancer and this may underlie the opposite imprinting of these two loci (Bartolomei *et al.*, 1993). Results of allelic expression analysis and Northern blotting in our series of WTs have been consistent with this: WTs that show biallelic *H19* hypermethylation also show biallelic *IGF2* mRNA expression, a finding that has been documented more extensively by Feinberg and co-workers (Steenman *et al.*, 1994). However, because these data are correlative, a proof of enhancer competition will have to come from studies in transgenic and deletion mice (Bartolomei *et al.*, 1993).

The finding of *H19* inactivation in a majority of WTs and the correlation of *H19* silencing with biallelic expression of *IGF2* is consistent with a model in which both genes might contribute to Wilms' tumorigenesis, as a tumor suppressor and tumor promoter, respectively. However, some significant problems need to be worked out concerning both genes. In terms of *H19*, the most obvious problem is that we lack a biochemical basis for understanding its tumor suppressor activity as observed in transfection assays. Also, although our finding of localized hypermethylation at the *H19* locus in WT patients is highly suggestive of a primary role for this gene as a tumor suppressor in the natural evolution of WTs, it is conceivable that other 11p15.5 genes, outside of the restricted area that we have mapped, might be inactivated by a similar epigenetic mechanism. In fact, long-range methylation mapping of 11p15.5 DNA in non-neoplastic tissues of WT patients, using the method which we have already applied to the region of DNA immediately flanking *H19*, would seem to be a promising approach to further testing of the '*H19* hypothesis' and simultaneously searching for other 11p15.5 genes that might be specifically inactivated in WT patients as part of a possible regional switch in 11p15.5 epigenotype (Côté, this volume).

In terms of *IGF2*, most WTs express high levels of its mRNA, regardless of the presence or absence of biallelic expression; the finding of low or undetectable immunoreactive IGF-II peptide in WTs (Haselbacher *et al.*, 1987; Baccarini *et al.*, 1993), despite the high levels of its mRNA, is difficult to reconcile with an autocrine growth-stimulating role for this gene product in the fully developed tumors. Consistent with this, high *IGF2* expression is not required for the proliferation of the more mature epithelial component of WTs (Moulton *et al.*, 1994). *IGF2* overexpression might well play a role at an earlier stage of Wilms' tumorigenesis, as for example in the expression of the nephrogenic precursor cell pool in patients with BWS. Additional studies in this very active field can be expected to quickly clarify these issues.

References

Baccarini, P., Fiorentino, M., D'Errico, A., Mancini, A. M. & Grigioni, W. F. (1993). Detection of anti-sense transcripts of the insulin-like growth factor-2 gene in Wilms' tumor. *Am. J. Pathol.* **143**, 1535–42.

Bartolomei, M. S., Webber, A. L., Brunkow, M. E. & Tilghman, S. M. (1993). Epigenetic mechanisms underlying the imprinting of the mouse *H19* gene. *Genes Devel.* **7**, 1663–73.

Bartolomei, M. S., Zemel, S. & Tilghman, S. M. (1991). Parental imprinting of the mouse *H19* gene. *Nature* **351**, 153–5.

Brannan, C. I., Dees, E. C., Ingram, R. S. & Tilghman, S. M. (1990). The product of the *H19* gene may function as an RNA. *Molec. Cell Biol.* **10**, 28–36.

Brunkow, M. E. & Tilghman, S. M. (1991). Ectopic expression of the *H19* gene in mice causes prenatal lethality. *Genes Devel.* **5**, 1092–101.

Davis, R. L., Weintraub, H. & Lassar, A. B. (1987). Expression of a single transfected cDNA converts fibroblasts to myoblasts. *Cell* **51**, 987–1000.

Ferguson-Smith, A. C., Sasaki, H., Cattanach, B. M. & Surani, M. A. (1993). Parental-origin-specific epigenetic modifications of the mouse *H19* gene. *Nature* **362**, 751–5.

Fidler, A. E., Maw, M. A., Eccles, M. R. & Reeve, A. E. (1992). Trans-sensing hypothesis for origin of Beckwith–Wiedemann syndrome. *Lancet* **339**, 243.

Giannoukakis, N., Deal, C., Paquette, J., Goodyer, C. G. & Polychronakos, C. (1993). Parental genomic imprinting of the human *IGF2* gene. *Nature Genet.* **4**, 98–101.

Glaser, T., Housman, D., Lewis, W. H., Gerhard, D. & Jones, C. (1989). A fine-structure deletion map of human chromosome 11p: analysis of J1 series hybrids. *Somat. Cell molec. Genet.* **15**, 477–501.

Goshen, R., Rachmilewitz, J., Schneider, T., de Groot, N., Ariel, I., Palti, Z. & Hochberg, A. (1993). The expression of the *H19* and *IGF2* genes during human embryogenesis and placental development. *Molec. Reprod. Devel.* **34**, 374–9.

Han, D. K. & Liau, G. (1992). Identification and characterization of developmentally regulated genes in vascular smooth muscle cells. *Circulation Res.* **71**, 711–19.

Hao, Y., Crenshaw, T., Moulton, T., Newcomb, E. & Tycko, B. (1993). Tumour-suppressor activity of *H19* RNA. *Nature* **365**, 764–7.

Haselbacher, G. K., Irminger, J.-C., Zapf, J., Ziegler, W. H. & Humbel, R. E. (1987). Insulin-like growth factor II in human adrenal pheochromocytomas and Wilms tumors: Expression at the mRNA and protein level. *Proc. Natl. Acad. Sci. USA* **84**, 1104–6.

Li, E., Beard, C., & Jaenisch, R. (1993). Role for DNA methylation in genomic imprinting. *Nature* **366**, 362–5.

Mannens, M., Devilee, P., Bliek, J., Mandjes, I., de Kraker, J., Heyting, C., Slater, R. M. & Westerveld, A. (1990). Loss of heterozygosity in Wilms' tumors, studied for six putative tumor suppressor regions, is limited to chromosome 11. *Cancer Res.* **50**, 3279–83.

Moulton, T., Crenshaw, T., Hao, Y., Moosikasuwan, J., Lin, N., Dembitzer, F., Hensle, T., Weiss, L., McMorrow, L., Loew, T., Kraus, W., Gerald, W. & Tycko, B. (1994). Epigenetic lesions at the *H19* locus in Wilms' tumor patients. *Nature Genet.* **7**, 440–7.

Ogawa, O., Eccles, M. R., Szeto, J., McNoe, L. A., Yun, K., Maw, M. A., Smith, P. J. & Reeve, A. E. (1993). Relaxation of insulin-like growth factor II gene imprinting implicated in Wilms' tumour. *Nature* **362**, 749–51.

Ohlsson, R., Hedborg, F., Holmgren, L., Walsh, C. & Ekström, T. J. (1994). Overlapping patterns of *IGF2* and *H19* expression during human development: biallelic *IGF2* expression correlates with a lack of *H19* expression. *Development* **120**, 361–8.

Ohlsson, R., Nyström, A., Pfeifer-Ohlsson, S., Töhönen, V., Hedborg, F., Schofield, P., Flam, F. & Ekström, T. J. (1993). *IGF2* is parentally imprinted during human embryogenesis and in the Beckwith–Wiedemann syndrome. *Nature Genet.* **4**, 94–7.

Pachnis, V., Brannan, C. I. & Tilghman, S. M. (1988). The structure and expression of a novel gene activated in early mouse embryogenesis. *EMBO J.* **7**, 673–81.

Pal, N., Wadey, R. B., Buckle, B., Yeomans, E., Pritchard, J. & Cowell, J. K. (1990). Preferential loss of maternal alleles in sporadic Wilms' tumor. *Oncogene* **5**, 1665–8.

Poirier, F., Chan, C.-T. J., Timmons, P. M., Roberson, E. J., Evans, M. J. & Rigby, P. W. J. (1992). The murine *H19* gene is activated during embryonic stem cell differentiation *in vitro* and at the time of implantation in the developing embryo. *Development* **13**, 1105–14.

Rachmilewitz, J., Gileadi, O., Eldar-Geva, T., Schneider, T., de-Groot, N. & Hochberg, A. (1992a). Transcription of the *H19* gene in differentiating cytotrophoblasts from human placenta. *Molec. Reprod. Devel.* **321**, 196–202.

Rachmilewitz, J., Goshen, R., Ariel, I., Schneider, T., de Groot, N., & Hochberg, A. (1992b). Parental imprinting of the human *H19* gene. *FEBS Lett.* **309**, 25–8.

Rainier, S., Johnson, L., Dobry, C. J., Ping, A. J., Grundy, P. E. & Feinberg, A. P. (1993). Relaxation of imprinted genes in human cancer. *Nature* **362**, 747–9.

Richard, C. W. III, Boehnke, M., Berg, D. J., Lichy, J. H., Meeker, T. C., Hauser, E., Myers, R. M. & Cox, D. R. (1993). A radiation hybrid map of the distal short arm of human chromosome 11, containing the Beckwith–Wiedemann and associated embryonal tumor disease loci. *Am. J. Hum. Genet.* **52**, 915–21.

Schroeder, W. T., Chao, L.-Y., Dao, D. T., Strong, L. C., Pathak, S., Riccardi, V. M., Lewis, W. K. & Saunders, G. F. (1987). Nonrandom loss of maternal chromosome 11 alleles in Wilms' tumors. *Am. J. Hum. Genet.* **40**, 413–20.

Steenman, M. J. C., Rainier, S., Dobry, C. J., Grundy, P., Horon, I. L. & Feinberg, A. P. (1994). Loss of imprinting of *IGF2* is linked to reduced expression and abnormal methylation of *H19* in Wilms' tumors. *Nature Genet.* **7**, 433–9.

Tartof, K. & Henikoff, S. (1991). Trans-sensing effects from Drosophila to humans. *Cell* **65**, 201–3.

Tycko, B. (1994). Genomic imprinting: mechanism and role in human pathology. *Am. J. Pathol.* **144**, 431–43.

Weksberg, R., Shen, D. R., Fei, Y. L., Song, Q. L. & Squire J. (1993). Disruption of insulin-like growth factor-2 imprinting in Beckwith–Wiedemann syndrome. *Nature Genet.* **5**, 143–50.

Wiles, M. V. (1988). Isolation of differentially expressed human cDNA clones: similarities between mouse and human embryonal stem cell differentiation. *Development* **104**, 403–13.

Williams, J. C., Brown, K. W., Mott, M. G. & Maitland, N. J. (1989). Maternal allele loss in Wilms' tumor. *Lancet* **i**, 283–4.

Zhang, Y., Shields, T., Crenshaw, T., Hao, Y., Moulton, T. & Tycko, B. (1993). Imprinting of human *H19*: allele-specific CpG methylation, loss of the active allele in Wilms' tumor and potential for somatic allele switching. *Am. J. Hum. Genet.* **53**, 113–24.

Zhang, Y. & Tycko, B. (1992). Monoallelic expression of the human *H19* gene. *Nature Genet.* **1**, 40–4.

19

A domain of abnormal imprinting in human cancer

ANDREW P. FEINBERG

Introduction

Genomic imprinting is defined as parental-origin-specific differential gene expression (reviewed by Monk & Grant, 1990). In human cancer, there is some fairly old indirect evidence for a role for imprinting. A hydatidiform mole is an androgenetic intrauterine tumor caused by paternal uniparental disomy. Conversely, a complete ovarian teratoma, which can include teeth and hair, is parthenogenetic and caused by maternal uniparental disomy (Linder *et al.*, 1975). So, clearly, you need both your father's and your mother's chromosomes, not just a complete set, and an imbalance can lead to cancer. Recent molecular evidence for a role of genomic imprinting in cancer began with the observation of preferential loss of heterozygosity (LOH) of specific parental alleles (usually maternal) in several embryonal tumors (see Feinberg, 1993, for review). However, the mechanistic significance has been unclear despite abundant speculation in the literature.

Linkage of Beckwith–Wiedemann syndrome to a potentially imprinted region

Our studies of imprinting began with a story that derived from my 10% clinical responsibility as a geneticist. I was asked to see Riley, a two-month-old boy, because of his unusual appearance: macroglossia (enlarged tongue), midface hypoplasia caused by overgrowth of the occiput, and an ear crease (Fig. 19.1). He was born hypoglycemic, and this young man was very large, weighing 14 pounds (6.4 kg) and measuring 23 inches (58 cm) at birth. Riley had Beckwith–Wiedemann syndrome (BWS), which is characterized by both developmental overgrowth (with macroglossia in 95% of patients) and predisposition to cancer, a variety of so-called embryonal tumors of childhood, which are defined by the pathologist as caused by fetal material residual after birth. It was doubly

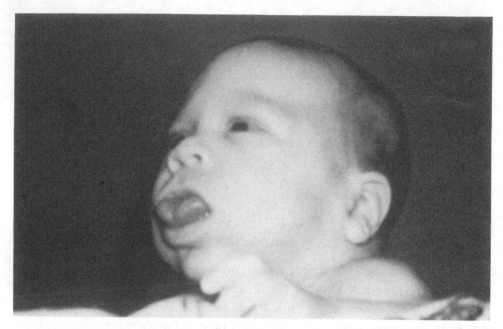

Fig. 19.1. Riley at age four months. Note the clinical stigmata of Beckwith–Wiedemann syndrome (BWS): macroglossia, midface hypoplasia, and characteristic ear creases. The child also had a WT, which was cured by surgery and chemotherapy. Use of photograph and first name with permission of the family.

gratifying to see this patient, first because it led to a very interesting area of research in our laboratory. Second, when we made the diagnosis on this patient, we recommended that he have an ultrasound examination of the kidneys, which detected a Wilms' tumor (WT). It had barely invaded the capsule, requiring chemotherapy and surgery, which cured his cancer. There is a very high cure rate of WT if diagnosed at an early stage of disease. What was particularly unusual was that Riley's aunt had had part of her tongue resected because it interfered with speech and eating.

Thus, Riley came from a rare family with BWS. It had earlier been reported that Wilms' tumors show LOH of chromosome 11p (Fearon *et al.*, 1984); Tony Reeve, on his sabbatical in my laboratory, mapped LOH to 11p15 (Reeve *et al.*, 1989), rather than 11p13, which harbors the *WT1* gene. A. J. Ping, Mike Boehnke and I therefore performed genetic linkage analysis on this and a second family, to see whether BWS maps to either 11p15 or 11p13. The second family included two siblings, one of whom had died earlier, and again we recommended ultrasound examination on the surviving child. A neuroblastoma was diagnosed in this child; she was also cured of her tumor.

Using polymorphic markers from both 11p13 and 11p15, we mapped *BWS* near the *insulin* gene on 11p15 with a high lod score (Ping *et al.*, 1989). Thus, our working hypothesis was that the *BWS* gene and the '*WT2*' gene within the second domain of LOH were identical, as both mapped to 11p15. We now believe that the genetics are even more complicated, as will be described later. However, it was interesting that some families with BWS had shown transmission ratio distortion, with increased penetrance when the gene is inherited from the mother (Viljoen & Ramesar, 1992). Genes on bands 11p15 and 15q11–12 map to adjacent regions of mouse chromosome 7 (Davisson *et al.*, 1991); band 15q11–12 harbors the Prader–Willi syndrome gene, which appears to be imprinted (Nicholls *et al.*, 1989). Thus, the localization of *BWS* to 11p15 provided an early clue that the gene might be part of a conserved imprinted region.

An unusual distribution of germline translocations in patients with BWS

As a first step toward isolating the *BWS* gene, we focused on cell lines from several patients with germline chromosomal rearrangements, as such patients have provided an enormous boon to isolating genes for other genetic disorders. Linda Kalikin in our laboratory, using cosmids mapped to 11p15, generated sequence-tagged sites (STSs) from them and used these to isolate yeast artificial chromosomes (YACs). From these YACs, additional STSs were generated from end clones, which were used to generate YAC contigs for 11p15. In order to determine whether YACs spanned *BWS* breakpoints, we collaborated with Jan Hoovers and Marcel Mannens, who performed fluorescence *in situ* hybridization (FISH). We thus molecularly cloned in YACs, and subcloned in cosmids, six germline translocations from BWS patients. Our map of these breakpoints led to two surprising observations. First, the *BWS* breakpoints span a surprisingly large distance (>7 Mb), which would be extraordinary for a single gene (J. Hoovers, L. M. Kalikin *et al.*, unpublished). For example, it seems unlikely that the entire β-globin gene cluster is simply an interesting intron of the *BWS* gene. Second, some patients with BWS show balanced germline rearrangements and others have unbalanced duplications. By examination of published reports (Norman *et al.*, 1992; Tommerup *et al.*, 1993; Weksberg *et al.*, 1993a,b) and some additional detective work (J. Hoovers, L. M. Kalikin *et al.*, unpublished) it became clear that all of the balanced rearrangements from BWS patients were of maternal origin, and all of the unbalanced duplications were of paternal origin. This is consistent with Claudine Junien's observation of paternal uniparental disomy (UPD) in some BWS patients (Henry *et al.*, 1991). Thus there appears to be a difference between the maternal and paternal alleles of the *BWS* gene, i.e. it is imprinted.

Imprinting would also explain the very long distances between the breakpoints

in BWS patients with germline translocations. An imprinting model that recon-
ciles all of the data predicts that the paternal allele is normally active and the
maternal allele is inactive (Little *et al.*, 1991). Balanced rearrangements move
the maternal allele to another autosome, thereby activating it, giving two
functioning *BWS* genes and disease. Duplications are paternal, also giving two
working gene copies. Paternal uniparental disomy itself is compatible with either
a paternal-on or a maternal-off model, but the other data suggest that the former
is correct. It is most intriguing that the long distance between balanced rearrangements suggests that the gene can be controlled by a chromosomal domain
acting over many megabases.

Imprinting of *H19* and *IGF2*

While we were mapping *WT2* and *BWS*, several laboratories had described
imprinted genes in the mouse, including *IGF2* (DeChiara *et al.*, 1991) and *H19*
(Bartolomei *et al.*, 1991) on mouse chromosome 7, whose homologs both map to
11p15. There was also some indirect evidence that *H19* might be imprinted in
humans, in that it shows monoallelic expression (Zhang & Tycko, 1992) and it is
not expressed in hydatidiform moles, which are androgenetic (Rachmilewitz *et
al.*, 1992). However, monoallelic expression might not be parental-origin-
specific, and tumors do not necessarily reflect normal gene expression.

We decided to look specifically at whether *H19* shows parental-origin-specific
monoallelic expression by exploring a known transcribed polymorphism in the
gene (Zhang & Tycko, 1992). *IGF2* was more difficult to analyze because,
although there is a published *Apa*I polymorphism (Tadokoro *et al.*, 1991), its
informativeness is quite low. We studied a dinucleotide repeat in the *IGF2* gene
that is very large (> 800 bp). Indeed, it is impossible to see this polymorphism
unless you amplify with a labeled primer on either the 5' or 3' side, and then use a
restriction enzyme that cuts in the middle of the dinucleotide repeat. Using this
approach, we found five alleles that showed Mendelian segregation (Rainier *et
al.*, 1993, 1994).

As illustrated on the pedigree in Fig. 19.2, the daughter has inherited the **a** allele
of *H19* from her mother and the **b** allele from the father. In the RT+ lane, but not
the RT− lane, there is expression of only the maternal *H19* allele. We have seen
this in ten different samples of normal tissue in which we can identify the parental
origin (Rainier *et al.*, 1993; S. Rainier & A. P. Feinberg, unpublished).

IGF2 is reciprocally imprinted, as shown in Fig. 19.3. Here, the **a** allele is
inherited from the father and the **b** allele is inherited from the mother. Only the
paternally inherited **a** allele is expressed, as we have seen in all eight samples
examined (Rainier *et al.*, 1993; S. Rainier & A. P. Feinberg, unpublished).

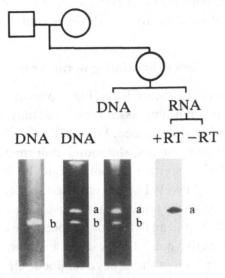

Fig. 19.2. Imprinting of human *H19* gene. The daughter has inherited the **a** allele from her mother, and the **b** allele from her father. Only the **a** allele is expressed as RNA (+RT lane). PCR and restriction enzyme digestion are as described in Rainier *et al.* (1993), from which the figure is reprinted with permission.

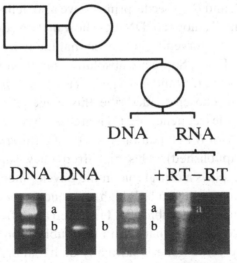

Fig. 19.3. Imprinting of human *IGF2* gene. The daughter has inherited the **a** allele from her father, and the **b** allele from her mother. Only the **a** allele is expressed as RNA (+RT lane). PCR and restriction enzyme digestion are as described in Rainier *et al.* (1993), from which the figure is reprinted with permission.

Thus, as in the mouse, both *H19* and *IGF2* are imprinted, with maternal *H19* expression and paternal *IGF2* expression (Rainier *et al.*, 1993).

Loss of imprinting in cancer

The expectation of most investigators, including us, was that abnormal imprinting leads to inactivation of a tumor suppressor gene. That may be true; we have data, described later, supporting such an idea. However, when Shirley Rainier in our laboratory looked at Wilms' tumors, she found abnormal gene activation. We examined *H19* and *IGF2*, as either or both might be involved in abnormal imprinting in cancer. Forty-two WTs were screened to identify those not having undergone LOH. RNA from the tumors was reverse-transcribed, and the cDNA was then amplified by PCR and analyzed for the presence of one or both alleles. Sixteen tumors were heterozygous. Of these, 11 expressed both maternal and paternal alleles of one or both of the genes examined. Of those tumors heterozygous for *IGF2*, 69% showed biallelic expression (Fig. 19.4) (Rainier *et al.*, 1993). Of tumors heterozygous for *H19*, 29% showed biallelic expression (Fig. 19.4) (Rainier *et al.*, 1993). It is quite important in scoring biallelic expression that one be sure that one is not just looking at contaminated DNA. We took care to use only poly (A$^+$) RNA and RT-specific primers; we also deliberately spiked one of our samples with a small amount of DNA to show that one detects a different pair of bands because of an intervening intron, so that the two alleles are different in size in the DNA and RNA. So we are absolutely sure that what we are seeing is biallelic expression of the *H19* and *IGF2* genes (Rainier *et al.*, 1993).

The term we have chosen to describe this epigenetic mutation is loss of imprinting, or LOI. The frequency of LOI is greater than that of LOH (30%) and much greater than that of WT1 mutations (5–10%) (Little *et al.*, 1992; S. Rainier & A. P. Feinberg, unpublished). This high frequency supports the idea that abnormal imprinting plays a causal role in the development of these tumors, as does the fact that it occurred at similarly high frequency in the earliest stage tumors.

Shortly after our paper was published, I received a call from a local newspaper reporter asking me to explain what was in this publication. I described that the paternal copy of the *IGF2* gene is normally active and the maternal copy is normally inactive. I told him that in tumors, both alleles are active, which might lead to overproduction of a growth factor. To my horror, the illustration shown in Fig. 19.5 appeared the next morning on the front page of the *Detroit Free Press*. The problem is that the reporter apparently decided that the maternal allele is abnormally activated in the germline, not just in the tumor (as we had observed). The newspaper thus said essentially that LOI was a germline event.

We therefore thought that we should determine whether what the newspaper

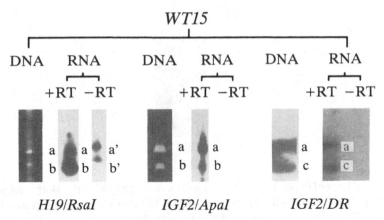

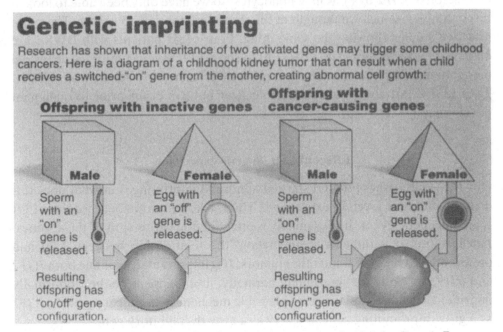

Fig. 19.4. LOI of *H19* and *IGF2* in a WT. In the first experiment, the −RT lane deliberately included DNA to demonstrate the different-sized fragments of DNA compared with RNA. Reprinted from Rainier *et al.* (1993), with permission.

Genetic imprinting

Research has shown that inheritance of two activated genes may trigger some childhood cancers. Here is a diagram of a childhood kidney tumor that can result when a child receives a switched-"on" gene from the mother, creating abnormal cell growth:

Offspring with inactive genes

Offspring with cancer-causing genes

Male

Female

Male

Female

Sperm with an "on" gene is released.

Egg with an "off" gene is released.

Sperm with an "on" gene is released.

Egg with an "on" gene is released.

Resulting offspring has "on/off" gene configuration.

Resulting offspring has "on/on" gene configuration.

Fig. 19.5. Genetic imprinting and LOI. An interpretation by the *Detroit Free Press* of our experiment demonstrating LOI in cancer, reported by Rainier *et al.* (1993). The artist assumed that the mutation was in the germline, which we confirmed as shown in Fig. 19.6. Reprinted with permission.

reported was correct, and it was (or, at least, LOI can occur early in development). In at least some patients with Beckwith–Wiedemann syndrome, we found biallelic expression of *IGF2* in non-tumor tissues. Figure 19.6 shows this in the non-tumor kidney of a BWS patient. We have not been able to detect

RT   +   −

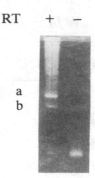

a
b

Fig. 19.6. Loss of imprinting in Beckwith–Wiedemann syndrome. Both alleles of
IGF2 are expressed (+RT lane) as shown by PCR amplication and restriction
enzyme digestion with ApaI.

expression of *IGF2* by PCR in lymphocytes, so we have only been able to look at
three samples, which we thought at the time were too few to report. There are
now two studies showing the same thing. Four of six patients with BWS were
observed by Weksberg *et al.* (1993a,b) to show LOI in non-tumor tissue, as did
one patient with developmental overgrowth described by Ogawa *et al.* (1994).
Thus LOI is not always secondary to cancer but can occur prior to malignant
development.

Effect of LOI on gene expression

Our RT–PCR assays for LOI showed abnormal imprinting, but what does this
do to quantitative levels of expression? This is a key question because since LOI
is an epigenetic event, it presumably is affecting the expression of these genes.
Furthermore, it is difficult to understand the relationship between LOI and
preferential LOH in WT and other tumors. It is important to examine both *IGF2*
and *H19*, as both are imprinted normally, both appear to be abnormally
imprinted in cancer, and there is a plausible mechanism in cancer for each, *IGF2*
as a growth-promoting gene and *H19* as a growth-inhibitory gene.

We were also concerned in performing these experiments that *IGF2* expression should not be compared to adjacent kidney, as normal kidney is em-
bryologically dissimilar to WT, and fetal kidney varies in level of expression of
IGF2. Indeed, although *IGF2* is widely assumed to be overexpressed in WT, that
has also been challenged (Scott *et al.*, 1985). We thus made a comparison of nine
tumors with LOI and five tumors without LOI or LOH, measuring *IGF2* and
H19 expression by Northern blot analysis. All filters were rehybridized with
GAPDH to control for RNA loading, and quantitative densitometry as well as

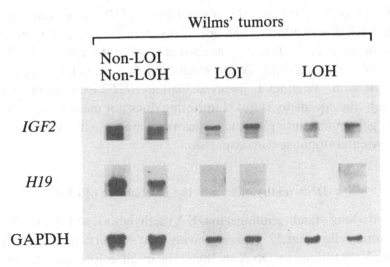

Fig. 19.7. Expression of *IGF2* and *H19* in tumors with LOI and LOH. Northern blot analysis, with GAPDH as a control for RNA loading. Note the marked reduction in *H19* expression in WTs with LOI of *IGF2*, as well as WTs with LOH, implying a common final pathway of LOI and LOH, and epigenetic inactivation of a growth suppressor gene. Reprinted from Steenman *et al.* (1994), with permission.

statistical analysis was performed. Figure 19.7 shows several examples of Wilms' tumors, comparing those with LOI to those without LOI or LOH, and Northern blots of all three genes. The average level of expression of *IGF2* and those tumors with loss of imprinting is twice that in tumors that have no LOI of LOH. However, there is so much variation in *IGF2* expression from tumor to tumor that this does not achieve statistical significance (Steenman *et al.*, 1994).

On the other hand, in all the tumors in which we see loss of imprinting of *IGF2* (about 70%), the level of *H19* expression is reduced on average about 80-fold. Thus *H19* expression is essentially abrogated in tumors with LOI of *IGF2* (Steenman *et al.*, 1994). Therefore, LOH of *IGF2* and *H19* are affected jointly by this epigenetic alteration. Thus LOI appears to be an epigenetic mechanism for inactivation of a tumor suppressor gene.

The first indirect molecular evidence suggesting a role for genomic imprinting in cancer was preferential allelic loss (reviewed in Feinberg, 1993), with Wilms' tumor showing preferential loss of the maternal allele (Schroeder *et al.*, 1987). The maternal allele is the one that normally expresses *H19*, so one would predict that *H19* is not expressed when there is maternal LOH. To investigate this possibility, we examined four tumors with LOH, and indeed *H19* showed negligible expression (Fig. 19.7). This suggests that LOI and LOH may share as a common final pathway, the abrogation of *H19* expression.

Thus, LOI of *IGF2* involves down-regulation of *H19* expression in addition to abnormal *IGF2* activation. Although I hope that semantic arguments do not obscure the science, I believe that the correct term for this epigenetic alteration is still 'loss of imprinting', which is by definition the loss of parental-origin-specific gene expression. Whether it involved biallelic *IGF2* expression or null *H19* expression, the specificity is lost. Imprinting does not mean absent expression. Indeed, 'gain of imprinting' would be incorrect, because it would imply acquisition of parental-origin-specific expression.

DNA methylation and the mechanism of LOI

I have had a long-standing interest in DNA methylation, which dates back to my postdoctoral fellowship 12 years ago with Bert Vogelstein, during which we discovered alterations in DNA methylation in all colorectal cancers and adenomas (Fig. 19.8) (Feinberg & Vogelstein, 1983; Goelz *et al.*, 1985). This usually involves hypomethylation, although we saw increased DNA methylation at some sites as well (Vogelstein *et al.*, 1985). Collaborating with Melanie Ehrlich, we later found an overall reduction in 5-methylcytosine in cancer as well as slightly increased methylation in patients predisposed to cancer (Feinberg *et al.*, 1988). These observations have been repeated by many other laboratories, with many other tumors, involving both increases and decreases of DNA methylation (reviewed in Jones *et al.*, 1992).

Thus, methylation seems to be important in cancer. It might also play an important role in imprinting, both because of the recent observation by several different laboratories of parental-origin-specific DNA methylation in the vicinity of imprinted genes (Stöger *et al.*, 1993; Ferguson-Smith *et al.*, 1993; Bartolomei *et al.*, 1993), and the remarkable observation by Jaenisch and his colleagues that knockout mice lacking a normal DNA methyltransferase show abnormal imprinting (Li *et al.*, 1993).

To investigate the relationship of DNA methylation to abnormal imprinting in cancer, we first examined the *H19* gene. Azim Surani and his colleagues had observed parental-origin-specific DNA methylation of a CpG island in the *H19* promoter, using parthenogenetic embryos maternally disomic for chromosome 7 (including *H19*) (Ferguson-Smith *et al.*, 1993). Using methylcytosine-sensitive restriction endonucleases, they observed tissue-invariant half-methylation in normal embryos, and hypomethylation in embryos maternally disomic for chromosome 7. Thus, the maternally derived chromosome is unmethylated and the paternal chromosome methylated at these sites.

We used a similar approach to examine the homologous region in humans. In this case, however, we had to employ other means to distinguish the two parental

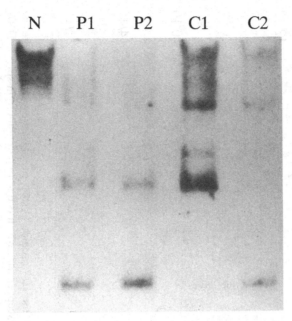

Fig. 19.8. Alterations in DNA methylation in colon cancer (C1, C2) and premalignant polyps (P1, P2), compared with normal mucosa from the same patient (N). DNA was digested with *Hpa*II and hybridized after Southern blotting with a growth hormone probe. Reprinted from Goelz *et al.* (1985), with permission.

chromosomes. As in the mouse, human DNA showed a cluster of methyl-cytosine sensitive sites in the promoter region of *H19*, representing a CpG island. This CpG island was half-methylated in all tissues that we examined, with the exception of sperm, which was hypomethylated (Fig. 19.9) (Steenman *et al.*, 1994). It was also shown in mice by Ferguson-Smith *et al.* (1993) that the sperm does not show this parental-origin-specific methylation, suggesting that, in both mouse and human, imprinting occurs after fertilization.

Is this half-methylation due to some cells being methylated and some cells not being methylated, or, alternatively in all cells is one chromosome methylated and the others not? This is a difficult question to sort out in humans, on whom experimental manipulations like those of Surani's laboratory on mice obviously cannot be performed. However, we could take advantage of the fact that some patients with Beckwith–Wiedemann syndrome have paternal uniparental disomy. Thus nature provides us with an experimental model system similar to that of Ferguson-Smith *et al.* (1993), but paternally rather than maternally disomic.

We therefore obtained blood specimens from 25 BWS patients and their parents, and identified four with uniparental disomy. In all four of these

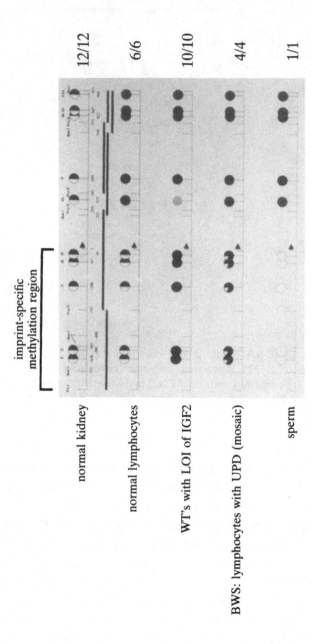

Fig. 19.9. Methylation pattern of a CpG island in the *H19* promoter (start site shown by arrow). Note the hemimethylation (half-filled circles) in all tissues except sperm, which is due to parental-origin-specific DNA methylation, as shown by examination of DNA from patients with paternal uniparental disomy (UPD). WTs with LOI acquire a paternal methylation pattern on the maternal chromosome. Reprinted from Steenman *et al.* (1994), with permission.

individuals, the *H19* CpG island was methylated. This CpG island methylation was not due to BWS itself, because most BWS patients without UPD were hemimethylated at this locus, the exception being patients with constitutional LOI. The degree of methylation was approximately 80% in UPD, consistent with approximately 80% somatic mosaicism for UPD seen in all of these patients in our hands and in the literature (Fig. 19.9) (Steenman *et al.*, 1994). Therefore, the paternal allele is methylated and the maternal allele is unmethylated in man. This parental-origin-specific, tissue-independent methylation did not extend outside of the CpG island in *H19*, with the body of the gene showing more typical expression-dependent methylation (Steenman *et al.*, 1994).

As described earlier, LOI of *IGF2* was linked to down-regulation of *H19* in all cases. Consistent with this observation, in 9 of 9 tumors in which we saw loss of imprinting of *IGF2*, we also observed abnormal methylation of the CpG island of the *H19* gene. The same was true of the minority of BWS patients with LOI of *IGF2* in non-tumor tissue (Fig. 19.8) (Steenman *et al.*, 1994). Thus, loss of imprinting in WT involves a large domain of 11p15, with changes in DNA methylation and gene expression involving both *IGF2* and *H19*.

A model of LOI in cancer

Putting all these data together, I offer the model shown in Fig. 19.10. Normally, on the paternal chromosome there is an active *IGF2* gene and an inactive *H19* gene. The opposite is true on the maternal chromosome, with inactive *IGF2* and active *H19*. Thus there is at least one balanced effect on cell growth, albeit not acting on the same targets, but with a growth-promoting gene on one chromosome and a growth-inhibiting gene on the other (Steenman *et al.*, 1994).

There are at least three abnormalities occurring together on the maternally derived chromosome in tumors with LOI: (i) abnormal expression of *IGF2*; (ii) abnormal down-regulation of *H19*; and (iii) abnormal methylation of the *H19* promoter. Thus, there is an unchecked growth effect from both chromosomes. Furthermore, there is a large domain in which an epigenotype that was previously maternal has been reversed to a paternal type (Steenman *et al.*, 1994). This idea is consistent with evolutionary hypotheses that predict a growth-stimulatory role for genes expressed specifically by the paternal chromosome, and a growth-stimulatory role for genes expressed specifically by the maternal chromosome (Haig & Graham, 1991). LOI of *H19* on the maternal chromosome, when it occurs, could occur independently or could be influenced by events on the paternal chromosome. Note that other as yet unidentified 11p15 genes could be involved in this imprint-related effect on cell growth.

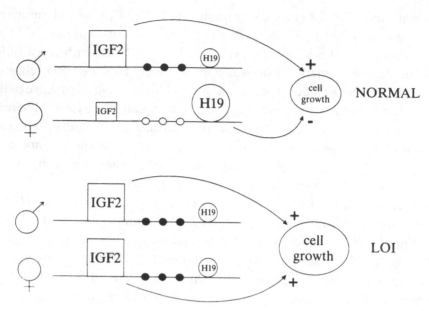

Fig. 19.10. A domain of abnormal imprinting in human cancer and methylation of the *H19* promoter in Wilms' tumor. In normal cells, the paternal *IGF2* and maternal *H19* genes are expressed (large boxes). CpG islands in the *H19* promoter are methylated on the paternal allele (filled circles). In tumors with LOI, the maternal chromosome acquires a paternal epigenotype, with *IGF2* expressed, *H19* transcriptionally silent, and a paternal pattern of methylation of the *H19* CpG island. LOI of *H19* on the maternal chromosomes, when it occurs, could arise independently or could be influenced by events on the paternal chromosome. Reprinted from Steenman *et al.* (1994), with permission.

One of the implications of this model that particularly interests us is whether or not one might be able to manipulate DNA methylation in somatic cells to restore a normal pattern of gene expression, at least in part. Given that DNA methyltransferase-deficient mice are hypomethylated at the *H19* CpG island and show LOI of *H19* (Li *et al.*, 1993), perhaps one can influence the imprint in somatic cells experimentally. Along these lines, Jones *et al.* (1993) induced expression of *IGF2* in maternally disomic mouse cells with 5-azacytidine. We are currently attempting to restore *H19* expression and/or inhibit *IGF2* expression experimentally in tumors with LOI using 5-azacytidine.

An additional tumor suppressor gene on 11p15

Although inhibition of *H19* expression may play a role in tumorigenesis, and *H19* has been shown to confer growth-inhibitory properties on tumor cells (Hao *et al.*, 1993), other experiments from our laboratory suggest the existence of another tumor suppressor gene on 11p15. Direct expression cloning of suppressor genes in manageable vectors is usually impossible, because growth suppression is normally selected against. We recently developed a strategy for transferring subchromosomal transferable fragments (STFs) intermediate in size between YACs and chromosomes, described in detail by Koi *et al.* (1993).

Our strategy involves three steps: (i) transfection of a mammalian selectable marker gene into mouse cells containing a single independently selectable human chromosome; (ii) chromosome transfer by microcell fusion, followed by double selection for both the human chromosome and the marker gene; and (iii) isolation of individual marker-containing chromosomal subfragments by irradiated microcell transfer from the pooled hybrid panel. Unlike conventional radiation hybrids, each resulting fragment can then be transferred independently to mammalian cells, by virtue of the selectable marker gene.

Using STFs, we were able to localize an 11p15 tumor suppressor gene that caused growth arrest of RD rhabdomyosarcoma cells *in vitro*. This gene was localized to a 3 Mb region of 11p15, between the β-globin gene cluster and the region of *IGF2* and *H19* (Koi *et al.*, 1993). Thus, several STFs containing DNA in this region caused *in vitro* growth arrest of RD cells into which it was introduced, but had no effect on cervical or lung cancer cells; and STFs outside this region had no effect on RD cell growth *in vitro* or *in vivo*. The STFs also enabled us to delimit the candidate region to a relatively small size, map the region, and isolate a large number of cosmid and phage clones from it.

Thus, we have found that a tumor suppressor gene on 11p15 mapped by LOH is distinct from *H19*. Furthermore, we have molecularly cloned a balanced chromosomal translocation from a rhabdoid tumor (TM87-16; note that G401, historically described as a WT (Karnes *et al.*, 1991) and suppressed by chromosome 11, was actually found to be a rhabdoid tumor on re-examination (Garvin *et al.*, 1993)). The breakpoint in TM87-16 is also within the STF, and also outside the region of (and centromeric to) *IGF2* and *H19* (J. Hoovers, L. M. Kalikin *et al.*, unpublished). The distinct tumor suppressor gene on 11p15 may be involved in a number of common malignancies that do not occur in BWS, since, for example, 80% of lung cancer patients show loss of heterozygosity for 11p15 (Weston *et al.*, 1991), as do half of metastatic breast cancers (Takita *et al.*, 1992).

Some questions to be answered

The discovery of abnormal imprinting in cancer raises two new areas of investigation: the role of abnormal imprinting in cancer, and whether tumors can be used to better understand the mechanism and function of normal imprinting. We are

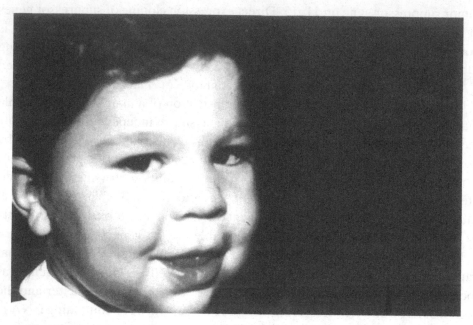

Fig. 19.11. Riley at age four years. Compare with Fig. 19.1. Note the loss of most stigmata of BWS. He has also largely outgrown the risk of malignancy, indicating the development as well as tissue-specificity of BWS.

asking some of the following questions regarding the role of imprinting in cancer. (i) How ubiquitous is LOI in cancer? Preliminary data from our laboratory suggest that LOI occurs in many embryonal tumors (S. Rainier & A. P. Feinberg, unpublished), and Suzuki *et al*. (1994) have recently observed LOI in 47% of lung cancers. (ii) Are other imprinted genes affected in cancer? (iii) Is the imprinting information irretrievably lost in tumors, or is it possible to restore a normal imprint experimentally or therapeutically? (iv) Does LOI involve alterations in target sequences, aside from changes in DNA methylation, and/or are *trans*-acting factors responsible?

The study of tumors may also provide a novel approach to understanding normal genomic imprinting. For example, they may provide a way to examine higher-order chromatin structure of imprinted and non-imprinted chromosomes. Toward this end, we have recently developed a stable diploid immortalized cell line from a female Indian muntjac deer, whose only native chromosomes are 1,2 and X. By generating monochromosome hybrids containing a 'maternal' or 'paternal' human chromosome 11, one can purify virtually unlimited quantities of either chromosome to homogeneity by using sucrose gradient centrifugation, because of the 10-fold difference in size between the human and muntjac chromosomes (Lee *et al*., 1994). In addition, tumor cells provide the opportunity for manipulation of DNA methylation *in vitro* and *in vivo*, as has been done with MatDi7 mouse cells, but with a greater variety of cell types showing normal imprinting or LOI.

As genomic imprinting appears to break classical Mendelian rules, we should perhaps not be surprised that tumors show abnormal imprinting, given their great genetic plasticity and adaptability. At the same time, we should not forget that the process of imprinting itself is under genetic control, and genetic abnormalities in tumors may provide insights into the mechanisms responsible. Finally, cancer biology may help us to understand the role of genomic imprinting in normal development. One of the most interesting features of Beckwith–Wiedemann syndrome is its developmental specificity. Thus, children are at risk of cancer in a relatively narrow developmental window; they appear to outgrow most of the clinical stigmata of the disease with time, as is evident from Riley's photograph at age 4 (Fig. 19.11). Thus, genomic imprinting may be important in the normal expansion of specific cell lineages, and tumors may arise from disturbances in the control of that process.

Acknowledgements

This work was supported by the National Institutes of Health. I thank Joanne Furman for preparing the manuscript.

References

Bartolomei, M. S., Webber, A. L., Brunkow, M. E. & Tilghman, S. M. (1993). Epigenetic mechanisms underlying the imprinting of the mouse *H19* gene. *Genes Devel.* 7, 1663–73.

Bartolomei, M., Zemel, S. & Tilghman, S. M. (1991). Parental imprinting of the mouse *H19* gene. *Nature* **351**, 153–5.

Davisson, M. T., Lalley, P. A., Peters, J., Doolittle, D. P., Hillyard, A. L. & Searle, A. G. (1991). Report of the comparative committee for human, mouse and other rodents. *Cytogenet. Cell Genet.* **58**, 1152–89.

DeChiara, T. M., Robertson, E. J. & Efstratiadis, A. (1991). Parental imprinting of the mouse insulin-like growth factor-II gene. *Cell* **64**, 849–59.

Fearon, E. R., Vogelstein, B. & Feinberg, A. P. (1984). Somatic deletion and duplication of genes on chromosome 11 in Wilms' tumors. *Nature* **309**, 176–8.

Feinberg, A. (1993). Genomic imprinting and gene activation in cancer. *Nature Genet.* **4**, 110–13.

Feinberg, A. P., Gehrke, C. W., Kuo, K. C. & Ehrlich, M. (1988). Reduced genomic 5-methylcytosine content in human colonic neoplasia. *Cancer Res.* **48**, 1159–61.

Feinberg, A. P. & Vogelstein, B. (1983). Hypomethylation distinguishes genes of some human cancers from their normal counterparts. *Nature* **301**, 89–92.

Ferguson-Smith, A. C., Sasaki, H., Cattanach, B. M. & Surani, M. A. (1993). Parental-origin-specific epigenetic modification of the mouse H19 gene. *Nature* **362**, 751–5.

Garvin, A. J., Re, G. G., Tarnowski, B. I., Hazen-Martin, D. J. & Sens, D. A. (1993). The G401 cell line, utilized for studies of chromosomal changes in Wilms' tumor, is derived from a rhabdoid tumor of the kidney. *Am. J. Pathol.* **142**, 375–80.

Goelz, S. E., Vogelstein, B., Hamilton, S. R. & Feinberg, A. P. (1985). Hypomethylation of DNA from benign and malignant human colon neoplasms *Science* **228**, 187–90.

Haig, D. & Graham, D. (1991). Genomic imprinting and the strange case of the insulin-like growth factor II receptor. *Cell* **64**, 1045–6.

Hao, Y., Crenshaw, T., Moulton, T., Newcomb, E. & Tycko, B. (1993). Tumor-suppressor activity of H19 RNA. *Nature* **365**, 764–7.

Henry, I., Bonaitijk-Pellie, C., Chehensse, V., Beldjord, C., Schwarz, C., Utermann, G. & Junien, C. (1991). Uniparental paternal disomy in a genetic cancer-predisposing syndrome. *Nature* **351**, 665–7.

Jones, P. A., Rideout, W. M. III, Shen, J.-C., Spruck, C.H. & Tsai, Y. C. (1993). Methylation, mutation and cancer. *Bioessays* **14**(1), 33–6.

Karnes, P. S., Tran, T. N., Cui, M. Y., Bogenmann, E., Shimada, H. & Ying, K. L. (1991). Establishment of a rhabdoid tumor cell line with a specific chromosomal abnormality, 46, XY, t(11,22)(p15.5; q11.23). *Cancer Genet. Cytogenet.* **56**, 31–8.

Koi, M., Johnson, L. A., Kalikin, L. M., Little, P. F. R., Nakamura, Y. & Feinberg, A. P. (1993). Tumor cell growth arrest caused by subchromosomal transferable DNA fragments from human chromosome 11. *Science* **260**, 361–4.

Kreidberg, J. A., Sariola, H., Loring, J. M., Maeda, M., Pelletier, J., Housman, D. & Jaenisch, R. (1993). WT-1 is required for early kidney development. *Cell* **74**, 679–91.

Lee, J.-Y., Koi, M., Stanbridge, E. J., Oshimura, M., Kumamoto, A. T. & Feinberg, A. P. (1994). Simple purification of human chromosomes to homogeneity using muntjac hybrid cells. *Nature Genet.* **7**, 29–33.

Li, E., Beard, C. & Jaenisch, R. (1993). Role for DNA methylation in genomic imprinting. *Nature* **366**, 362–5.

Linder, D., McCaw, B., Kaiser, X. & Hecht, F. (1975). Parthenogenetic origin of benign ovarian teratomas. *New Engl. J. Med.* **292**, 63–6.

Little, M., van Heyningen, V. & Hastie, N. (1991). Dads and disomy and disease. *Nature* **351**, 609–10.

Little, M. H., Prosser, J., Condie, A., Smith, P. J., van Heyningen, V. & Hastie, N. D. (1992). Zinc finger point mutations within the WT1 gene in Wilms' tumor patients. *Proc. Natl. Acad. Sci. USA* **89**, 4791–5.

Monk, M. & Grant, M. (1990). Preferential X-chromosome inactivation, DNA methylation and imprinting. *Development* (Supplement), 55–62.

Nicholls, R. D., Knoll, J. H. M., Butler, M. G., Karam, S. & Lalande, M. (1989) Genetic imprinting suggested by maternal heterodisomy in nondeletion Prader-Willi syndrome. *Nature* **342**, 281–5.

Norman, A. M., Read, A. P., Clayton-Smith, J., Andrews, T. & Donnai, D. (1992). Recurrent Wiedemann–Beckwith syndrome with inversion of chromosome (11) (p11.2p15.5). *Am. J. med. Genet.* **42**(4), 638–41.

Ogawa, O., Becroft, D. M., Morison, I. M., Eccles, M. R., Skeen, J. E.,, Mauger, D. C. & Reeve, A. E. (1994). Constitutional relaxation of insulin-like growth factor II gene imprinting associated with Wilms' tumour and gigantism. *Nature Genet.* **5**(4), 408–12.

Pelletier, J., Bruening, W., Kashtan, C. E., Mauer, S. M., Manivel, J. C., Striegel, J. E., Houghton, D. C., Junien, C., Habib, R. *et al.* (1991). Germline mutations in the Wilms' tumor suppressor gene are associated with abnormal urogenital development in Denys-Drash syndrome. *Cell* **67**, 437–47.

Ping. A. J., Reeve, A. E., Law, D. J., Young, M. R., Boehnke, M. & Feinberg, A. P. (1989). Genetic linkage of Beckwith–Wiedemann syndrome to 11p15. *Am. J. Hum. Genet.* **44**, 720–3.

Rachmilewitz, J., Goshen, R., Ariel, I., Schneider, T., de Groot, N. & Hochberg, A. (1992). Parental imprinting of the human H19 gene. *FEBS Lett.* **309**(1), 25–8.

Rainier, S., Dobry, C. J. & Feinberg, A. P. (1994). Dinucleotide repeat polymorphism in the human insulin-like growth factor II (IGF2) gene on chromosome 11. *Hum. molec. Genet.* **3**, 384.

Rainier, S., Johnson, L. A., Dobry, C. J., Ping, A. J., Grundy, P. E. & Feinberg, A. P. (1993). Relaxation of imprinted genes in human cancer. *Nature* **362**, 747–9.

Reeve, A. E., Sih, S. A., Raizis, A. M. & Feinberg, A. P. (1989). Loss of allelic heterozygosity at a second locus on chromosome 11 in sporadic Wilms' tumor cells. *Molec. Cell Biol.* **9**(4), 1799–803.

Schroeder, W. T., Chao, L.-Y., Dao, D. D., Strong, L. C., Pathak, S., Riccardi, V., Lewis, W. H. & Saunders, G. F. (1987). Nonrandom loss of maternal chromosome 11 alleles in Wilms' tumors. *Am. J. Hum. Genet.* **40**, 413–20.

Scott, J., Cowell, J. & Robertson, M. E. (1985). Insulin-like growth factor-II gene expression in Wilms' tumour and embryonic tissues. *Nature* **317**, 260–2.

Steenman, M. J. C., Rainier, S., Dobry, C. J., Grundy, P., Horon, I. & Feinberg, A. P. (1994). Loss of imprinting of IGF2 is linked to reduced expression and abnormal methylation of H19 in Wilms' tumor. *Nature Genet.* **7**, 433–9.

Stöger, R., Kubicka, P., Liu, C.-G., Kafri, T., Razin, A., Cedar, H. & Barlow, D. P. (1993). Maternal-specific methylation of the imprinted mouse *Igf2r* locus identifies the expressed locus as carrying the imprinting signal. *Cell* **73**, 61–71.

Suzuki, H., Ueda, R., Takahashi, T. & Takahashi, T. (1994). Altered imprinting in lung cancer. *Nature Genet.* **6**, 332–33.

Tadokoro, K., Fujii, H., Inoue, T. & Yamada, M. (1991). Polymerase chain reaction (PCR) for detection of ApaI polymorphism at the insulin-like growth factor II gene (IGF2). *Nucleic Acids Res.* **19**(24), 6967.

Takita, K. I., Sato, T., Mijagi, M., Watatani, M., Akiyama, F., Sakamoto, G., Kasumi, F., Abe, R. & Nakamura, Y. (1992). Correlation of loss of alleles on the short arms of chromosomes 11 and 17 with metastasis of primary breast cancer to lymph nodes. *Cancer Res.* **52**, 3914–17.

Tommerup, N., Brandt, C. A., Pederson, S., Bolund, L. & Kamper, J. (1993). Sex dependent transmission of Beckwith–Wiedemann syndrome associated with a reciprocal translocation t (9, 11)(p11.2, p15.5). *J. med. Genet.* **30**, 958–61.

Viljoen, D. & Ramesar, R. (1992). Evidence for paternal imprinting in familial Beckwith–Wiedemann syndrome. *J. med. Genet.* **29**(4), 221–5.

Vogelstein, B., Fearon, E. R., Hamilton, S. R. & Feinberg, A. P. (1985). Use of restriction fragment length polymorphisms to determine the clonal origin of human tumors. *Science* **227**, 642–5.

Weksberg, R., Shen, D. R., Fei, Y. L., Song, Q. L. & Squire, J. (1993a). Disruption of insulin-like growth factor 2 imprinting in Beckwith–Wiedemann syndrome. *Nature Genet.* **5**, 143–50.

Weksberg, R., Teshima, I., Williams, B. R., Greenberg, C. R., Pueschel, S. M., Chernos, J. E., Fowlow, S. B., Hoyme, E., Anderson, I. J. & Whiteman, D. A. (1993b). Molecular characterization of cytogenetic alterations associated with the Beckwith–Wiedemann syndrome (BWS) phenotype refines the localization and suggests the gene for BWS is imprinted. *Hum. molec. Genet.* **2**(5), 549–56.

Weston, A., Wiley, J. C., Modali, R., Sugimura, H., McDowell, E. M., Resau, J., Light, B., Haugen, A., Mann, D. L., Trump, B. F. & Harris, C. C. (1991). Differential DNA sequence deletions from chromosomes 3, 11, 13, and 17 in squamous-cell carcinoma, large-cell carcinoma, and adenocarcinoma of the human lung. *Proc. Natl. Acad. Sci. USA* **86**, 5099–103.

Zhang, Y. & Tycko, B. (1992). Monoallelic expression of the human H19 gene. *Nature Genet.* **1**, 40–4.

V

Genomic imprinting and the Prader–Willi syndrome

20

Parent-of-origin-specific DNA methylation and imprinting mutations on human chromosome 15

BERNHARD HORSTHEMKE, BÄRBEL DITTRICH AND
KARIN BUITING

Summary

The Prader–Willi/Angelman syndrome region on human chromosome 15 contains several loci that are subject to parent-of-origin-specific gene expression and DNA methylation. We have identified a *Hpa*II site and a *Cfo*I site at the D15S63 locus, which are methylated on the maternal chromosome and unmethylated on the paternal chromosome. These differences can be employed for rapid diagnostic testing of patients suspected of having Prader–Willi or Angelman syndrome. Recently, several patients with apparently normal chromosomes but abnormal methylation patterns have been identified. These patients appear to have a defect in the imprinting process. We propose that the Prader–Willi/Angelman syndrome region contains an imprinting center, which regulates chromatin structure, DNA methylation and gene expression. Mutations in this center may prevent the resetting of the imprint in the germline and disturb the expression of imprinted genes in this region.

Introduction

Prader–Willi syndrome (PWS) and Angelman syndrome (AS) are distinct neurogenetic syndromes (Table 20.1). Although both syndromes are usually sporadic, familial recurrence has been observed in several AS families (Clayton-Smith et al., 1992; Meijers-Heijboer et al., 1992; Wagstaff et al., 1992, 1993) and in a very few PWS families (Lubinsky et al., 1987; Burke et al., 1987; Ishikawa et al., 1987; Örstavik et al., 1992; Reis et al., 1994). Cytogenetic observations and molecular studies have identified 15q11–13 as the critical chromosomal region for both syndromes (Ledbetter et al., 1981; Kaplan et al., 1987; Magenis et al., 1987; Pembrey et al., 1989). The strict parental bias in the origin of deletions and uniparental disomy (see Table 20.1) suggests that the PWS gene(s) is(are)

295

Table 20.1. *Clinical and genetic findings in PWS and AS*

	PWS	AS
clinical signs	neonatal hyopotonia	microcephalus
	hypogonadism	jerky movements
	hyperphagia and obesity	no speech
	short stature	abnormal EEG
	small hands and feet	severe mental retardation
	craniofacial dysmorphism	compulsive laughing behavior
	mental retardation	hypopigmentation
	hypopigmentation	
genetic lesions	pat. deletion 15q11–13 (70%)	mat. deletion 15q11–13 (70%)
(frequency)	maternal disomy (28%)	paternal disomy (2%)
	others (2%)	others (28%)

expressed from the paternal chromosome only and that the AS gene(s) is(are) expressed from the maternal chromosome only (Knoll *et al.*, 1989; Nicholls *et al.*, 1989; Malcolm *et al.*, 1991). Whereas all the available data are compatible with the assumption that AS is caused by a single gene, PWS may be a contiguous gene syndrome (see below).

The critical PWS/AS region in 15q11–13 (Fig. 20.1) has recently been cloned in overlapping yeast artificial chromosome clones (Mutirangura *et al.*, 1993). Most of the patients with PWS or AS have a deletion of 4–5 Mb. Detailed molecular studies of translocation breakpoints (Wagstaff *et al.*, 1991) and breakpoints in patients with atypical deletions (Saitoh *et al.*, 1992; Buiting *et al.*, 1993) suggest that the PWS genes are centromeric to D15S174 and that the AS gene is telomeric to D15S174. Whereas the gene for AS is still unknown, three genes have been identified which are paternally expressed and possibly involved in PWS: *SNRPN* (Özcelik *et al.*, 1992; Glenn *et al.*, 1993b; Nakao *et al.*, 1994) and *PAR5* and *PAR1* (Sutcliffe *et al.*, 1994). The *SNRPN* gene encodes the small nuclear ribonucleoprotein N, which is involved in the splicing of RNA in the brain. The function of *PAR5* and *PAR1* remains to be elucidated.

Parent-of-origin-specific DNA methylation in 15q11–13

The mechanisms underlying parent-of-origin-specific gene expression are unknown, but chromatin compaction (Ferguson-Smith *et al.*, 1993), replication timing (Izumikawa *et al.*, 1991; Kitsberg *et al.*, 1993; Knoll *et al.*, 1994) and DNA methylation (Driscoll *et al.*, 1992; Dittrich *et al.*, 1992; Glenn *et al.*, 1993b;

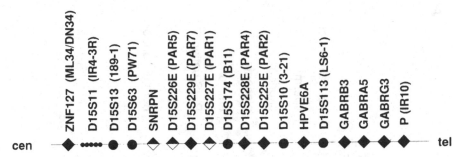

Fig. 20.1. Locus order in 15q11–13. The common deletion region in PWS and AS extends from the zinc finger gene *ZNF127* to the pigmentation gene *P* and comprises 4–5 Mb (not drawn to scale). Circle, anonymous probe; diamond, gene; half-filled diamond, gene known to be imprinted; *SNRPN*, small nuclear ribonucleoprotein N; HPVE6A, E6-associated protein; GABRB3, GABA$_A$ (γ-aminobutyric acid) receptor β3 subunit; GABRA5, α5 subunit; GABRG3, γ3 subunit.

Buiting *et al.*, 1994) may be involved. Driscoll *et al.* (1992) have reported parent-of-origin-specific DNA methylation at the *ZNF127* (ML34/DN34) locus. Glenn *et al.* (1993b) and Buiting *et al.* (1994) have found that a DNA sequence in intron 5 of the *SNRPN* gene is methylated on the paternal chromosome, but unmethylated on the maternal chromosome. We have focused our studies on the D15S63 locus, which maps 130 kb proximal of *SNRPN* (Buiting *et al.*, 1993) and is defined by the anonymous microdissection clone PW71 (Buiting *et al.*, 1990).

PW71 is located on a 6.6 kb genomic *Hind*III fragment. Hybridization of *Hind*III + *Hpa*II-digested DNA from peripheral blood of normal individuals reveals a 6.6 kb and a 4.7 kb fragment (Fig. 20.2A). In *Hind*III + *Cfo*I-digested DNA, PW71 hybridizes to a 6.6 kb and 3.4 kb fragment. AS deletion and disomy patients lack the 6.6 kb fragment. Thus, this band represents the maternal allele. PWS patients lack the smaller fragments, which represent the paternal allele. These results suggest that a *Hpa*II site and a *Cfo*I site close to PW71 are methylated on the maternal chromosome and unmethylated on the paternal chromosome (Dittrich *et al.*, 1992, 1993).

The *Hpa*II site is part of a solitary long terminal repeat (LTR) of human endogenous retroviruses (Dittrich *et al.*, 1993). The LTR may be derived from a retrovirus that integrated into the germline during evolution and was lost again by unequal crossing over at the LTRs, leaving behind the solitary LTR. It is unclear whether the LTR promotes the expression of a nearby gene and whether parent-of-origin-specific DNA methylation of the LTR modulates this process. In mouse and rat, there are examples of genes that are under the control of a solitary LTR. These are the mouse intracisternal A-particle promoted placental gene (*MIPP*) (Chang-Yeh *et al.*, 1991) and the rat oncomodulin gene (Furter

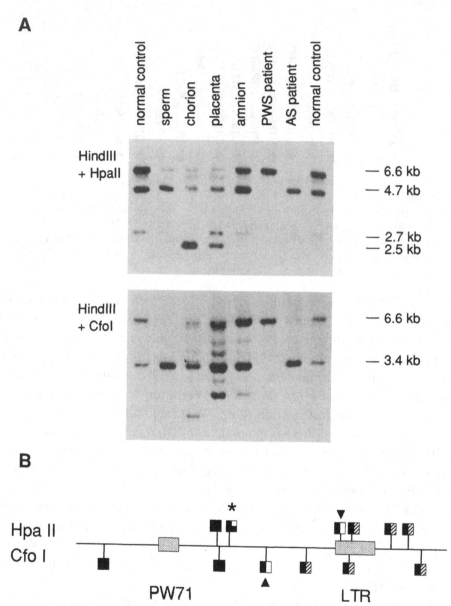

Fig. 20.2. D15S63 methylation pattern. (A) DNA samples were digested with *Hind* III + *Hpa* II or *Hind* III + *Cfo* I and probed with PW71. The PWS patient has a paternally derived 15q11–13 deletion. The AS patient has a maternally derived 15q11–13 deletion. (B) Map of the 6.6 kb *Hind* III fragment containing PW71 and the solitary LTR (dotted boxes). The boxes at the restriction enzyme sites indicate their methylation status in blood cell DNA. Left half, maternal copy; right half, paternal copy. Filled box, methylated; half-filled box, methylated in 80% of cells; open box, unmethylated; hatched box, methylation status unknown; asterisk, variable site. The arrowheads indicate the sites that are subject to parent-of-origin-specific DNA methylation. (Modified from Dittrich *et al.*, 1993.)

et al., 1989). Interestingly, these genes are preferentially expressed in the placenta. Their methylation status has not been determined.

It is also possible that the methylation imprint at the D15S63 locus has no functional significance at all, but represents an evolutionary reminiscence. Barlow (1993) has pointed out that the imprinting process may have evolved from a host defense mechanism that serves to neutralize invading DNA. The D15S63 LTR most probably is the remains of a retrovirus that invaded the germline. It is of interest to note that in this case, and in all cases of parent-specific transgene methylation, it is always the maternal locus that is methylated.

It is unclear why one *Hpa*II site at the D15S63 locus is imprinted and others are not (Fig. 20.2B). It is possible that the DNA surrounding the LTR *Hpa*II site contains an imprinting signal. Interestingly, the Rsv-Ig-myc transgene displaying parent-of-origin-specific methylation and expression in the mouse contains an LTR of the Rous sarcoma virus (Chaillet *et al.*, 1991). In this case it has been demonstrated that the transgene itself and not the insertion site determines the methylation pattern. It is possible that the Rsv-LTR contains a sequence that is recognized as an imprinting signal. Recently, such a signal in the mouse *Igf2r* gene has been identified (Stöger *et al.*, 1993). It has no homology to the sequences containing the imprinted *Hpa*II and *Cfo*I sites at the D15S63 locus (Dittrich *et al.*, 1993).

As shown in Fig. 20.2A, sperm DNA has the 4.7 kb *Hind*III+*Hpa*II and the 3.4 kb *Hind*III+*Cfo*I band only, i.e. the adult paternal methylation pattern (Dittrich *et al.*, 1993). This suggests that the paternal D15S63 imprint is fully developed by the final stage of spermatogenesis. This is similar to the development of the maternal Rsv-Ig-myc and *Igf2r* imprints, which are fully established by the final stage of oogenesis (Chaillet *et al.*, 1991; Stöger *et al.*, 1993), but in contrast to the paternal Rsv-Ig-myc transgene methylation imprint, which is acquired only by day 6.5 of embryogenesis (Chaillet *et al.*, 1991). As we cannot obtain sufficient amounts of oocyte DNA, we cannot study the development of the maternal D15S63 imprint. Extraembryonic tissues (Fig. 20.2A), tumor cells and lymphoblastoid cell lines (not shown) are hypomethylated at the D15S63 locus.

Despite numerous studies, the mechanisms linking DNA methylation and gene expression remain to be elucidated. It is possible that enhancer or promoter activity is inhibited by DNA methylation, because transcription factors may not bind to their methylated target sequences. Other enhancers or promoters may be activated by methylation, because some transcription factors may preferentially bind to methylated DNA or to other factors bound to methylated DNA. Likewise, the activity of silencers and repressors may be regulated by DNA methylation. (For a review on the role of DNA methylation in the regulation of transcription see Eden & Cedar, 1994.)

Diagnostic applications

The parent-of-origin-specific DNA methylation at the D15S63 (PW71) locus can be used for rapid diagnostic testing of patients suspected of having PWS or AS (Dittrich *et al.*, 1992, 1993; Buiting *et al.*, 1994). Lack of the paternal band is diagnostic for PWS. Lack of the maternal band is diagnostic for AS. In contrast to the clear Southern patterns obtained with PW71, the DN34/ML34 and the *SNRPN* bands are not completely specific for the paternal and maternal alleles, but differ only in intensity in PWS and AS patients. This suggests that at these two loci only a small fraction of blood cells displays parent-of-origin-specific DNA methylation. Therefore, DN34/ML34 and *SNRPN* methylation is less useful for a diagnostic testing.

   The D15S63 methylation test has several advantages over cytogenetic analysis or DNA polymorphism studies. It detects both deletions and uniparental disomy, does not require parental DNA samples, and is informative in each case. The availability of a rapid diagnostic test is of great clinical importance, because in newborns and young infants these syndromes are difficult to diagnose by clinical examination only. Among 65 newborns with severe hypotonia, for example, we have detected 29 patients with PWS (Gillessen-Kaesbach *et al.*, 1995). It should be noted, however, that the methylation test does not provide any information on the nature of the genetic lesion. This information can be obtained only by additional tests. Knowledge about the specific etiology of PWS or AS in a given patient is important for accurate estimates about the recurrence risk.

Imprinting mutations in the Prader–Willi and Angelman syndromes

In the course of diagnostic testing, we and others have identified several PWS and AS patients with apparently normal chromosomes of biparental origin, but an abnormal methylation pattern (Glenn *et al.*, 1993a; Reis *et al.*, 1994; Buiting *et al.*, 1994). Five such families are shown in Fig. 20.3. Although all the patients have two copies of the D15S63 locus, as shown by microsatellite or dosage analysis, the PWS patients in families S and O lack the paternal *Hind*III + *Hpa*II band and the AS patients in families D, W and K lack the maternal *Hind*III + *Hpa*II band (Reis *et al.*, 1994). Similar findings were made in two other PWS patients (14-3 and S12) (Buiting *et al.*, 1994). Abnormal methylation at the ML34/DN34 locus was observed in the AS patients and the PWS sibs of family O.

   Southern blot hybridization of the patients' DNA with a cDNA clone for *SNRPN* revealed the presence of two copies in the AS patients, the sibs of family O, patient 14-3 and patient S12. In contrast, the sibs of family S were found to

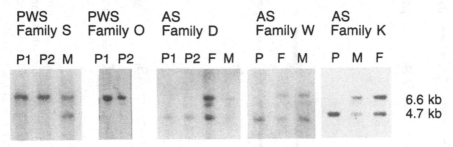

Fig. 20.3. Southern blot analysis of the D15S63 methylation. DNA was digested with *Hind* III + *Hpa* II and probed with PW71. The 6.6 kb band represents the maternal methylation imprint, and the 4.7 kb band represents the paternal methylation imprint. Although the patients have two copies of D15S63, the PWS patients lack the 4.7 kb band and the AS patients lack the 6.6 kb band. P, P1, P2, patients; M, mother; F, father. (Reprinted from Reis *et al.*, 1994; © The American Society of Human Genetics.)

have a microdeletion encompassing *SNRPN* but none of the flanking markers (Buiting *et al.*, 1994). Using a cosmid probe and fluorescence *in situ* hybridization, Sutcliffe *et al.* (1994) have identified a small deletion proximal to *SNRPN* in family O. It is not clear whether this deletion includes 5' regulatory sequences of *SNRPN*.

The observation of an aberrant methylation imprint in these families is highly suggestive of the presence of imprinting mutations. As the methylation patterns in 15q11–13 appear to be correlated with the expression status of the PWS and AS gene(s), the finding of a maternal methylation imprint on a paternal chromosome and a paternal methylation imprint on a maternal chromosome suggests that, in the patients described here, both copies of the PWS and AS genes, respectively, have been silenced by the imprinting process. Aberrant imprinting may result from a mutation that acts either in *cis* or in *trans* on the PWS and AS genes. Since all the patients described here exhibit a classical phenotype, the mutation does not disturb the imprinting in general, but affects the PWS and AS genes specifically.

A *cis* effect resulting from a mutation or subtle chromosomal rearrangement within or close to the critical PWS/AS region is likely, because the PWS and AS sibs share the same paternal and maternal chromosomes, respectively. Tentative evidence for a *cis* effect was found in the PWS patients S and O, who have a microdeletion close to the D15S63 locus. In these patients, deletion of all or part of the *SNRPN* gene and/or neighboring genes may be the cause of PWS. However, it is more likely that a deletion of the *SNRPN* gene is not sufficient for typical PWS. Almost all patients have a large deletion or uniparental disomy. We are not aware of any patient with typical PWS and a *SNRPN* point mutation. It is

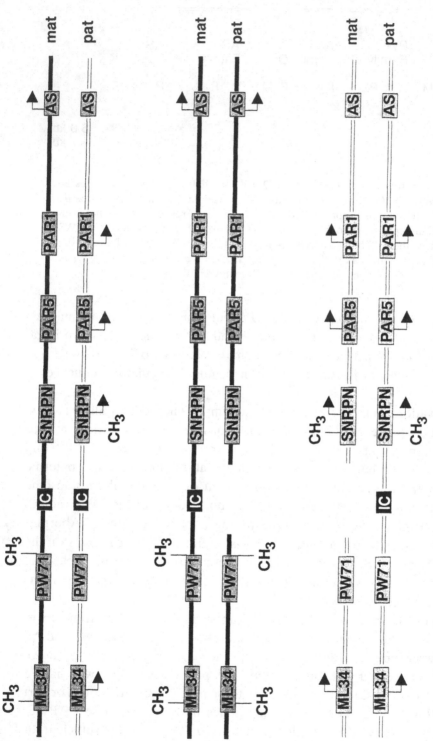

Fig. 20.4. Imprinting center hypothesis. The imprinting center (IC) regulates the chromatin structure, DNA methylation and gene activity in the PWS/AS region. In normal individuals (upper part of figure), the maternal chromosome has a heterochromatoid region (thick line) from which the AS gene is transcribed (arrow). The paternal chromosome has a euchromatoid region (thin lines) from which the PWS genes are transcribed (arrows). In some PWS and AS families, a deletion or mutation of the imprinting center in a parent has prevented the resetting of the imprint in the germline. Consequently, both chromosomes of the patient have a heterochromatoid domain, which silences the PWS genes (middle part of figure), or a euchromatoid domain, which silences the AS gene (bottom part of figure).

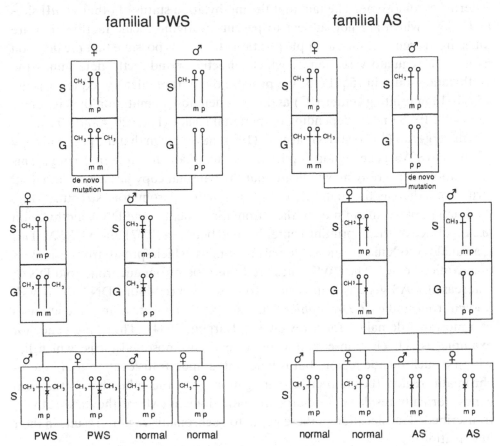

Fig. 20.5. Imprinting mutation model in familial PWS and AS. In somatic cells, the maternal chromosome 15 is methylated and the paternal chromosome 15 is unmethylated at the D15S63 locus. The imprint is reset in the germline. Sperm cells carry only the paternal PW71 methylation imprint (Dittrich *et al.*, 1993). Oocytes are assumed to carry the maternal methylation imprint. A *de novo* mutation in 15q11–13 in the grandmaternal germline results in failure to reset the imprint in the paternal germline (left-hand side of diagram). The phenotypically normal father will transmit this chromosome to 50% of his offspring. As the PWS gene(s) on this chromosome remain(s) silent, the children will have PWS. In analogy, a grandpaternal germline mutation transmitted through a normal female carrier will lead to familial recurrence of AS (right-hand side of diagram). X, mutation; S, somatic cells; G, germline cells; m, maternal; p, paternal. (Reprinted from Reis *et al.*, 1994; © The American Society of Human Genetics.)

possible that the full PWS phenotype requires the inactivation of additional genes, by deletion, uniparental disomy or – as suggested by our findings – aberrant imprinting.

It is unclear why the microdeletions change the methylation imprint on the paternal chromosome. The fact that the methylation status of other *Hpa*II sites at D15S63 which are not subject to parent-of-origin-specific methylation are unchanged argues against a simple position effect. It is possible that the deletion includes a regulatory sequence, which directly or indirectly determines the methylation status in 15q11–13. We propose that this regulatory sequence is the 15q11–13 imprinting center (IC) and that a deletion or mutation of this center can cause PWS or AS, depending on parental legacy (Figs. 20.4 and 20.5).

Kitsberg *et al.* (1993) and Knoll *et al.* (1994) have shown that the paternal copy of the PWS/AS gene region replicates earlier than the maternal copy. This replication asynchrony may indicate that the paternal copy has a euchromatoid structure, whereas the maternal copy has a heterochromatoid structure (Fig. 20.4, upper part). In our model, the chromatin structure and DNA methylation are regulated by the imprinting center located between PW71 and *SNRPN*. This is an analogy to X inactivation in female mammals, which spreads from a single X inactivation center. The PWS genes are transcribed from euchromatoid DNA, whereas the AS gene is transcribed from heterochromatoid DNA. It is well known from studies in *Drosophila* that transcriptional states can correlate with chromosomal domains (for a review see Karpen, 1994). The *white* gene, for example, is actively transcribed at its normal chromosomal locus, which lies within a euchromatic region, but is inactivated upon translocation to a hetero-chromatic region (position-effect variegation). On the other hand, the *light* genes normally reside in a heterochromatic domain, where they are actively transcribed. Translocation of these genes to euchromatic regions results in their inactivation.

In the PWS and AS families discussed above, an imprinting center mutation in a parent may have prevented the resetting of the imprint in the germline (Fig. 20.5). Consequently, both chromosomes of the patient have a heterochromatoid domain, which silences the PWS genes (Fig. 20.4, middle part), or a eu-chromatoid domain, which silences the AS gene (Fig. 20.4, bottom). From this model we would predict (i) that the maternal and paternal copies of 15q11–13 replicate synchronously in these patients and (ii) that these AS patients have a deletion or mutation in the same region that is deleted in the PWS patients, i.e. proximal to *SNRPN*. These predictions are currently being tested.

The nature of the putative imprinting center remains to be elucidated. Detailed mapping of the breakpoints in the patients discussed above should make it possible to narrow down the location of the imprinting center to a few kilobases. In view of the analogy of the imprinting process to the X inactivation process, it may be possible to identify homologous DNA sequences. The molecular identification of the imprinting center will be a major step forward in understanding genomic imprinting in 15q11–13 and other chromosome regions.

Acknowledgements

Part of this work was supported by the Deutsche Forschungsgemeinschaft. We thank S. Groβ and S. Kaya-Westerloh for expert technical assistance, and Drs D. Abeliovich, M. Anvret, G. Gillessen-Kaesbach, M. Guitart, D. H. Ledbetter, E. Passarge, A. Reis and W. P. Robinson for collaboration.

References

Barlow, D. P. (1993). Methylation and imprinting: From host defense to gene regulation? *Science* **260**, 309–10.

Buiting, K., Dittrich, B., Groβ, S., Greger, V., Lalande, M., Robinson, W. P., Mutiranagura, A., Ledbetter, D. & Horsthemke, B. (1993). Molecular definition of the Prader–Willi syndrome chromosome region and orientation of the *SNRPN* gene. *Hum. molec. Genet.* **2**, 1991–4.

Buiting, K., Dittrich, B., Robinson, W. P., Guitart, M., Abeliovich, D., Lerer, I. & Horsthemke, B. (1994). Detection of aberrant DNA methylation in unique Prader–Willi syndrome patients and its diagnostic implications. *Hum. molec. Genet.* **3**, 893–5.

Buiting, K., Neumann, M., Lüdecke, H. J., Senger, G., Claussen, U., Antich, J., Passarge, E. & Horsthemke, B. (1990). Microdissection of the Prader–Willi syndrome chromosome region and identification of potential gene sequences. *Genomics* **6**, 521–7.

Burke, C. M., Kouseff, B. G., Gleeson, M., O'Connell, B. M. & Devlin, J. G. (1987). Familial Prader–Willi syndrome. *Arch. int. Med.* **147**, 673–5.

Chaillet, J. R., Vogt, T. F., Beier, D. R. & Leder, P. (1991). Parental-specific methylation of an imprinted transgene is established during gametogenesis and progressively changes during embryogenesis. *Cell* **66**, 77–83.

Chang-Yeh, A., Mold, D. E. & Huang, R. C. (1991). Identification of a novel murine IAP-promoted placenta-expressed gene. *Nucleic Acids Res.* **19**, 3667–72.

Clayton-Smith, J., Webb, T., Robb, S. A., Dijkstra, I., Willems, P., Lam, S., Chen, X.-J. *et al.* (1992). Further evidence for dominant inheritance at the chromosome 15q11–13 locus in familial Angelman syndrome. *Am. J. Hum. Genet.* **44**, 256–60.

Dittrich, B., Buiting, K., Groβ, S. & Horsthemke, B. (1993). Characterization of a methylation imprint in the Prader–Willi syndrome region. *Hum. molec. Genet.* **2**, 1995–9.

Dittrich, B., Robinson, W. P., Knoblauch, H., Buiting, K., Schmidt, K., Gillessen-Kaesbach, G. & Horsthemke, B. (1992). Molecular diagnosis of the Prader–Willi and Angelman syndromes by detection of parent-of-origin-specific DNA methylation in 15q11–13. *Hum. Genet.* **90**, 313–15.

Driscoll, D. J., Waters, M. F., Williams, C. A., Zori, R. T., Glenn, C. C., Avidano, K. M. & Nicholls, R. D. (1992). A DNA methylation imprint, determined by the sex of the parent, distinguishes the Angelman and Prader–Willi syndromes. *Genomics* **13**, 917–24.

Eden, S. & Cedar, H. (1994). Role of DNA methylation in the regulation of transcription. *Curr. Opin. Genet. Devel.* **4**, 255–9.

Ferguson-Smith, A. C., Sasaki, H., Cattanach, B. M. & Surani, M. A. (1993). Parental-origin-specific epigenetic modification of the mouse *H19* gene. *Nature* **362**, 751–5.

Furter, C. S., Heizmann, C. & Berchthold, M. W. (1989). Isolation and analysis of a rat genomic clone containing a long terminal repeat with high similarity to the oncomodulin mRNA leader sequence. *J. biol. Chem.* **264**, 18276–79.

Gillessen-Kaesbach, G., Gross, S., Kaya-Westerloh, S., Passarge, E. & Horsthemke, B. (1995). DNA methylation based testing of 450 patients suspected of having Prader–Willi syndrome. *J. med. Genet.* **32**, 88–92.

Glenn, C. C., Nicholls, R. D., Robinson, W. P., Saitoh, S., Nikawa, N., Schinzel, A., Horsthemke, B. & Driscoll, D. J. (1993a). Modification of 15q11–13 DNA methylation imprints in unique Angelman and Prader–Willi patients. *Hum. molec. Genet.* **9**, 1377–82.

Glenn, C. C., Porter, K. A., Jong, M. T. C., Nicholls, R. D. & Driscoll, D. J. (1993b). Functional imprinting and epigenetic modification of the human SNRPN gene. *Hum. molec. Genet.* **2**, 2001–5.

Ishikawa, T., Kanayama, M. & Wada, Y. (1987). Prader–Willi syndrome in two siblings: One with normal karyotype, one with a terminal deletion of distal Xq. *Clin. Genet.* **32**, 295–9.

Izumikawa, Y., Naritomi, K. & Hirayama, K. (1991). Replication asynchrony between homologs 15q11.2: Cytogenetic evidence for genomic imprinting. *Hum. Genet.* **87**, 1–5.

Kaplan, L. C., Wharton, R., Elias, E., Mandell, F., Donlon, T. & Latt, S. A. (1987). Clinical heterogeneity associated with deletions in the long arm of chromosome 15: report of 3 new cases and their possible significance. *Am. J. med. Genet.* **28**, 45–53.

Karpen, G. H. (1994). Position-effect variegation and the new biology of heterochromatin. *Curr. Opin. Genet. Devel.* **4**, 281–91.

Kitsberg, D., Selig, S., Brandeis, M., Simon, I., Keshet, I., Driscoll, D. J., Nicholls, R. D. & Cedar, H. (1993). Allele-specific replication timing of imprinted gene regions. *Nature* **364**, 459–63.

Knoll, J. H. M., Cheng, S.-D. & Lalande, M. (1994). Allele specificity of DNA replication timing in the Angelman/Prader-Willi syndrome imprinted chromosomal region. *Nature Genet.* **6**, 41–6.

Knoll, J. H. M., Nicholls, R. D., Magenis, R. E., Graham, J. M., Jr., Lalande, M. & Latt, S. A. (1989). Angelman and Prader–Willi syndrome share a common chromosome 15 deletion but differ in parental origin of the deletion. *Am. J. med. Genet.* **32**, 285–90.

Ledbetter, D., Riccardi, V. M., Airhart, S. D., Strobel, R. J., Keenan, B. S. & Crawford, J. D. (1981). Deletions of chromosome 15 as a cause of the Prader–Willi syndrome. *New Engl. J. Med.* **304**, 325–9.

Lubinsky, M., Zellweger, H., Greenswag, L., Larson, G., Hansmann, I. & Ledbetter, D. (1987). Familial Prader–Willi syndrome with apparently normal chromosomes. *Am. J. med. Genet.* **28**, 37–43.

Magenis, R. E., Brown, M. G., Lacy, D. A., Budden, S. & LaFranchi, S. (1987) Is Angelman syndrome an alternate result of del(15)(q11q13)? *Am. J. med. Genet.* **28**, 829–38.

Malcolm, S., Clayton-Smith, J., Nichols, M., Robb, S., Well, T., Armour, J. A. L., Jeffreys, A. J. *et al.* (1991). Uniparental paternal disomy in Angelman's syndrome. *Lancet* **337**, 694–7.

Meijers-Heijboer, E. J., Sandkuijl, L. A., Brunner, H. G., Smeets, H. J. M., Hoogeboom, A. J. M., Deelen, W. H., van Hemel, J. O. *et al.* (1992). Linkage analysis with chromosome 15q11–13 markers shows genomic imprinting in familial Angelman syndrome. *J. med. Genet.* **29**, 853–7.

Mutirangura, A., Jayakumar, A., Sutcliffe, J. S., Nakao, M., McKinney, M. J., Buiting, K., Horsthemke, B. *et al.* (1993). A complete YAC contig of the Prader–Willi/Angelman chromosome region (15q11-q13) and refined localization of the SNRPN gene. *Genomics* **18**, 546–52.

Nakao, M., Sutcliffe, J. S., Durtschi, B., Mutirangura, A., Ledbetter, D. H. & Beaudet, A. L. (1994). Imprinting analysis of three genes in the Prader–Willi/Angelman region: SNRPN, E6-associated protein, and PAR-2 (D15S225E). *Hum. molec. Genet.* **3**, 309–15.

Nicholls, R. D. (1993). Genomic imprinting and candidate genes in the Prader–Willi and Angelman syndromes. *Curr. Opin. Genet. Devel.* **3**, 445–56.

Nicholls, R. D., Knoll, J. H. M., Butler, M. G., Karam, S. & Lalande, M. (1989). Genetic imprinting suggested by maternal heterodisomy in non-deletion Prader–Willi syndrome. *Nature* **342**, 281–5.

Örstavik, K. H., Tangsrud, S. E., Kiil, R., Hansteen, IL, Steen-Johnson, J., Cassidy, S. B., Marony, A. *et al.* (1992). Prader–Willi syndrome in a brother and sister without cytogenetic or detectable molecular genetic abnormality at chromosome 15q11q13. *Am. J. med. Genet.* **44**, 534–8.

Özcelik, T., Leff, S., Robinson, W., Donlon, T., Lalande, M., Sanjines, E., Schinzel, A. & Francke, U. (1992). Small nuclear ribonucleoprotein polypeptide N (SNRPN), an expressed gene in the Prader–Willi syndrome critical region. *Nature Genet.* **2**, 265–9.

Pembrey, M., Fennell, S. J., van den Berghe, J., Fitchett, M., Summers, D., Butler, L., Clarke C. *et al.* (1989) The association of Angelman's syndrome with deletions within 15q11–13. *J. med. Genet.* **26**, 73–7.

Reis, A., Dittrich, B., Greger, V., Buiting, K., Lalande, M., Gillessen-Kaesbach, G., Anvret, M. & Horsthemke, B. (1994). Imprinting mutations suggested by abnormal DNA methylation patterns in familial Angelman and Prader–Willi syndromes. *Am. J. Hum. Genet.* **54**, 741–7.

Saitoh, S., Kubota, T., Ohta, T., Jinno, Y., Niikawa, N., Sugimoto, T., Wagstaff, J. *et al.* (1992). Familial Angelman syndrome caused by imprinted submicroscopic deletion encompassing GABA$_A$ receptor β_3-subunit gene. *Lancet* **339**, 366–7.

Stöger, R., Kubicka, P., Liu, C. G., Kafri, T., Razin, A., Cedar, H. & Barlow, D. P. (1993). Maternal-specific methylation of the imprinted mouse *Igf2r* locus identifies the expressed locus as carrying the imprinting signal. *Cell* **73**, 61–71.

Sutcliffe, J. S., Nakao, M., Mutirangura, A., Christian, S., Ledbetter, D. H. & Beaudet, A. L. (1994). Physical mapping and isolation of expressed sequences in the Prader–Willi/Angelman critical region of chromosome 15q11-q13. In: Report of the Second International Workshop on Human Chromosome 15 Mapping. *Cytogenet. Cell Genet.* **67**, 1–22.

Wagstaff, J., Knoll, J. H. M., Fleming, J., Kirkness, E. F., Martin-Gallardo, A., Greenberg, F., Graham J. M., Jr., Menninger, J., Ward, D., Venter, C. & Lalande, M. (1991). Localization of the gene encoding the GABA$_A$ receptor β_3 subunit to the Angelman/Prader–Willi region of human chromosome 15. *Am. J. Hum. Genet.* **49**, 330–7.

Wagstaff, J., Knoll, J. H. M., Glatt, K. A., Shugart, Y. Y., Sommer, A. & Lalande, M. (1992). Maternal but not paternal transmission of 15qq11-q13-linked nondeletion Angelman syndrome leads to phenotypic expression. *Nature Genet.* **1**, 291–4.
Wagstaff, J., Shugart, Y. Y. & Lalande, M. (1993). Linkage analysis in familial Angelman syndrome. *Am. J. Hum. Genet.* **53**, 105–12.

Note added in proof, December 1994

As predicted in this chapter, our group and Dr Nicholls' group have recently found mutations between D15S63 and *SNRPN* in AS imprinting mutation families (Buiting, K., Saitoh, S., Groβ, S., Dittrich, B., Schartz, S., Nicholls, R. D. & Horsthemke, B. (1995). Inherited microdeletions in the Angelman and Prader–Willi syndromes define an imprinting center on human chromosome 15. *Nature Genet.* **9**, 395–400.

21

The SNRPN gene and Prader–Willi syndrome

UTA FRANCKE, JULIE A. KERNS AND JOSEPH GIACALONE

Clinical and cytogenetic features of Prader–Willi (PWS) and Angelman (AS) syndromes

Recognized as a clinical entity in 1956, PWS was named after Andrea Prader, a pediatric endocrinologist in Zürich who, together with his colleagues A. Labhart and H. Willi, described nine patients with obesity, short stature, cryptorchidism and oligophrenia, following transient severe hypotonia in the newborn period (Prader *et al.*, 1956). The etiology of the condition remained unknown for decades. The majority of cases are sporadic with an estimated recurrence risk of less than 0.1% (Cassidy, 1987). It was hypothesized early that a primary developmental defect in the hypothalamus could be responsible for the clinical findings (Table 21.1). Starting in 1976, various abnormalities involving chromosome 15 were reported, including Robertsonian and reciprocal translocations, both balanced and unbalanced, isochromosomes for the long arm, and additional small metacentric markers derived from chromosome 15. These rare and inconsistent karyotypic abnormalities did not suggest a straightforward hypothesis of PWS being due to a distinct chromosomal imbalance. In 1981, high resolution chromosome banding studies revealed small interstitial deletions of the 15q11–q13 region in a large proportion of PWS patients (Ledbetter *et al.*, 1981, 1982). Cases with apparently normal karyotypes were speculated to have submicroscropic deletions or somatic mosaicism.

The unique pathogenetic relationship between the apparent chromosome 15 deletion and the PWS phenotype was challenged when, in 1987, an identical deletion was reported in patients with a congenital disorder quite different from PWS (Magenis *et al.*, 1987). The features of Angelman syndrome (AS), named after the author of the first report in 1965, include microcephaly, jerky movements, seizures, a peculiar face with prominent chin, large mouth with protruding tongue, absence of speech, and inappropriate laughter (Angelman, 1965).

309

Table 21.1. *Criteria for clinical diagnosis of PWS*

Major criteria
  1. Neonatal/infantile central hypotonia
  2. Feeding problems/failure to thrive in infancy
  3. Rapid weight gain after 12 months
  4. Facial features: narrow bifrontal diameter, almond-shaped eyes
  5. Hypogonadism
  6. Mild/moderate developmental delay
  7. Hyperphagia

Minor criteria
  1. Decreased fetal movement; infantile lethargy, improving with age
  2. Behavior problems; obsessive/compulsive, rigid, stubborn
  3. Sleep disturbance/apnea
  4. Short stature by age 15
  5. Hypopigmentation
  6. Small hands and feet for height age
  7. Narrow hands with straight ulnar border
  8. Esotropia, myopia
  9. Thick viscous saliva
 10. Speech articulation defects
 11. Skin picking

Other findings
  1. High pain threshold
  2. Decreased vomiting
  3. Temperature control problems
  4. Scoliosis and/or kyphosis
  5. Early adrenarche
  6. Osteoporosis
  7. Unusual skill with jigsaw puzzles
  8. Normal neuromuscular studies
  9. Lack of spermatogenesis

Source: Modified from Holm *et al.* (1993).

Mental retardation is more severe in AS than in PWS patients. The fact that the dysmorphic, neurologic and behavioral findings are strikingly distinct excludes the possibility that the two entities represent extreme ends of a spectrum of overlapping microdeletions. The deletions of the 15q11–q13 region in PWS and AS appear cytogenetically similar, if not identical (Magenis *et al.*, 1990).

Prader–Willi and Angelman syndromes involve oppositely imprinted genes

This puzzle was solved when it was discovered that deletions in PWS always involve the paternally derived chromosome 15 (Butler & Palmer, 1983) whereas deletions in AS involve the maternally derived copy (Magenis *et al.*, 1990). Furthermore, in many PWS individuals with structurally and numerically normal karyotypes, both copies of 15 are maternally derived with no paternal copy present (uniparental disomy, UPD) (Nicholls *et al.*, 1989). In AS, a very small fraction of cases has paternal UPD. This is not surprising: maternal disomy is thought to arise by 'disomic rescue' of a conceptus with trisomy 15, and the meiotic origin of any non-disjoined chromosome is predominantly maternal (Cassidy *et al.*, 1992; Purvis-Smith *et al.*, 1992). Classically affected cases with neither deletion nor UPD are extremely rare for PWS but constitute about 30% of patients with AS. It is likely, therefore, that PWS is a true microdeletion syndrome that requires the silencing or deletion of more than one locus normally expressed only from the paternally derived chromosome 15, whereas a single deleted or mutant gene on the maternally derived chromosome could suffice to generate the AS phenotype, owing to loss of expression of an exclusively maternally expressed gene.

Molecular delineation of minimal deletion regions for PWS and AS

An interesting question with respect to the mechanism of monoallelic expression due to parent-of-origin-specific imprinting is whether the oppositely imprinted genes responsible for PWS and AS are intermingled, alternating or confined to distinct subregions. In the majority of PWS and AS cases the deletions are quite similar at the molecular level and extend from a breakpoint proximal to the molecular marker D15S9 (derived from an expressed gene *ZNF127*) (Driscoll *et al.*, 1992) to a breakpoint distal to marker D15S12 (representing the non-imprinted *P* locus involved in tyrosinase-positive oculocutaneous albinism) (Gardner *et al.*, 1992) (Fig. 21.1). These common deletions, estimated to span 3–5 megabase pairs, are detectable by high-resolution banding cytogenetic analysis (Labidi & Cassidy, 1986; Magenis *et al.*, 1990).

The discovery of a few unusual patients, who appear to have the full syndrome in the presence of submicroscopic deletions, has allowed the subdivisions of the region into a PWS minimal deletion region (PWCR) and a distally adjacent Angelman chromosome region (ANCR) (Fig. 21.1). In a three-generation Japanese family, a woman who inherited a submicroscopic deletion from her father was phenotypically normal and did not have any features of PWS, but her three children, who inherited her chromosome 15 with the deletion, were

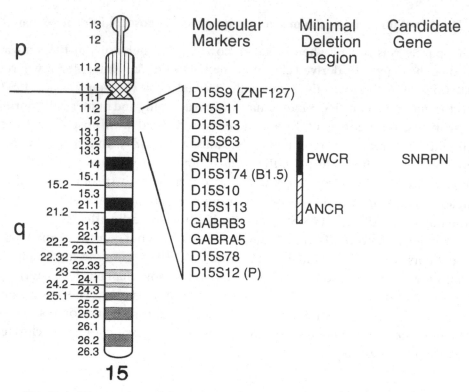

Fig. 21.1. The common deletion region (15q11.2–q13.1) in Prader–Willi and Angelman syndromes, with ideogram of human chromosome 15 from Francke (1994) and order of molecular markers within the deletion from Buiting *et al.* (1993). The minimal deletion region for Prader–Willi syndrome (PWCR) extends from a breakpoint near D15S63 (PW71) to D15S174 (B1.5; Greger *et al.*, 1993) and the Angelman syndrome region (ANCR) from D15S174 to a breakpoint within GABRB3, the gene for the β$_3$-GABA$_A$ receptor (Wagstaff *et al.*, 1991). *SNRPN* is the only candidate gene encoding a defined protein that has been identified so far within either PWCR or ANCR.

affected with AS (Hamabe *et al.* 1991; Saitoh *et al.*, 1992). The deletion in this family delimits the ANCR. The proximal deletion junction fragment D15S174 (clone pB1.5) demarcates the distal border of the PWCR (Greger *et al.*, 1993). The proximal border of the PWCR is defined by a PWS patient with another partial deletion (PW63) (Robinson *et al.*, 1991). Based on analysis of a yeast artificial chromosome contig, the size of the PWCR has been estimated as 320 kb (Buiting *et al.*, 1993).

Mapping of the gene for small nuclear ribonucleoprotein polypeptide N (*SNRPN*) to the PWS minimal deletion region and to the homologous region on mouse chromosome 7

The first gene encoding a defined protein that was mapped to the PWCR was *SNRPN*, the gene for small nuclear ribonucleoprotein particle (snRNP)-associated polypeptide SmN (or N) (Özçelik *et al.*, 1992). Processing of primary RNA transcripts is carried out by nuclear structures, called spliceosomes, that consist of several snRNPs and other proteins (Guthrie, 1991). A single snRNP (U snRNP) contains a small nuclear RNA molecule of type U1, U2, U4, U5 or U6 and up to 10 different proteins. The autoimmune antiserum anti-Sm, found in patients with systemic lupus erythematosus (Lerner & Steitz, 1979), reacts with several snRNP-associated proteins, such as the ubiquitous B and the neuron-specific N polypeptides. The *SNRPN* gene encoding the N protein has been cloned by three different groups (McAllister *et al.*, 1988; Li *et al.*, 1989; Rokeach *et al.*, 1989). The predicted polypeptide sequence of N is highly similar to that of B, which is encoded by the *SNRPB* gene on human chromosome 20 (Schmauss *et al.*, 1992; our unpublished results).

Whereas Schmauss *et al.* (1992) reported an assignment of the *SNRPN* gene to chromosome 4, our laboratory (Özçelik *et al.*, 1992) has mapped *SNRPN* to chromosome 15, and further to region 15pter–q14, by studying our somatic cell hybrid mapping panels. A processed pseudogene (*SNRPNP1*) was identified and mapped to chromosome 6, region pter–p21. By using DNA from exceptional PWS and AS patients with partial 15q12 deletions for comparative dosage blotting experiments, we were able to map the *SNRPN* gene to the PWCR and to exclude it from the ANCR (Fig. 21.1) (Özçelik *et al.*, 1992). The mouse homolog *Snrpn* was similarly mapped to mouse chromosome 7 by Southern analysis of rodent × mouse somatic cell hybrid panels, and a processed pseudogene was identified and mapped to mouse chromosome 14 (Özçelik *et al.*, 1992). Mapping by interspecies backcross analysis further refined the location of the *Snrpn* gene to a chromosome 7 region of known homology with the human 15q11.2–q12 region (Leff *et al.*, 1992).

The *SNRPN* gene is imprinted in mouse

A sequence polymorphism that distinguishes between the *Snrpn* transcripts of *Mus musculus* and *M. spretus* was exploited in an RNase protection assay to study allele-specific expression in offspring of interspecies crosses. Results of crosses in both directions confirmed that in the mouse brain the *Snrpn* gene is expressed exclusively from the paternal allele, as one would expect for a gene

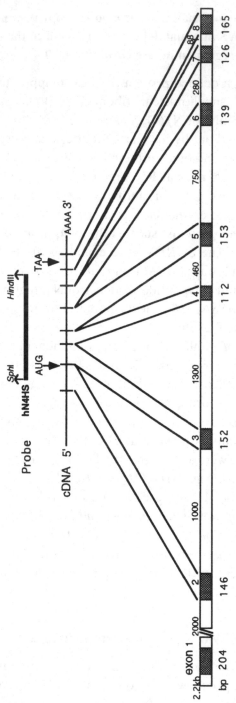

Fig. 21.2. Structure of the human *SNRPN* gene (updated from Özçelik *et al.*, 1992, and from Schmauss *et al.*, 1992). The initiation codon AUG is in exon 2 and the first amino acid codon in exon 3. Additional 5′ exons are under investigation.

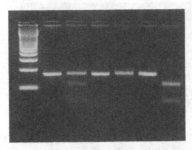

Fig. 21.3. C/T sequence polymorphism in exon 2 of the *SNRPN* gene, detected by *Bst*UI cleavage of PCR products. The 171 bp product was generated from PCR primers within exon 2 as described by Giacalone & Francke (1994). Lane 1, size markers, 100 bp ladder; lane 2, human DNA sample A, uncut; lane 3, sample A, *Bst*UI digested; lane 4, human DNA sample B, uncut; lane 5, sample B, *Bst*UI digested; lane 6, human DNA sample C, uncut; lane 7, sample C, *Bst*UI digested. Sample A is heterozygous C/T, sample B is homozygous T/T and sample C is homozygous C/C.

involved in the PWS phenotype (Leff *et al.*, 1992). Subsequently, the region of mouse chromosome 7 that is inserted into the X chromosome in Cattanach's translocation *Is(In7;X)1Ct* (Francke & Nesbitt, 1971) and contains the region homologous to the PWS/AS deletion region was tested for imprinting effects (Cattanach *et al.*, 1992). Differential recovery was observed for the maternal duplication offspring only. The *Snrpn* gene was not expressed in these maternal UPD mice, who suffered early postnatal death, possibly associated with reduced suckling activity. Paternal duplication mice were indistinguishable from normal littermates. These data suggest that maternal duplication of the central region of chromosome 7 could represent a mouse model for PWS, but they do not allow one to estimate how many genes besides *Snrpn* might be responsible for the phenotypic effects. In fact, the region of mouse chromosome 7 that is maternally duplicated in these *Is1Ct*-derived mice involves bands C to E (Nesbitt & Francke, 1973). Thus, it is four times the size of the PWS/AS deletion region and contains genes that have homologs on human chromosomes other than 15.

The *SNRPN* gene is imprinted in human fetal brain and cell lines

To determine whether *SNRPN* is also uniparentally expressed in humans, we have searched for polymorphisms within the transcribed region. PCR amplification and sequencing of the 8 characterized exons (Fig. 21.2) from ten unrelated human control samples yielded a single polymorphism. In the 5′ untranslated

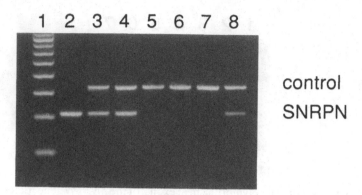

Fig. 21.4. *SNRPN* expression detected by amplification of reverse-transcribed RNA. Lane 1, 100 bp ladder; lane 2, human fibroblast control; lane 3, human uncultured leukocyte control; lane 4, human lymphoblastoid cell line control; lanes 5 and 6, lymphoblastoid cell lines from deletion PWS patients; lane 7, fresh leukocytes from non-deletion PWS patient; lane 8, lymphoblastoid cell line from deletion AS patient. The control primers amplify a lymphocyte-specific gene product present in lanes 2–8. *SNRPN* primers were derived from exons 3 and 4 and are separated by a 1300 bp intron (primers C and D described by Özçelik *et al.*, 1992). No amplification was observed in the absence of reverse transcriptase.

region at position 55 of exon 2 of the published cDNA sequence (Schmauss *et al.*, 1989), a C or a T is present at equal frequency within the sequence CC C/T GCG (Giacalone & Francke, 1994). The level of heterozygosity was 50% in the 104 individuals tested by us and also in the 36 fetal samples tested by Reed & Leff (1994). The presence of a C in this position generates a *BstU*I site (CGCG) that allowed us to develop a PCR–RFLP assay for this polymorphism (Giacalone & Francke, 1994) (Fig. 21.3). When applied to RT–PCR products of total mRNA from tissues, this assay should detect uniparental *SNRPN* expression in any heterozygous individual. By direct sequencing of RT–PCR products, mono-allelic expression was demonstrated in 18 brain RNAs, and the expressed allele was shown to be of paternal origin in four informative samples (Reed & Leff, 1994). These data are consistent with reported observations on lack of ectopic expression of *SNRPN*, detectable only by RT–PCR in cell lines from normal individuals, in transformed lymphoblasts and in fibroblasts from PWS patients (Glenn *et al.*, 1993; Nakao *et al.*, 1994). As shown in Fig. 21.4, no amplification product is obtained with *SNRPN*-specific primers from RNA of deletion PWS lymphoblastoid cell lines or leukocytes from a non-deletion PWS patient, whereas normal cells and deletion AS lymphoblasts express *SNRPN* mRNA.

Mutation search in non-deleted PWS patients with biparental inheritance

By virtue of its location in the PWCR and its uniparental expression from the paternal chromosome, *SNRPN* is the first, and so far the only, candidate gene for the etiology of the PWS phenotype. To evaluate whether *SNRPN* is solely responsible for the PWS phenotype, we need to find a mutation in the paternally derived copy of the gene in a classically affected PWS patient without a chromosome abnormality. Unfortunately, PWS in the absence of either deletion or UPD is extremely rare, possibly because the *SNRPN* gene does not constitute a large target for mutational events. The 1.6 kb cDNA contains 720 nucleotides that encode 240 amino acids and are distributed over 7 coding exons (Fig. 21.2). The total genomic size, including at least three 5' non-coding exons (U. Francke, unpublished data), is less than 25 kb.

In a Scandinavian family (Orstavik *et al.*, 1992), two siblings were diagnosed with PWS after the first child had died from severe hypotonia in the newborn period. Cytogenetic studies were normal and UPD was excluded for markers spanning the region. Through Dr Maria Anvret, our laboratory has obtained DNA samples from the affected sibs and both parents. When dosage blotting revealed no deletion or rearrangement of the *SNRPN* gene with a probe spanning exons 2–7 (Özçelik *et al.*, 1992), we carried out exon-by-exon amplification and DNA sequencing. The entire coding sequence was found to be normal in one affected child and in both parents, and all three samples were heterozygous for the C/T polymorphism in exon 2. These results rule out an intragenic deletion or a point mutation of the *SNRPN* gene in this family. We were unable to obtain additional DNA samples for methylation studies or live cells for expression studies.

Likewise, patients with some features of PWS, but not meeting the diagnostic criteria (Table 21.1) (Holm *et al.*, 1993), have been studied for *SNRPN* deletions or gene rearrangements, with negative results (Özçelik *et al.*, 1992). In one such case, the *SNRPN* coding exons have also been sequenced, but no mutation was found (J. P. Giacalone, G. Fekete & U. Francke, unpublished data).

Parent-of-origin-specific methylation at CpG sites: a manifestation of imprinting?

Methylation differences have been evaluated with probes throughout the common PWS/AS deletion region (Driscoll *et al.*, 1992). Consistent differences in the PWS critical region were first found with probe PW71 (locus D15S63), which recognizes a sequence of unknown function located 130 kb centromeric to the 5' end of the *SNRPN* gene (Dittrich *et al.*, 1993). Similarly, a *Hpa*II site and a *Hha*I site in intron 5 of the *SNRPN* gene are resistant to digestion in leukocyte DNA from deletion AS patients (paternal gene present) and are partly cleaved in DNA from PWS deletion patients (maternal chromosome only) (Glenn *et al.*, 1993). The conclusion was made that there is a methylated site (or sites) in intron 5 of the paternally derived *SNRPN* allele. The significance of these observations is difficult to determine, as *SNRPN* is not normally expressed in leukocytes to any detectable degree on Northern blots (in contrast to the spurious or ectopic expression detectable in normal EBV-transformed lymphoblasts or fibroblasts by the highly sensitive RT–PCR method). Most recently, Reis *et al.* (1994) have presented evidence for altered methylation patterns at sites that were biparentally present in two PWS families and suggested that localized small deletions can affect methylation and gene expression in *cis* over considerable chromosomal distances.

In order to evaluate the role of differential methylation at the *SNRPN* locus by a systematic approach, our laboratory has cloned and almost completely sequenced the entire *SNRPN* gene, including all introns and flanking sequences. The number and position of all potentially methylatable CpG sites is being determined; more than 26 recognition sites for seven different methylation-sensitive enzymes have been identified so far. We intend to study the methylation status of these CpG sites in fresh leukocyte DNA from PWS and AS deletion patients and their parents, as well as in DNA from human fetal brains where *SNRPN* is highly expressed, in the hope that expression data can be correlated directly with the methylation status of specific sites within and around the *SNRPN* locus at different stages of development.

SNRPN as a candidate gene for PWS phenotype

SNRPN is an attractive candidate gene based on functional considerations. It is the only known protein component of snRNP splicing particles that shows tissue-specific and developmental regulation of expression as demonstrated by Northern and Western blotting. *In situ* hybridization studies have demonstrated high levels of *SNRPN* expression in neurons of all areas of the brains studied, with particularly high concentration in the primary olfactory cortex, hippocampus, hypothalamic and brain stem nuclei, and spinal cord (Schmauss *et al.*, 1992; Horn *et al.*, 1992; Grimaldi *et al.*, 1993). Non-neuronal cells in brain do not express *SNRPN*. The only other mammalian tissues where *SNRPN* is expressed, albeit at lower levels, are pituitary gland and heart. Expression has also been reported in cultured cell lines, such as PC12 cells (pheochromocytoma); TT cells (medullary thyroid carcinoma); Raji cells; embryonal stem cells; and embryonal carcinoma cell lines (McAllister *et al.*, 1989; Schmauss *et al.*, 1989; Sharpe *et al.*, 1990).

When considering any possible effects of loss of *SNRPN* expression, one has to take into account the *SNRPB* gene, which (in humans only) gives rise to two alternatively spliced products, B and B', that only differ at the carboxy-terminal end (VanDam *et al.*, 1989). The amino acid sequences of B and N are 93% identical. B is ubiquitously expressed and considered a core protein of U snRNPs. In the heart, where both N and B are expressed, their relative levels – low N and high B – remain constant throughout development (Grimaldi *et al.*, 1993). In the brains of mice and rats there is a developmental shift, with exclusive expression of B in early embryonic life. N expression starts in late gestation and keeps increasing as B expression is down-regulated. In adult neurons, the B snRNP core protein is completely replaced by N (Grimaldi *et al.*, 1993). The functional significance of this developmental- and cell-type-specific switch is unknown. By using monoclonal antibodies, Huntriss *et al.* (1993) have investigated the localization of N and B polypeptides within snRNP particles in cell lines and tissues. When N was expressed at low levels and B was also present, N was detected only in U2 snRNPs and B in both U1 and U2 snRNPs. When N was present at high levels, replacing B as in neuronal cells, it was found to be incorporated into both U1 and U2 snRNPs.

The neuron-specific expression of *SNRPN* suggested that N-containing snRNP particles may have a brain-specific function, e.g. neuron-specific splicing of differentially spliced genes such as the calcitonin/calcitonin gene-related peptide (CGRP) transcript (McAllister *et al.*, 1988; Li *et al.*, 1989). Co-occurrence of CGRP production and N expression in some tissues and cell lines made this hypothesis attractive, but recently Delsert & Rosenfeld (1992) have presented experimental evidence that N is neither sufficient nor required for the neuron-specific CGRP splicing decision. Similarly, tissue-specific splicing of NCAM and SRC did not correlate with the presence of N (Horn & Latchman, 1993).

Because N is replacing the ubiquitous B in neuronal cells, it must be involved in carrying out all the splicing functions rather than having a limited role in neuron-specific alternative splicing events. One speculation about the pathogenetic mechanism of *SNRPN* deficiency assumes that, in the absence of *SNRPN* expression, no N-containing snRNPs would be made. The absence of these particles might not affect all of the central nervous system neurons equally but may be particularly important for areas of the hypothalamus, where centers responsible for the regulation of muscle tone, growth, appetite control, temperature control and pain sensitivity, all systems affected in PWS, are located (Table 21.1). In another possible scenario, lack of *SNRPN* expression would have a detrimental effect on overall brain function that could be overcome if *SNRPB* were re-expressed or never turned off in neuronal tissues. Coordinate regulation of two unlinked gene loci is a distinct possibility. If there were such a (hypothetical) feed-back loop, *SNRPB* expression may not be turned off in the absence of a functional *SNRPN* gene. To test this hypothesis it will be necessary to obtain PWS brain tissues, to study the experimental mouse model with maternal duplication of central chromosome 7 (Cattanach *et al.*, 1992), or await the arrival of an *Snrpn* knock-out mouse.

Although *SNRPN* is a promising candidate gene for the hypothalamic manifestations, most PWS patients have deletions that extend far beyond the PWCR and include many more genes. In addition, the concept of the 320 kb PWCR as containing all relevant genes has to be regarded with caution, because a localized structural change could have a long-range effect on the behavior of the entire region. This region is known to behave differently with respect to the timing of replication on the maternal and the paternal chromosome 15 in cells from normal individuals (Kitsberg *et al.*, 1993). Genes outside of the deleted PWCR whose pattern of methylation, replication and expression has been altered by the deletion may contribute to the phenotype. It will be necessary, therefore, to identify all genes in the region that are potentially involved before accepting the hypothesis that *SNRPN* is a major, or the only, player in the pathogenesis of PWS.

Acknowledgements

We thank Rachel Wevrick for figures and critical reading of the manuscript. The work was supported by NIH research grants and the Howard Hughes Medical Institute.

References

Angelman, H. (1965). 'Puppet Children': a report of three cases. *Devel. Med. Child Neurol.* **7**, 681–8.

Buiting, K., Dittrich, B., Groß, S., Greger, V., Lalande, M., Robinson, W., Mutirangura, A., Ledbetter, D. & Horsthemke, B. (1993). Molecular definition of the Prader–Willi syndrome chromosome region and orientation of the SNRPN gene. *Hum. molec. Genet.* **2**, 1991–4.

Butler, M. G. & Palmer, C. G. (1983). Parental origin of chromosome 15 deletion in Prader–Willi syndrome. (Letter.) *Lancet* **i**, 1285–6.

Cassidy, S. B. (1987). Recurrence risk in Prader–Willi syndrome. *Am. J. med. Genet.* **28**, 59–60.

Cassidy, S. B., Lai, L.-W., Erickson, R. P., Magnuson, L., Thomas, E., Gendron, R. & Herrmann, J. (1992). Trisomy 15 with loss of the paternal 15 as a cause of Prader–Willi syndrome due to maternal disomy. *Am. J. Hum. Genet.* **51**, 701–8.

Cattanach, B. M., Barr, J. A., Evans, E. P., Burtenshaw, M., Beechey, C. V., Leff, S. E., Brannan, C. I., Copeland, N. G., Jenkins, N. A. & Jones, J. (1992). A candidate mouse model for Prader–Willi syndrome which shows an absence of Snrpn expression. *Nature Genet.* **2**, 270–4.

Delsert, C. D. & Rosenfeld, M. G. (1992). A tissue-specific small nuclear ribonucleoprotein and the regulated splicing of the calcitonin/calcitonin gene-related protein transcript. *J. biol. Chem.* **267**, 14576–9.

Dittrich, B., Buiting, K., Groβ, S. & Horsthemke, B. (1993). Characterization of a methylation imprint in the Prader–Willi syndrome chromosome region. *Hum. molec. Genet.* **2**, 1995–9.

Driscoll, D. J., Waters, M. F., Williams, C. A., Zori, R. T., Glenn, C. C., Avidano, K. M. & Nicholls, R. D. (1992). A DNA methylation imprint, determined by the sex of the parent, distinguishes the Angelman and Prader–Willi syndromes. *Genomics* **13**, 917–24.

Francke, U. (1994). Digitized and differentially shaded human chromosome ideograms for genomic applications. *Cytogenet. Cell Genet.* **65**, 206–19.

Francke, U. & Nesbitt, M. (1971). Cattanach's translocation: Cytological characterization by quinacrine mustard staining. *Proc. Natl. Acad. Sci. USA* **68**, 2918–20.

Gardner, J. M., Nakatsu, Y., Gondo, Y., Lee, S., Lyon, M. F., King, R. A. & Brilliant, M. H. (1992). The mouse pink eyed dilution gene: association with human Prader–Willi and Angelman syndromes. *Science* **257**, 1121–4.

Giacalone, J. & Francke, U. (1994). Single nucleotide dimorphism in the transcribed region of the SNRPN gene at 15q12. *Hum. molec. Genet.* **3**, 379–80.

Glenn, C. C., Porter, K. A., Jong, M. T. C., Nicholls, R. D. & Driscoll, D. J. (1993). Functional imprinting and epigenetic modifications of the human SNRPN gene. *Hum. molec. Genet.* **2**, 2001–5.

Greger, V., Woolf, E. & Lalande, M. (1993). Cloning of the breakpoints of a submicroscopic deletion in an Angelman syndrome patient. *Hum. molec. Genet.* **2**, 921–4.

Grimaldi, K., Horn, D. A., Hudson, L. D., Therenghi, G., Barton, P., Polak, J. M. & Latchman, D. S. (1993). Expression of the SmN splicing protein is developmentally regulated in the rodent brain but not in the rodent heart. *Devel. Biol.* **156**, 319–23.

Guthrie, G. (1991). Messenger RNA splicing in yeast: clues to why the spliceosome is a ribonucleoprotein. *Science* **253**, 157–63.

Hamabe, J., Kuroki, Y., Imaizumi, K., Sugimoto, T., Fukushima, Y., Yamaguchi, A., Izumikawa, Y. & Niikawa, N. (1991). DNA deletion and its parental origin in Angelman syndrome patients. *Am. J. med. Genet.* **41**, 64–8.

Holm, V. A., Cassidy, S. B., Butler, M. G., Hanchett, J. M., Greenswag, L. R., Whitman, B. Y. & Greenberg, F. (1993). Prader–Willi syndrome: consensus diagnostic criteria. *Pediatrics* **91**, 398–402.

Horn, D. A. & Latchman, D. S. (1993). The tissue specific SmN protein does not influence the alternative splicing of endogenous N-Cam and C-SRC RNAs in transfected 3T3 cells. *Molec. Brain Res.* **19**, 181–7.

Horn, D. A., Suburo, A., Terenghi, G., Hudson, L. D., Polak, J. M. & Latchman, D. S. (1992). Expression of the tissue specific splicing protein SmN in neuronal cell lines and in regions of the brain with different splicing capacities. *Molec. Brain Res.* **16**, 13–19.

Huntriss, J. D., Latchman, D. S. & Williams, D. G. (1993). The snRNP core protein SmB and tissue-specific SmN protein are differentially distributed between snRNP particles. *Nucleic Acids. Res.* **21**, 4047–53.

Kistberg, D., Selig, S., Brandeis, M., Simon, I., Driscoll, D. J., Nicholls, R. D. & Cedar, H. (1993). Allele specific replication timing of imprinted gene regions. *Nature* **364**, 459–63.

Labidi, F. & Cassidy, S. B. (1986). A blind prometaphase study of Prader–Willi syndrome: frequency and consistency in interpretation of del 15q. *Am. J. Hum. Genet.* **39**, 452–60.

Ledbetter, D. H., Mascarello, J. T., Riccardi, V. M., Harper, V. D., Airhart, S. D. & Strobel, R. J. (1982). Chromosome 15 abnormalities and the Prader–Willi syndrome: a follow-up report of 40 cases. *Am. J. Hum. Genet.* **34**, 278–85.

Ledbetter, D. H., Riccardi, V. M., Airhart, S. D., Strobel, R. J., Keenan, B. S. & Crawford, J. D. (1981). Deletions of chromosome 15 as a cause of the Prader–Willi syndrome. *New Engl. J. Med.* **304**, 325–9.

Leff, S. E., Brannan, C. I., Reed, M. L., Özçelik, T., Francke, U., Copeland, N. G. & Jenkins, N. A. (1992). Maternal imprinting of the mouse *Snrpn* gene and conserved linkage homology with the human Prader–Willi syndrome region. *Nature Genet.* **2**, 259–64.

Lerner, M. R. & Steitz, J. A. (1979). Antibodies to small nuclear RNAs complexed with proteins are produced by patients with systemic lupus erythematosus. *Proc. Natl. Acad. Sci. USA* **76**, 5495–9.

Li, S., Klein, E. S., Russo, A. F., Simmons, D. M. & Rosenfeld, M. G. (1989). Isolation of cDNA clones encoding small nuclear ribonucleoparticle-associated proteins with different tissue specificities. *Proc. Natl. Acad. Sci. USA* **86**, 9778–82.

Magenis, R. E., Brown, M. G., Lacy, D. A., Budden, S. & LaFranchi, S. (1987). Is Angelman syndrome an alternate result of del(15)(q11q13)? *Am. J. med. Genet.* **28**, 829–38.

Magenis, R. E., Fejel-Toth, S., Allen, L. J., Black, M., Brown, M. G., Budden, S., Cohen, R., Friedman, J. M., Kalousek, D., Zonana, J., Lacy, D., LaFranchi, S., Lahr, M., Macfarlane, J. & Williams, C. P. S. (1990). Comparison of the 15q deletions in Prader–Willi and Angelman syndromes: Specific regions, extent of deletions, parental origin, and clinical consequences. *Am. J. med. Genet.* **35**, 333–49.

McAllister, G., Amara, S. G. & Lerner, M. R. (1988). Tissue specific expression and cDNA cloning of small nuclear ribonucleoprotein-associated polypeptide N. *Proc. Natl. Acad. Sci. USA* **85**, 5296–300.

McAllister, G., Roby-Shemkovitz, A., Amara, S. G. & Lerner, M. R. (1989). cDNA sequence of the rat U snRNP-associated protein N: description of a potential Sm epitope. *EMBO J.* **8**, 1177–81.

Nakao, M., Sutcliffe, J. S., Burtschi, B., Mutirangura, A., Ledbetter, D. H. & Beaudet, A. L. (1994). Imprinting analysis of three genes in the Prader–Willi/Angelman region: SNRPN, E6-associated protein, and PAR-2 (D15S225E). *Hum. molec. Genet.* **3**, 309–15.

Nesbitt, M. & Francke, U. (1973). A system of nomenclature for band patterns of mouse chromosomes. *Chromosoma* **41**, 145–58.

Nicholls, R. D., Knoll, J. H. M., Butler, M. G., Karam, S. & Lalande, M. (1989). Genetic imprinting suggested by maternal heterodisomy in non-deletion Prader–Willi syndrome. *Nature* **342**, 281–5.

Orstavik, K. H., Tangsrud, S. E., Kiil, R., Hansteen, I.-L., Steen Johnsen, J., Cassidy, S. B., Martony, A., Anvret, M., Tommerup, N. & Brondum-Nielsen, K. (1992).

Prader–Willi syndrome in a brother and sister without cytogenetic or detectable molecular genetic abnormality at chromosome 15q11q13. *Am. J. med. Genet.* **44**, 534–8.

Özçelik, T., Leff, S., Robinson, W., Donlon, T., Lalande, M., Sanjines, E., Schinzel, A. & Francke, U. (1992). Small nuclear ribonucleoprotein polypeptide N (SNRPN), an expressed gene in the Prader–Willi syndrome critical region. *Nature Genet.* **2**, 265–9.

Prader, A., Labhart, A. & Willi, H. (1956). Ein Syndrom von Adipositas, Kleinwuchs, Kryptorchidismus und Oligophrenie nach myatonieartigem Zustand im Neugeborenenalter. *Schweiz. med. Wschr.* **86**, 1260–1.

Purvis-Smith, S. G., Saville, T., Manass, S., Yip, M.-Y., Lam-Po-Tang, P. R. L., Duffy, B., Johnston, H., Leigh, D. & McDonald, B. (1992). Uniparental disomy 15 resulting from 'correction' of an initial trisomy 15. (Letter.) *Am. J. Hum. Genet.* **50**, 1348–50.

Reed, M. & Leff, S. E. (1994). Maternal imprinting of human SNRPN, a gene deleted in Prader–Willi syndrome. *Nature Genet.* **6**, 163–7.

Reis, A., Dittrich, B., Greger, V., Buiting, K., Lalande, M., Gillessen-Kaesbach, G., Anvret, M. & Horsthemke, B. (1994). Imprinting mutations suggested by abnormal DNA methylation patterns in familial Angelman and Prader–Willi syndromes. *Am. J. Hum. Genet.* **54**, 741–7.

Robinson, W. P., Bottani, A., Yagang, X., Balakrishman, J., Binkert, F., Machler, M., Prader, A. & Schinzel, A. (1991). Molecular, cytogenetic and clinical investigations of Prader–Willi syndrome patients. *Am. J. Hum. Genet.* **49**, 1219–34.

Rokeach, L. A., Jannatipour, M., Haselby, J. A. & Hoch, S. O. (1989). Primary structure of a human small nuclear ribonucleoprotein polypeptide as deduced by cDNA analysis. *J. biol. Chem.* **264**, 5024–30.

Saitoh, S., Kubota, T., Ohta, T., Jinno, Y., Niikawa, N., Sugimoto, T., Wagstaff, J. & Lalande, M. (1992). Familial Angelman syndrome caused by imprinted submicroscopic deletion encompassing GABA$_A$ receptor β_3 subunit gene. *Lancet* **339**, 366–7.

Schmauss, C., Brines, M. L. & Lerner, M. R. (1992). The gene encoding the small nuclear ribonuclear protein-associated protein N is expressed at high levels in neurons. *J. biol. Chem.* **267**, 8521–9.

Schmauss, C., McAllister, G., Ohosone, Y., Hardin, J. A. & Lerner, M. R. (1989). A comparison of snRNP-associated Sm-autoantigens: human N, rat N and human B/B'. *Nucleic Acids Res.* **17**, 1733–43.

Sharpe, N. G., Williams, D. G. & Latchman, D. S. (1990). Regulated expression of the small nuclear ribonucleoprotein particle SmN in embryonic stem cell differentiation. *Molec. Cell Biol.* **10**, 6817–20.

VanDam, A. I., Winkel, A. I., Ziglstra-Baalbergen, J., Smeenk, R. & Cuypers, H. T. (1989). Cloned human snRNP proteins B and B' differ only in their carboxy terminal part. *EMBO J.* **8**, 3853–60.

Wagstaff, J., Knoll, H. M., Fleming, J., Kirkness, E. F., Martin-Gallardo, A., Greenberg, F., Graham, J. M., Menninger, J., Ward, D., Venter, J. C. & Lalande, M. (1991). Localization of the gene encoding the GABA$_A$ receptor β3 subunit to the Angelman/Prader–Willi region of human chromosome 15. *Am. J. Hum. Genet.* **49**, 330–7.

VI

Imprinting: a search for new genes and unifying principles

22

Use of chromosome rearrangements for investigations into imprinting in the mouse

BRUCE M. CATTANACH, JACKY BARR AND JANET JONES

Introduction

Mouse genetic studies using chromosome rearrangements to generate maternal (Mat Di) and paternal disomies (Pat Di) or equivalent duplications (Mat Dp and Pat Dp) of specific chromosome segments have contributed substantially to the recognition of imprinting in mammals and have since provided means of investigating the phenomenon (Cattanach & Kirk, 1985; Cattanach, 1986, 1991; Searle & Beechey, 1990; Cattanach & Beechey, 1990a). Specifically, such studies have demonstrated the following points.

(1) It is not the whole genome that is imprinted but seemingly only certain genes that lie within ten defined chromosomal regions ('imprinting regions') distributed over six different chromosomes.
(2) Maternal or paternal duplication of these genes results in characteristic 'imprinting' phenotypes, which range from early embryonic and mid-gestation lethalities to phenotypic anomalies detectable before and/or after birth. With almost the whole genome now screened, a total of 15 such imprinting effects have been recognized.
(3) Imprinting is a one-generation effect.
(4) Imprinting can involve either maternal or paternal copies of affected genes.

It was further clear from such work that imprinting is a germline event, perhaps relating to the imprinting of chromosomes that occurs in certain insects (Crouse, 1960; Brown & Nelson-Rees, 1961) to cause differential chromosome behaviors according to parental origin (Cattanach, 1991). Thus, it is evident from the imprinting effects observed in the mouse that, as in the insects, the phenomenon plays a role in development. In addition, as with the hetero-chromatic behavior of chromosomes seen in some insects, evidence of

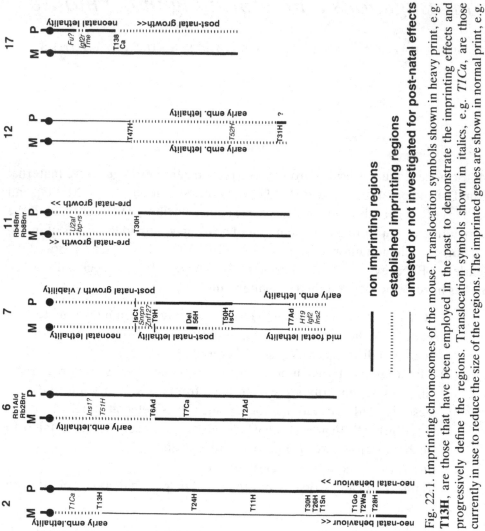

Fig. 22.1. Imprinting chromosomes of the mouse. Translocation symbols shown in heavy print, e.g. **T13H**, are those that have been employed in the past to demonstrate the imprinting effects and progressively define the regions. Translocation symbols shown in italics, e.g. *T1Ca*, are those currently in use to reduce the size of the regions. The imprinted genes are shown in normal print, e.g. H19.

asynchronous chromatin replication has recently been implicated in mammalian imprinting (Kitsberg *et al.*, 1993). Inactivation of genes (gene repression) was considered the developmental consequence of the germline imprints. Evidence of repression of maternal or paternal copies of some genes has since been demonstrated (*Igf2*, DeChiara, *et al.*, 1990; *Igf2r*, Barlow *et al.*, 1991; *H19*, Bartolomei *et al.*, 1991; *Snrpn*, Leff *et al.*, 1992; Cattanach *et al.*, 1992; *Ins1*, *Ins2*, Giddings *et al.*, 1994; *U2afbp-rs*, Hatada *et al.*, 1993; Hayashizaki *et al.*, 1994), all of which are located within the imprinting regions (Fig. 22.1).

In this chapter we summarize further work currently being conducted at Harwell using the Di/Dp system. We also review some of our recent findings on known imprinted genes, which clearly add complexity to our understanding of imprinting, and we describe our attempts to identify other genes that are subject to imprinting. Finally, we introduce a new mutant of potential value for imprinting investigations.

Reduction in size of the imprinting regions

The use of Robertsonian and reciprocal translocations to generate maternal/ paternal disomies, and equivalent duplications respectively, has been described in detail elsewhere (Cattanach & Kirk 1985; Cattanach & Beechey, 1990b) and need not be repeated here. It should however be noted that the Mat/Pat Di and Mat/Pat Dp genotypes lack the corresponding Pat/Mat chromosomes/ chromosome region; this is crucial to their use in gene expression studies. In such animals with parental chromosome imbalance, imprinting is detected by developmental abnormalities (Fig. 22.1).

Most of the imprinting regions are relatively large, up to 30% of individual chromosomes, but this size merely represents the paucity of suitable transloca- tions involving these chromosomes. However, where a number of suitable translocations are distributed along the length of a chromosome, the imprinting regions can be reduced in size to levels that make detailed gene mapping feasible, so facilitating identification of the specific genes involved. This has been achieved most effectively for the distal Chr 2 region (Fig. 22.1). This region has been reduced to the area bounded by the T1Wa and T28H breakpoints and is calculated to comprise about 7.5 Mb. Detailed mapping has been conducted by Jo Peters at Harwell. On the basis of this work and appraisal of the homologous human segment in human Chr 20q, she has deduced that at least 22 genes must lie within the region. However, none of the 15 investigated so far has shown any evidence of imprinting.

At Harwell, searches continue for new translocations, which may prove of use for narrowing down the size of the imprinting regions further. Some examples of these are indicated (in italics) in Fig. 22.1. It may be further noted that small segments within the central Chr 7 and distal Chr 12 imprinting regions are now shown not to be involved in imprinting. In the case of central Chr 7, this has been indicated by the normal inheritance of a deletion within the region (Tease & Fisher, 1994). In the case of distal Chr 12, the situation is somewhat complicated. In studies with the T31H translocation several years ago, Beechey *et al.* (1980) reported that mice with paternal monosomy for the region distal to the break-point were viable. This rules out the possibility that this region is responsible for the Pat Dp dist 12.T31H embryonic lethality. However, skeletal abnormalities were noted in these animals, and this is reminiscent of the defects seen in androgenetic/normal neonatal chimeras (Mann *et al.*, 1990). The possibility of imprinting in the extreme distal region cannot therefore be ruled out; more than a single imprinting effect may be associated with Chr 12.

As a further point of interest regarding the definition of the imprinting regions, it should be noted that in Fig. 22.1 the T9H breakpoint is now shown to be distal to that for IsCt. Cytogenetic and linkage studies (Searle & Beechey, 1974; Beechey, 1993; E. P. Evans, personal communication) had suggested the reverse order (Cattanach *et al.*, 1992), but new imprinting studies with *Snrpn* (J. A. Barr, unpublished; J. Mann, personal communication) have indicated that this im-printed gene (see later) must lie proximal to T9H, not distal. This establishes that a region of mouse Chr 7 that is homologous with that spanned by the human Prader–Willi and Angelman Chr 15 deletions must lie between the T9H and IsCt breakpoints; it also opens up the possibility that the postnatal imprinting effect associated with Pat Dp prox7.T9H represents the mouse model of Angelman syndrome, just as the Mat Dp cen7.IsCt effect may represent the mouse model of Prader–Willi syndrome (Cattanach *et al.*, 1992).

Dosage effects and imprinting

The presence of only single non-functional copies of genes is likely to be responsible for most of the observed imprinting effects, but in the case of the lethality associated with maternal duplication for the region of Chr 7 distal to the T7Ad breakpoint (Mat Dp dist7.T7Ad), an excess of *H19* rather than an absence of *Igf2* may be responsible. For some other imprinting regions it has proved possible to determine whether the absence of one parental copy, or the presence of two, is responsible for the effects observed, even without knowledge of the actual genes involved. This is achievable whenever chromosome imbalance of the regions can be created. Thus, the knowledge that animals with two maternal copies and one paternal copy of the central region of Chr 7 (Cattanach, 1961) do not show the imprinting neonatal lethality characteristic of Mat Dp central

Is1Ct

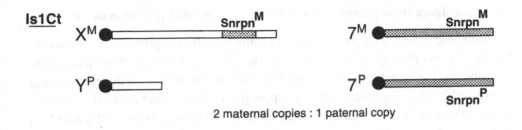

2 maternal copies : 1 paternal copy

T1Go

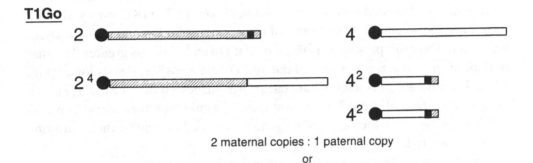

2 maternal copies : 1 paternal copy

or

1 maternal copy : 2 paternal copies

■ = distal Chr 2 imprinting region

Fig. 22.2. Chromosome imbalance obtainable with IsCt and T1Go. IsCt: Chromosomally unbalanced mice carrying two maternal copies and one paternal copy of the central region of Chr 7, including the imprinted gene *Snrpn*, can readily be generated. The effects are best studied in males to avoid the consequences of X inactivation. Such males are retarded, presumably owing to their chromosome imbalance, but do not show the imprinting lethality seen with Mat Dp cen7. Animals with two paternal copies and one maternal copy can also be generated as XO females (not shown).

T1Go: Heterozygotes for the translocation occasionally produce tertiary trisomics (as shown), these having three copies of the distal Chr 2 imprinting region. Single cases of mice with two maternal copies and one paternal copy, and the reciprocal type, have been identified; neither showed the imprinting effect.

(cen)7.IsCt, establishes that it is the absence of a paternal copy, rather than the presence of two maternal copies, that causes this specific imprinting effect (Fig. 22.2); this conclusion is consistent with the obseved maternal repression of the candidate locus for the effect (*Snrpn*; see later). Likewise, animals with either two material copies and one paternal copy of distal Chr 2, or the reciprocal, exhibit normal phenotypes (Beechey & Peters, 1994); the single additional Pat or Mat region prevents the imprinting phenotypes (Fig. 22.2). It is clear that different genes must be responsible for the two imprinting effects, despite their seemingly 'opposite' characteristics (Fig. 22.1).

Evidence from phenotypes on timing of imprinted gene expression

As indicated in Fig. 22.1, Mat Dp prox11 animals show a growth retardation at birth, whereas Pat Dp animals demonstrate an overgrowth. Although the gene responsible has not yet been identified, its time of action in development is suggested by developmental studies upon the growth effects. On the basis of masses taken at birth, weaning and adult ages, the growth rates of the Mat Dp, Pat Dp and normal classes do not differ significantly throughout postnatal development (Fig. 22.3). The size differences are therefore established by birth and are only maintained postnatally. However, from 12.5 to 18 days of gestation, differences between the growth rates of the normal, Mat Dp and Pat Dp classes were seen. Over this period, growth of the Pat Dp embryos was greater than that of their normal sibs, whereas that of the Mat Dp embryos was clearly lower (Fig. 22.3). Extrapolating each set of data backwards suggested that the divergence in growth rates starts at about 7.6 days gestation. It would therefore seem likely that this is the time when the responsible gene is switched on and/or the imprinting effect is initiated.

Placental mass correlated with embryo mass, but the divergence was detected later than that for the embryos. This suggests that embryo size determines placental size and therefore that the imprinted gene responsible for the growth differentials operates in the embryo rather than in the placenta. Based on such clues on the time and place of action of the gene responsible for the proximal Chr 11 imprinting effect, no obvious candidate as yet presents itself.

Expression and imprinting studies on candidate genes

The Di/Dp system has been used at Harwell to investigate the time and tissue distribution of imprinting repression for three genes that have been identified as subject to imprinting, *U2afbp-rs* in proximal Chr 11, and *Snrpn* and *Znf127* in central Chr 7 (Fig. 22.1). *Gabrb3*, which lies close to *Znf127* and *Snrpn*, has also been studied for evidence of imprinting.

U2af binding protein related sequence, U2afbp-rs

U2afbp-rs was identified by restriction landmark genome scanning (Hatada *et al.*, 1993; Hayashizaki *et al.*, 1994) as a gene possibly subject to imprinting; this appeared to be confirmed by the observation of monoallelic paternal expression in reciprocal cross F$_1$ hybrid mice (Hayashizaki *et al.*, 1994). Significantly, they also mapped the gene to a proximal position in Chr 11, i.e. within the proximal Chr 11 imprinting region (Fig. 22.1). The protein may involve mRNA splicing, as does *Snrpn*.

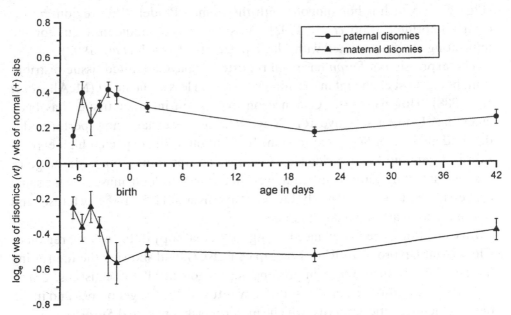

Fig. 22.3. Pre- and postnatal growth rates of Mat Di and Pat Di mice.

We have performed RT–PCR using several primers and sequences supplied by Dr Hayashizaki to show essentially ubiquitous expression of *U2afbp-rs* during embryonic development and in a wide range of adult tissues, with the highest levels of expression in the brain. However, although maternal imprinting repression was anticipated in Mat Dp prox11 mice, we have, as yet, been unable to demonstrate it; *U2afbp-rs* was expressed in all adult and fetal tissues. The discordance with the evidence obtained in the hybrid animals (Hatada *et al.*, 1993; Hayashizaki *et al.*, 1994) is remarkable. It remains to be seen whether technical factors are responsible or whether the discordant results could perhaps be attributable to parental gene dosage. As of now it would seem unlikely that *U2afbp-rs* is in any way involved with the Chr 11 imprinting phenotype. As the data stand they suggest yet a further degree of complexity to investigations into imprinting.

Small nuclear ribopolypeptide N, Snrpn

Snrpn encodes SmN, a polypeptide associated with RNA splicing (Li *et al.*, 1989; McAllister *et al.*, 1989). The human homolog, *SNRPN*, lies within the minimum critical region of Chr 15 for the Prader–Willi syndrome (Özçelik *et al.*, 1992) and, as an imprinting gene (Reed & Leff, 1994), is the current candidate locus for the syndrome. The mouse gene lies within the central segment of Chr 7

(Fig. 22.1), which is homologous with the human Prader–Willi region, and is clearly imprinted (Leff *et al.*, 1992). As such, it is a candidate locus for the imprinting effect associated with Mat Dp cen7 (Cattanach *et al.*, 1992).

The expression of *Snrpn* has been reported to have a limited tissue distribution, being most abundant in the adult brain, with less in the heart (McAllister *et al.*, 1988). However, little evidence on expression in other tissues has been available. Using a sensitive RT–PCR technique, we have now performed a detailed analysis of *Snrpn* expression. In addition to the expected high expression in brain and heart, evidence of expression was found in a wide range of tissues, including lung, liver, kidney, spleen and skeletal muscle. The same expression pattern was seen in brain, heart and liver of 12.5 – 18.5 day fetuses and in brain and heart of 9.5 day embryos.

Investigation of neonatal mice lacking a paternal copy of the central region of Chr 7 (Mat Dp prox7.T50H or Mat Dp cen7.IsCt), and showing the imprinting lethality, established *Snrpn* imprinting repression in all these tissues. *Snrpn* repression was also seen in 12.5 – 18.5 day fetuses of these genotypes and in 9.5 day parthenogenetic embryos, which similarly lack a paternal *Snrpn* allele.

In view of the observation of Latham *et al.* (1994) that the maternal repression of *Igf2* is not seen in 2-cell–4.5 day parthenogenetic embryos, we were particularly interested to determine whether or not this would be true for *Snrpn*. However, the gene was not found to be expressed in normal preimplantation embryos, confounding the investigation. We therefore do not know whether the imprinting of *Snrpn* is a two-step process of original germline imprint followed by gene repression at some stage of embryonic development, as indicated for *Igf2* (Latham *et al.*, 1994). It is clear from the data obtained, however, that the imprinting repression of *Snrpn* is seen wherever and whenever the gene is normally expressed.

Zinc finger protein 127, Znf127

The gene for the human zinc finger protein, *ZNF127*, lies close to *SNRPN* but outside the minimum critical region for Prader–Willi syndrome (Özçelik *et al.*, 1992). Nevertheless, methylation studies have suggested that the locus is imprinted (Driscoll *et al.*, 1992). The mouse homolog, *Znf127*, also lies close to *Snrpn* in central Chr 7.

In collaborative studies with Nicholls and using similar technologies to those employed with *Snrpn*, we have found evidence of *Znf127* expression in brain, heart, kidney, liver, spleen and skeletal muscle of normal adult mice and in postimplantation embryos 8.5 days and older.

In embryonic and neonatal mice lacking a paternal copy of the central region

Table 22.1. *Comparison of* Snrpn *and* Znf127 *imprinting in Mat Dp cen7 tissues*

| Tissue | Imprinting of: | |
	Snrpn	*Znf127*
Neonates		
brain	yes	yes
spleen	yes	no
kidney	yes	no
liver	yes	no
heart	yes	yes
lung	yes	no
skeletal muscle	yes	no
12.5–18.5 d embryos		
head	yes	yes
liver	yes	no
heart	yes	n.t.[a]

[a] n.t., Not tested.

of Chr 7 (Mat Dp prox7.T50H or Mat Dp cen7.IsCt), evidence of *Znf127* maternal repression was indicated in brain and heart but, significantly, there was no evidence of repression in liver or spleen. Overall, therefore, the locus appears to be imprinted in the mouse as indicated in humans, but the imprinting is tissue-specific.

The latter finding contrasts with ubiquitous imprinting seen with the closely linked *Snrpn* (Table 22.1). The discord between *Znf127* and *Snrpn* imprinting is surprising in that the two genes are closely linked and both show maternal allele repression. Their different developmental profiles therefore suggest either that *Snrpn* and *Znf127* receive different germline imprinting signals or, if they receive the same germline signal, their subsequent imprinting repression is not co-regulated, differing in the various tissues.

The γ-aminobutyric acid receptor, Gabrb3

A third gene that lies within the Prader–Willi critical region is *GABRB3*. We have shown that the mouse homolog *Gabrb3*, which again lies in the central region of Chr 7 close to *Snrpn*, is not subject to imprinting (Cattanach *et al.*, 1992). It is therefore clear that, as with the proximal Chr 17 (*Tme*) imprinting regions (Barlow *et al.*, 1991), the imprinting within central Chr 7 does not involve contiguous blocks of genes, but only certain ones within the localized region of chromatin.

Screening for further imprinted genes

Critical for full investigation of imprinting is identification of the genes involved throughout the whole genome; it would seem likely that these will be located within the imprinting regions. Insofar as all the imprinting effects discovered have involved growth and development, it has been anticipated that members of growth factor families located within the regions would be good candidates. Examination of the mouse and human linkage maps pertaining to the imprinting regions has revealed a number of likely candidates for the various effects. These include;

(1) *Erbb*, which maps to the proximal mouse Chr 11 region and potentially could affect growth, while the human homolog maps to Chr 7, the maternal disomy for which causes an intrauterine growth retardation (Spence *et al.*, 1988; Voss *et al.*, 1989; Spotila *et al.*, 1992);

(2) the *Erbb* embryonic ligand, *Tgfa*, which maps to mouse Chr 6; and

(3) two other genes that map within the Chr 11 region, *Lif* and the *Rel* oncogene.

Evidence of differential parental gene expression of each of these genes has been investigated in whole embryos of various ages without indications of imprinting being found. However, in view of the more recent findings with some of the known imprinted genes (*Igf2*, *Snrpn*, *Znf127*) it may be necessary to verify the above conclusion for individual tissues. That *Tgfa* showed no evidence of imprinting ultimately proved unremarkable when it was mapped outside the Chr 6 imprinted region and further shown to be responsible for the *wal* mutation (Luetteke *et al.*, 1993; Mann *et al.*, 1993), which clearly does not show an imprinting inheritance.

An alternative approach

A current difficulty with the above approach is that the imprinting regions are, with the exception of distal Chr 2, as yet too large for detailed mapping and hence for identifying those genes within them that are subject to imprinting. More effective for indentifying and investigating imprinting genes are deletions that show parent-of-origin phenotypic effects. In humans, the classic examples are the series of small deletions in Chr 15q which give rise to the Prader–Willi and Angelman syndromes when inherited through the fathers and mothers, respectively. As indicated earlier, these have allowed the critical regions to be progressively defined and the candidate loci within them identified. *SNRPN* was identified in this way. In the mouse, the minimum critical region defined by the proximal Chr 17 T^{hp} and t^{lub2} deletions (Johnson, 1974, 1975; Winking & Silver, 1984) results in the *Tme* imprinting lethality (Fig. 22.1). The small size of the region permitted identification of candidate genes, one of which, *Igf2r*, has shown evidence of imprinting (Barlow *et al.*, 1991). We now describe what may prove to be a further example of this phenomenon, although it has not yet been established whether a deletion is involved. It was first recognized as a dominant mutation in a radiation experiment designed to detect deletions (Cattanach *et al.*, 1993; Cattanach & Evans, 1994). Exceptionally, the dominant inheritance was only seen with transmission through males. The mutation therefore showed an imprinting inheritance (Hall, 1990).

The mutation, denoted minute (*Mnt*), causes a proportionately normal but severely growth retarded phenotype (*ca.* 50% of normal). Exceptionally, with this degree of effect, the viability is near-normal. The small size is immediately obvious at birth and persists throughout to adulthood. *Mnt* embryos are also detectable on the basis of size at least as far back as 13 days' gestation. Doming of the skull is a further regular phenotypic effect. This can be clearly seen at birth and persists to adulthood. The imprinting nature of the mutation is illustrated by the simple dominant inheritance exhibited when transmitted through males, but the absence of both the size and head characteristics of the mutant phenotype when transmitted through females (Fig. 22.4). Failure of expression, rather than of transmission, is established by the reappearance of affected young among the progeny of about half the sons of such females. The combined phenotype of growth retardation plus domed skull strongly suggests that *Mnt* represents a multilocus deletion, but cytogenetic studies have so far been negative (E.P. Evans, personal communication).

We anticipate that *Mnt* will map within an imprinting region in which maternal duplication results in some form of imprinting phenotype. Proximal Chr 11 was the first obvious candidate in view of the imprinting growth effects (Fig. 22.1). However, *Mnt* has not shown linkage with either of the proximal Chr 11 visible markers *wa2* and *vt*. A second candidate region was distal Chr 7, and specifically the *Igf2* locus, as the null mutation of this gene shows an imprinting inheritance identical to that of *Mnt*. However, preliminary RT-PCR analysis has suggested the presence of *Igf2* transcripts in fetal *Mnt* tissues. Hence, the *Igf2* locus may not be involved. Growth reduction is associated with the maternal proximal Chr 7 imprinting lethality (Searle & Beechey, 1990), making it the next possible candidate region. Linkage tests to check these regions are currently in progress. Thereafter, the other possible imprinting regions are proximal Chr 2, proximal

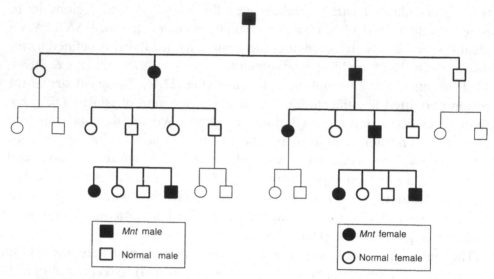

Fig. 22.4. Diagrammatic representation of the imprinting inheritance of the *Mnt* mutation.

Chr 6 and distal Chr 12 (Fig. 22.1). For each of the latter regions it would have to be assumed that the observed imprinting lethalities are attributable to genes outside of the putative *Mnt* deletion.

Whatever the exact location and actual nature of the *Mnt* mutation, it should provide a valuable new tool for imprinting studies.

Acknowledgements

We thank D. Papworth for statistical assistance and advice. The work was supported in part by a National Radiation Protection Board grant.

References

Barlow, D. P., Stöger, R., Hermann, B. G., Saito, K. & Schweifer, N. (1991). The mouse insulin-like growth factor type-2 receptor is imprinted and closely linked to the *Tme* locus. *Nature* **349**, 84–7.

Bartolomei, M. S., Zemel, S. & Tilghman, S. M. (1991). Parental imprinting of the mouse H19 gene. *Nature* **351**, 153–5.

Beechey, C. V. (1993). Maps of chromosome anomalies in the mouse. *Mouse Genome* **91**, 81–101.

Beechey, C. V., Kirk, M. & Searle, A. G. (1980). A reciprocal translocation induced in an oocyte and affecting fertility in male mice. *Cytogenet. Cell Genet.* **27**, 129–46.

Beechey, C. V. & Peters, J. (1994). Dosage effects of the distal chromosome 2 imprinting region. *Mouse Genome* **92**, 353–4.

Brown, S. W. & Nelson-Rees, W. A. (1961). Radiation analysis of a lecanoid genetic system. *Genetics* **46**, 983–1007.

Cattanach, B. M. (1961). A chemically-induced variegated-type position effect in the mouse. *Z. Vererbungs.* **92** 165–82.

Cattanach, B. M. (1986). Parental origin effects in mice. *J. Embryol. exp. Morphol.* **97**, 137–50.

Cattanach, B. M. (1991). Chromosome imprinting and its significance for mammalian development. In *Genome Analysis*, vol. 2, ed. K. Davies & S. Tilghman, pp. 41–71. New York: Cold Spring Harbor Laboratory Press.

Cattanach, B. M., Barr, J. A., Evans, E. P., Burtenshaw, M. D., Beechey, C. V., Leff, S. E., Brannan, C. I., Copeland, N. G., Jenkins, N. A. & Jones, J. (1992). A candidate mouse model for Prader–Willi syndrome which shows an absence of Snrpn expression. *Nature Genet.* **2**, 270–4.

Cattanach, B. M. & Beechey, C. V. (1990a). Chromosome imprinting phenomena in mice and indications in man. In *Chromosomes Today*, vol. 10, ed. K. Fredga, B. A. Kihlman & M. D. Bennett, pp. 135–48. London: Unwin Hyman.

Cattanach, B. M. & Beechey, C. V. (1990b). Autosomal and X chromosomal imprinting. In *Genomic Imprinting (Development* (Suppl.)), ed. M. Monk & A. Surani, pp. 63–72. Cambridge: The Company of Biologists.

Cattanach, B. M., Burtenshaw, M. D., Rasberry, C. & Evans, E. P. (1993). Large deletions and other gross forms of chromosome imbalance compatible with viability and fertility in the mouse. *Nature Genet.* **3**, 56–61.

Cattanach, B. M. & Evans, E. P. (1994). Radiation-induced large deletions and other gross forms of chromosome imbalance in the mouse. In *Radiation Protection: Molecular mechanisms in radiation mutagenesis and carcinogenesis*, ed. K. H. Chadwick, R. Cox, H. P. Leenhouts & J. Thacker, pp. 93–100. Luxembourg: European Commission.

Cattanach, B. M. & Kirk, M. (1985). Differential activity of maternally and paternally derived chromosome regions in mice. *Nature* **315**, 496–8.

Crouse, H. V. (1960). The controlling element in sex chromosome behaviour in *Sciara*. *Genetics* **45**, 1429–3.

DeChiara, T. M., Efstratiadis, A. & Robertson, E. J. (1990). A growth deficiency phenotype in heterozygous mice carrying an insulin-like growth factor II gene disrupted by targetting. *Nature* **345**, 78–80.

Driscoll, D. J., Waters, M. F., Williams, C. A., Zori, R. T., Glenn, C. C., Avidano, K. M. & Nicholls, R. D. (1992). A DNA methylation imprint, determined by the sex of the parent, distinguishes the Angelman and Prader–Willi syndromes. *Genomics* **13**, 917–24.

Giddings, S. J., King, C. D., Harman, K. W., Flood, J. F. & Carnaghi, L. R. (1994). Allele specific inactivation of insulin 1 and 2, in the mouse yolk sac, indicates imprinting. *Nature Genet.* **6**, 310–13.

Hall, J. G. (1990). Genomic imprinting: Review and relevance to human diseases. *Am. J. Hum. Genet.* **46**, 857–73.

Hatada, I., Sugama, T. & Mukai, T. (1993). A new imprinted gene cloned by a methylation-sensitive genome scanning method. *Nucleic Acids Res.* **21**, 5577–82.

Hayashizaki, Y., Shibata, H., Hirotsune, S., Sugino, H., Okazaki, Y., Sasaki, N., Hirose, K., Imoto, H., Okuizumi, H., Muramatsu, M., Komatsubara, H., Shiroishi, T., Moriwaki, K., Katsuki, M., Hatano, N., Sasaki, H., Ueda, T., Mise, N., Takagi, N., Plass, C. & Chapman, V. M. (1994). Identification of an imprinted U2af binding protein related sequence on mouse chromosome II using the RLGS method. *Nature Genet.* **6**, 33–40.

Johnson, D. R. (1974). Hairpin-tail: A case of post-reductional gene action in the mouse egg? *Genetics* **76**, 795–805.

Johnson, D. R. (1975). Further observations on the hairpin-tail (T^{hp}) mutation in the mouse. *Genet. Res.* **24**, 207–13.

Kitsberg, D., Selig, S., Brandels, M., Simon, I., Keshet, I., Driscoll, D. J., Nicholls, R. D. & Cedar, H. (1993). Allele-specific replication timing of imprinted gene regions. *Nature* **364**, 459–63.

Latham, K. E., Doherty, A. S., Scott, C. D. & Schulz, R. M. (1994). *Igf2r* and *Igf2* gene expression in androgenetic, gynogenetic and parthenogenetic preimplantation mouse embryos: absence of regulation by genomic imprinting. *Genes Devel.* **8**, 290–9.

Leff, S. E., Brannan, C. I., Reed, M. L., Özçelik, T., Francke, U., Copeland, N. G. & Jenkins, N. A. (1992). Maternal imprinting of the mouse Snrpn gene and conserved linkage homology with the human Prader–Willi syndrome region. *Nature Genet.* **2**, 259–64.

Li, S., Klein, E. S., Russo, A. F., Simmons, D. M. & Rosenfeld, M. G. (1989). Isolation of cDNA clones encoding small nuclear ribonucleoparticle-associated proteins with different tissue specificities. *Proc. Natl. Acad. Sci. USA* **86**, 9778–82.

Luetteke, N. C., Qiu, T. H., Peiffer, R. L., Oliver, P., Smithies, O. & Lee, D. C. (1993). TFGα deficiency results in hair follicle and eye abnormalities in targeted and waved-1 mice. *Cell* **73**, 263–78.

Mann, G. B., Fowler, K. J., Gabriel, A., Nice, E. C., Williams, R. L. & Dunn, A. R. (1993). Mice with a null mutation of the TGFα gene have abnormal skin architecture, wavy hair, and curly whiskers and often develop corneal inflammation. *Cell* **73**, 249–61.

Mann, J. R., Gadi, I., Harbison, M. L., Abbondanzo, S. J. & Stewart, C. L. (1990). Androgenetic mouse embryonic stem cells are pluripotent and cause skeletal defects in chimeras: implications for genetic imprinting. *Cell* **62**, 251–60.

McAllister, G., Amara, S. G. & Lerner, M. R. (1988). Tissue-specific expression and cDNA cloning of small nuclear ribonucleoprotein-associated polypeptide N. *Proc. Natl. Acad. Sci. USA* **85**, 5296–300.

McAllister, G., Roby-Shemkovitz, A., Amara, S. G. & Lerner, M. R. (1989). cDNA sequence of the rat U snRNP-associated protein N: Description of a potential Sm epitope. *EMBO J.* **8**, 1177–81.

Özçelik, T., Leff, S., Robinson, W., Donlon, T., Lalande, M., Sanjines, E., Schinzel, A. & Francke, U. (1992). Small nuclear ribonucleoprotein polypeptide N (SNPRN), an expressed gene in the Prader–Willi syndrome critical region. *Nature Genet.* **2**, 265–9.

Reed, M. L. & Leff, S. E. (1994). Maternal imprinting of human SNRPN, a gene deleted in Prader–Willi syndrome. *Nature Genet.* **6**, 163–7.

Searle, A. G. & Beechey, C. V. (1974). Position of T9H on Chr 7 and assignment to Chr 15. *Mouse News Lett.* **50**, 40.

Searle, A. G. & Beechey, C. V. (1990). Genome imprinting phenomena on mouse chromosome 7. *Genet. Res.* **56**, 237–44.

Spence, J. E., Perciaccante, R. G., Greig, G. M., Williard H. F., Ledbetter, D. H., Hejtmancik, J. F., Pollack, M. S., O'Brein, W. E. & Beaudet, A. L. (1988) Uniparental disomy as a mechanism of human genetic disease. *Am. J. Hum. Genet.* **42**, 217–26.

Spotila, L. D., Sereda, L. & Prockop, D. J. (1992). Partial isodisomy for maternal chromosome 7 and short stature in an individual with a mutation at the COLIA2 locus. *Am. J. Hum. Genet.* **51**, 1396–405.

Tease, C. & Fisher, G. (1994). New deletions detected among the progeny of X-irradiated females. *Mouse Genome* **92**, 348.

Voss, R., Ben-Simon, E., Avital, A., Godfrey, S. Zlotogora, J., Dagan, J., Tikochinski, Y. & Hillel, J. (1989). Isodisomy of chromosome 7 in a patient with cystic fibrosis: Could uniparental disomy be common in humans? *Am. J. Hum. Genet.* **45**, 373–80.

Winking, H. & Silver, L. M. (1984). Characterization of a recombinant mouse *t*-haplotype that expresses a dominant lethal maternal effect. *Genetics* **108**, 1013–20.

23

A new imprinted gene, U2af-related sequence, *isolated by a methylation-sensitive genome scanning method*

TSUNEHIRO MUKAI, IZUHO HATADA, TETSUJI YAMAOKA,
KAZUNORI KITAGAWA, XU-DONG WANG, TAKAKO SUGAMA,
JUNICHI MASUDA AND JUN OGATA

Introduction

Although little is known about the precise mechanism involved in the imprinting process to date, recent studies have suggested an important role for DNA methylation in mammalian genome imprinting (Sasaki *et al.*, 1992; Bartolomei *et al.*, 1993; Ferguson-Smith *et al.*, 1993; Stöger *et al.*, 1993; Li *et al.*, 1993). In vertebrates, DNA methylation is observed exclusively in the 5-position of the cytosine residue, the site of which is on the CpG dinucleotides. If the methylation-sensitive restriction enzyme was used for screening such sites in F_1 progeny obtained under reciprocal crosses, it would be possible to distinguish between the methylated and unmethylated sites of each allele at a particular locus. It would be challenging if a method could be developed to search for any differentially methylated genes throughout the whole genome.

Recently, we have developed a new genome scanning method, restriction landmark genome scanning (RLGS), based on the concept termed 'restriction landmark', in which a restriction recognition site can be used as a landmark for scanning (Hatada *et al.*, 1991). RLGS uses direct labeling of restriction sites coupled with high-resolution, two-dimensional electrophoresis, by which the resulting restriction landmark can be detected as an autoradiographic spot. We applied this RLGS method to a search for restriction landmarks that are differentially methylated in the genome. Here, we first describe the development of the method by which one is able to scan for differentially methylated sites in the genome, and then the isolation and identification of a new imprinted gene. In fact we found five spots on the RLGS profile showing differential methylation in reciprocal crosses of mouse strains. One of these spots, spot 2, was chosen for further analysis because this spot was mapped on chromosome 11, which is known as an imprinted chromosome but from which no gene has been previously mapped. This new gene was named *U2af1-rs1* (originally named SP2 and renamed because several related genes have been isolated in mice and humans (unpublished results)). In addition, this gene is significantly homologous to the U2 small nuclear ribonucleoprotein auxiliary factor small subunit (Hatada *et al.*, 1993).

Materials and methods

Mouse resources

C57BL/6 and DBA2 mice were used to obtain a reciprocal cross.

Procedure for two-dimensional gel electrophoresis

Ten micrograms of genomic DNA was incubated for 30 min at 37 °C along with 10 units of DNA polymerase I in 50 mM Tris-HCl (pH 7.5), 100 mM NaCl, 10 mM MgCl$_2$, 10 mM dithiothreitol, 0.33 μM dGTPαS, 0.33 μM dCTPαS, 33 μM ddATP and 33 μM ddTTP. The reaction mixture was then heated at 65 °C for 30 min. The pretreated DNA was digested with 100 units of *Not*I (or *Bss*HII) for 60 min. The cleavage ends were filled in with 20 units of Sequenase version 2.0 (USB & Co. Ltd.) in the presence of 0.33 μM [α^{32}P]dGTP (3000 Ci mM^{-1}) and 0.33 μM [α^{32}P]dCTP (6000 Ci mM^{-1}) for 30 min at 37 °C in 50 mM Tris–HCl (pH 7.5), 100 mM NaCl, 10 mM MgCl$_2$, 10 mM dithiothreitol, 0.16 μM dGTPαS, 0.16 μM dCTPαS, 33 μM ddATPαS and 33 μM ddTTPαS. To stop the reaction, excess ddGTP and ddCTP (33 μM) were added. The labeled DNA was then digested by *EcoR*V and phenol-extracted. For first-dimensional electrophoresis, one microgram of the DNA was fractionated on a 50 cm × 20 cm × 0.1 cm agarose gel (0.8% Seakem GTG agarose, FMC) in TAM buffer (50 mM Tris–acetate, pH 7.5; 0.7 mM magnesium acetate) at 4.5 V cm^{-1} for 12 h. The DNA-containing portion of the gel was excised as a strip and soaked for 30 min in the *Mbo*I buffer. Thereafter, DNA was digested in the gel by 1500 units of *Mbo*I at 37 °C for 2 h. The cut-out gel was fused to a 50 cm × 50 cm × 0.1 cm polyacrylamide gel (5–6% polyacrylamide; acrylamide: bis-acrylamide, 29 : 1) by adding melted agarose to fill up the gap. Second-dimensional electrophoresis was carried out in TBE buffer at 8 V cm^{-1} for 6 h. After drying the gel, appropriate regions from the original gel were excised and autoradiographed for 3–10 days on a film (XAR-5, Kodak) at −80 °C using an intensifying screen (Quanta III, Dupont).

DNA cloning

Out of five candidates for spots on the RLGS profile showing differential methylation from reciprocal crosses of mouse strains, spot 2 was cloned for further analysis. For cloning RLGS spots, mouse genomic DNA was digested with *Not*I and *Eco*RV and run through electrophoresis. The 1.8–2.4 kb fragment expected to include spot 2 was cut out from the gel, and a *Not*I–*Eco*RV boundary library was constructed. Five micrograms of this library was digested with *Not*I and *Eco*RV and subjected to RLGS analysis together with labeled genomic DNA at the *Not*I site, as described in Materials and methods above. Spot 2 was cut out, eluted from the gel and cloned into pBluescript. To clone the whole genomic *SP2*, mouse liver DNA was digested with *Xba*I and the region around the 8.3 kb fragment was cut out from the gel to construct the λzap library. The *SP2* cDNA clone was isolated from the mouse brain λgt10 library.

The DNA clone corresponding to spot 2 was initially named *SP2*, and renamed *U2af1-rs1* for the reason described in the Introduction.

RT–PCR analysis

Total RNA prepared from the whole body of newborn mice was used for RT–PCR analysis. The mice used in this analysis were C57BL/10(B), *Mus mus molossinus* (M), (*M. m. molossinus* × C57BL/10) F_1 (MBF$_1$) and (C57BL/10 × *M. m. molossinus*) F_1 (BMF$_1$). The polymorphic site between C57BL/6 and *M. m. molossinus* was amplified by RT–PCR. The primers were 5′-TGTGGTACG-GCCAGCCTATG-3′ and 5′-GATCAGACATACTGCGGATA-3′.

In situ *hybridization*

Procedures for serial sectioning of the sample, labeling the probe RNA and hybridization have been described previously (Arai *et al.*, 1994). To prepare the RNA probe, 730 bp of the *Not*I–*Bgl*II fragment was subcloned into pBluescript. This plasmid DNA was linearized either with *Not*I to generate an antisense probe by T7 RNA polymerase, or with *Sal*I to generate a sense probe by T3 RNA polymerase.

Mapping U2af1-rs1 *and* -rs2

For mapping the *U2af1-rs1* gene, the *Rsa*I-digested DNA of BXD inbred strains was run in agarose gel to detect polymorphism between C57BL/6 and DBA2. Using *Rsa*I polymorphism, we determined the strain distribution pattern of the

BXD inbred strain. We also determined the chromosomal location of the *U2af1-rs2* gene by using interspecific backcross mapping. The progeny used for interspecific backcross were obtained from the UK Human Genome Mapping Project: (C57BL/6 × *Mus spretus*)F$_1$ × *M. spretus* (BMM) mice and (C57BL/6 × *M. spretus*)F$_1$ × C57BL/6 (BMB) mice. To discriminate between strains, length polymorphism was used. The primers used for length polymorphism were 5'-ACTCCAGCATTAACTGATGC-3' and 5'-TGCTAGCTAATGCTAT-CATG-3'.

Results

New strategy for genome scanning

RLGS is a method for detecting recognition sites so that restriction enzymes can create landmarks, which are scattered throughout the genome. The strategies for genome scanning are shown schematically in Fig. 23.1 (Hatada *et al.*, 1991). Chromosomal DNA is digested by restriction enzyme, labeling the cleaved DNA end. The resulting DNAs are then separated two-dimensionally by electrophoresis, followed by autoradiography. The strategies include the following.

(i) Blocking: in general, genomic DNA gives rise to non-specific cleaved ends, nicks and/or gaps through the DNA preparation. This causes high background radiation because of the incorporation of radio-isotopes into damaged sites in the labeling process. Such misincorporation can be avoided by blocking those sites enzymatically with new nucleotide analogs (ddYTP[αS]) because analogs are expected to protect their sites from exonucleolytic attack and/or the additional incorporation of the nucleotide at blocked ends.

(ii) Landmark cleavage: appropriate sites within the blocked DNA are digested by restriction enzymes, and are used as restriction landmark sites.

(iii) Labeling: the cleaved ends of genomic DNA are labeled with radio-isotopes (dXTP[α^{32}P]).

(iv) First fractionation: DNA digests are fractionated in one dimension by thin-layer agarose gel electrophoresis. This step is performed after fragmentation with a second restriction enzyme before electrophoresis.

(v) Second fractionation: DNA fragments in the agarose gel are fractionated in the second dimension by polyacrylamide gel electrophoresis. This step is performed after further fragmentation with the third restriction enzyme in the gel.

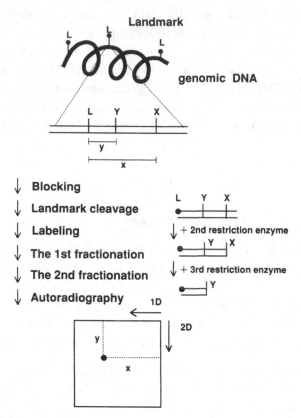

Fig. 23.1. Schematic presentation of genome scanning by two-dimensional gel electrophoresis (Hatada *et al.*, 1991). RLGS consists of: (i) blocking, (ii) landmark cleavage by the first restriction enzyme; (iii) labeling and fragmentation with the second restriction enzyme; (iv) first fractionation and fragmentation with the third restriction enzyme; (v) second fractionation; and (vi) autoradiography. L, landmark; x, distance from the landmark cleavage site that is generated by second enzyme digestion; y, distance from the landmark cleavage site generated by third enzyme digestion; shaded circle, labeled end; 1D and 2D, first- and second-dimensional, respectively.

(vi) Autoradiography: a typical profile of RLGS is shown in Fig. 23.2. Several thousand spots are clearly observed. We have confirmed that the position and intensity of each spot reflects its locus and is the exact copy number of the corresponding restriction site (Hatada *et al.*, 1991).

Search for parental-origin-specific CpG methylation by RLGS

This system is directly applicable to the search for differentially methylated sites if we use only the methylation-sensitive restriction endonuclease as a landmark

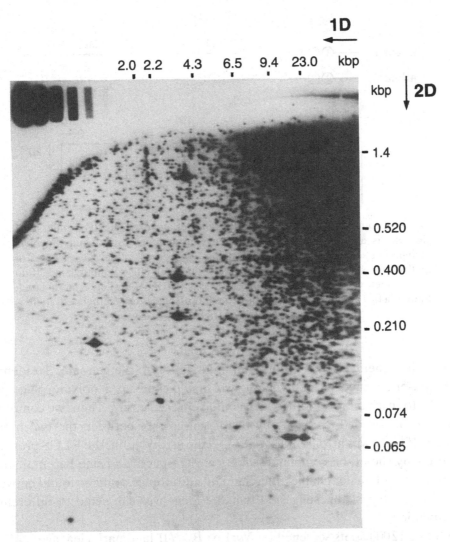

Fig. 23.2. Autoradiographic profile of RLGS analysis for mouse genomic DNA. Mouse genomic DNA was treated and developed two-dimensionally according to the experimental procedure. The cleavage restriction enzymes are: landmark cleavage by *Not*I, second cleavage by *Eco*RV, and third cleavage by *Mbo*I. The size marker is shown in kilobase pairs (kbp).

cleavage, this being sensitive to 5-methylcytosine in the CpG dinucleotide. Figure 23.3 shows the schematic representation of the relationship between the methylation status of each allele and the variation in spot intensity. If a locus is imprinted and one allele is methylated, the spot will be half as intense when compared with the surrounding spots where no allele is methylated.

We used a reciprocal cross of C57BL/6 and DBA2 mouse inbred strains to

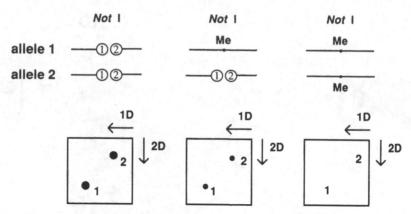

Fig. 23.3. Landmark cleavage of methylated sites and expected 2D profile. *Not*I cleavage is affected and results in change in spot intensity when the *Not*I recognition sequence is methylated at the CpG dinucleotide. Three types of methylation states are expected, depending on which allele is methylated. If no allele is methylated, there is a full-intensity spot (left); if one allele is methylated, there is a half-intensity spot (middle); and if both alleles are methylated, there is no spot (right).

screen the genetic loci for differential methylation in the genome. To identify parental-origin-specific methylation, we first picked up a polymorphic spot, specific for each inbred strain, which could be traced easily. Then, we compared the spot profile of F_1 progeny by reciprocal crosses between the two inbred strains. If there was no parental-origin-specific methylation, the RLGS profile of F_1 progeny should be completely identical, irrespective of one parental strain being male or female. On the other hand, if a difference could be found between two F_1 genotypes, this suggested that the locus was subjected to differential methylation.

Out of 12 000 spots screened by *Not*I or *Bss*HII landmark cleavage, 14% of them (1700 spots) were found to be polymorphic for either DBA2 or C57BL/6. We found five spots that appeared in one cross but not in the other. One of these spots, spot 2, specific to DBA2, appeared in one cross, (C57BL/6 × DBA2)F_1, but not in the opposite cross, (DBA2 × C57BL/6)F_1 (Fig. 23.4). This suggested that the DBA2 allele of spot 2 is demethylated in (C57BL/6 × DBA2)F_1 but methylated in (DBA2 × C57BL/6)F_1.

Cloning of a parental-origin-specific methylated spot

It is difficult to clone the spot DNA directly from the RLGS gel because numerous unlabeled DNA fragments exist together with the labeled spot. To

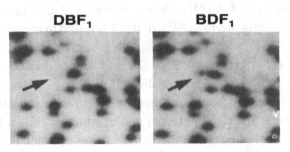

Fig. 23.4. The RLGS profile exhibiting the change in the spot intensity in F_1 progeny by reciprocal crosses. (DBA2 × C57BL/6)F_1 (DBF$_1$) and (C57BL/6 × DBA2)F_1 (BDF$_1$) progeny were used for RLGS analysis. The portion of the RLGS profile is presented where the spot intensity changed between DBF$_1$ and BDF$_1$. Arrow indicates spot 2. This spot disappeared in DBF$_1$, but appeared in BDF$_1$.

avoid cloning any non-specific DNA, the *Not*I-*Eco*RV boundary library was constructed and used for RLGS analysis to specifically clone spot 2. Two-dimensional gel electrophoresis of this library was performed together with a *Not*I labeled genomic DNA. Spot 2 was cut out from the gel and electro-eluted for cloning into pBluescript. To further clone the longer fragment of spot 2, we screened the boundary library using the eluted DNA fragment, and thus the 2.1 kb fragment of *Not*I–*Eco*RV, pSP2, was cloned.

We used pSP2 as a probe to examine the methylation status at the *Not*I site of genomic DNA between two reciprocal crosses ((DBA2 × C57BL/6)F_1 and (C57BL/6 × DBA2)F_1) by Southern hybridization. By a double digest with *Not*I and *Eco*RV, the 2.09 kb band corresponding to the demethylated fragment appeared in DBA2, whereas in C57BL/6 a 2.12 kb band appeared. This is due to DNA polymorphism between the two species. In (DBA2 × C57BL/6)F_1 (DBF$_1$) the 2.12 kb band was detected, whereas in (C57BL/6 × DBA2)F_1 (BDF$_1$) 2.09 kb band was detected, indicating that the *Not*I site is completely methylated on the maternal allele and demethylated on the paternal allele (Hatada *et al.*, 1993).

Parental imprinting of a new gene, SP2

SP2 DNA encoded 3.1 kb mRNA as shown by Northern blotting (Hatada *et al.*, 1993). Although this DNA was expressed ubiquitously in various tissues including brain, liver, heart, skeletal muscle, kidney, lung, testis, ovary and thymus, it was expressed predominantly in the brain. cDNA was cloned from the mouse brain library and its entire sequence was determined (2916 nucleotides; DDBJ, Genbank and EMBO accession no. D17407). As will be described in a later section two different types of cDNA have been cloned and sequenced. The first one, *SP2*, corresponding to spot 'pSP2' in this study and mapped on chromosome 11 (Hatada *et al.*, 1993), was examined for allele-specific expression. F_1 progeny of the reciprocal cross between C57BL/10 and *Mus musculus molossinus* was analyzed by RT–PCR, followed by digestion with a restriction enzyme to distinguish the *SP2* allele from each parent. The result indicated that *SP2* is expressed exclusively from the paternal allele, which is shown to be demethylated at the *Not*I site, but not from the maternal allele, which has been shown to be methylated (see Fig. 23.5).

The gene encoding the U2af-related sequence

Sequences of two types of cDNA, *SP2* and the other type, revealed open reading frames of 1284 and 1386 nucleotides corresponding to encoded proteins of 428 and 462 amino acids, respectively. *SP2* cDNA carried a long 5' non-coding sequence, including up to 1200 nucleotides, which contained a CpG island (Fig. 23.6). A homology search of both cDNAs with sequence databases revealed that these proteins had a significant similarity to U2 small nuclear ribonucleoprotein auxiliary factor small subunit (Fig. 23.7), and essential mammalian splicing factor (Zhang *et al.*, 1992). The extent of similarity is 31% with *SP2* and 36% with the other cDNA. The homology reaches up to more than 50% if we include the homologous amino acids in the comparison. Homology between *SP2* and the other type of cDNA was 73% (Yamaoka *et al.*, 1995). Accordingly, we renamed *SP2* as *U2af1-rs1* (U2af-related sequence) and the other cDNA as *U2af1-rs2*. *U2afbp-rs* corresponds to our *U2af1-rs1* (Hayashizaki *et al.*, 1994).

The gene structure and expression in the brain

To isolate a genomic clone corresponding to *U2af1-rs1* cDNA, a mouse genomic library was constructed from *Xba*I-digested DNA, which carries around 8.3 kb, because only one band was detected by Southern blotting. We isolated the genomic clone and sequenced around the mRNA coding region. The transcription initiation site was determined by 5' rapid amplification of cDNA ends (5' RACE) analysis. The comparison of the genomic sequence with the cDNA sequence revealed that *U2af1-rs1* gene is an intronless gene with an unusually long 5' non-coding sequence. There is a big CpG island spanning the region from the transcription initiation site to upstream of the translation initiation site. The *Not*I site, which was shown to be methylated in a parental-specific manner, was present in this 5' non-coding region. A highly repeated sequence was also observed in the same region. The unit of this repeated sequence is of the

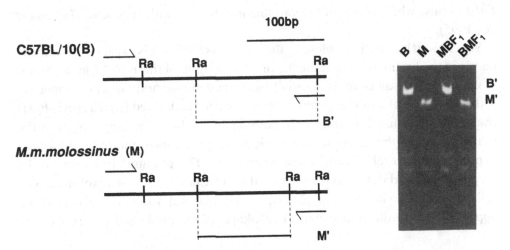

Fig. 23.5. Paternal expression of the *U2af1-rs1* gene. Total RNAs from C57BL/10 (B), *Mus m. molossinus* (M), (*M. m. molossinus* × C57BL/10)F₁ (MBF₁) and (C57BL/10 × *M. m. molossinus*)F₁ (BMF₁) were subjected to RT–PCR followed by cleavage with *Rsa*I. One of the *Rsa*I sites in the amplified region is polymorphic and distinguishable between C57BL/10 and *M. m. molossinus*. This gene is expressed from the allele of C57BL/10 in MBF1 and from the allele of *M. m. molossinus* in BMF1. B' and M' in the figure indicate the B- and M-specific fragment amplified by RT–PCR; Ra represents the site for *Rsa*I.

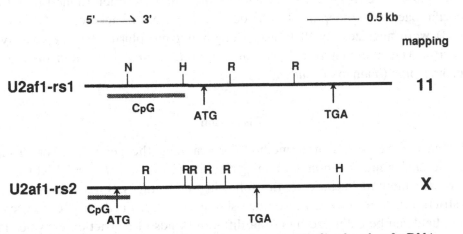

Fig. 23.6. Gene structure and mapping of mouse *U2af1-rs1* and *-rs2* cDNA. Dotted lines indicate CpG island. *U2af1-rs1* was mapped on chromosome 11 and *-rs2* on chromosome X. ATG and TGA indicate initiation and termination codons, respectively. N, *Not*I; H, *Hind*III; R, *Eco*RI.

*Fok*I family, which is one of the variable number of tandem repeats (Hatada *et al.*, 1995).

We showed by Northern blotting that *U2af1-rs1* mRNA is expressed predominantly in the brain. To determine the precise location of this mRNA in the brain, *in situ* hybridization analysis of serially sectioned mouse brain was performed. A 730 base region of a single-stranded antisense probe, derived from a *Not*I–*Bgl*II fragment, hybridized specifically in neurons throughout the gray matter of the brain, including the cerebral cortex, hippocampus, cauda putamen, thalamus, hypothalamus, cerebral cortex and brain stem. The pyramidal neurons in the hippocampus and dental gyrus showed the most intense signals. Non-neuronal cells, including glia, choroid plexus, ependyma and vascular cells, gave no appreciable hybridization signals (T. Mukai *et al.*, unpublished observation).

U2af1-rs1 *and* -rs2 *mapped on chromosomes 11 and X, respectively*

To determine the map position of these genes, we carried out a genetic mapping by a recombinant inbred (RI) strain analysis or an interspecific backcross analysis. In the case of *U2af1-rs1*, a set of 26 RI strains, derived from the BXD strain, was used. The strain distribution pattern of this allele was determined by Southern blotting using *Rsa*I polymorphism between C57BL/6 and DBA2 mice. The most similar pattern was obtained when the marker was assumed to be located between *Glns* and *Hba* on chromosome 11 (Hatada *et al.*, 1993). On the other hand, in *U2af1-rs2* the chromosomal location was determined by interspecific backcross mapping. DNAs derived from both backcrosses (BSS and BSB) were analyzed by PCR using length polymorphisms between the two species. The mapping results indicated that *U2af1-rs2* is located on the X chromosome (Yamaoka *et al.*, 1995).

Discussion

We have developed a new method for scanning the genome DNA, using restriction landmark genomic scanning (RLGS) (Hatada *et al.*, 1991). RLGS is a powerful method because of the following advantages. First, thousands of restriction landmarks can be scanned simultaneously. Furthermore, the scanning field can be extended by use of different kinds of restriction enzymes for landmark cleavage. Second, spot intensity reflects the copy number of the restriction landmark on the genome. Thus, not only the DNA amplification but also haploid and diploid genome DNA can be discriminated by this method. Third, this method can be applied to DNA from any organism without the use of any probe. Accordingly, this method is applicable to use in the genetic analysis of

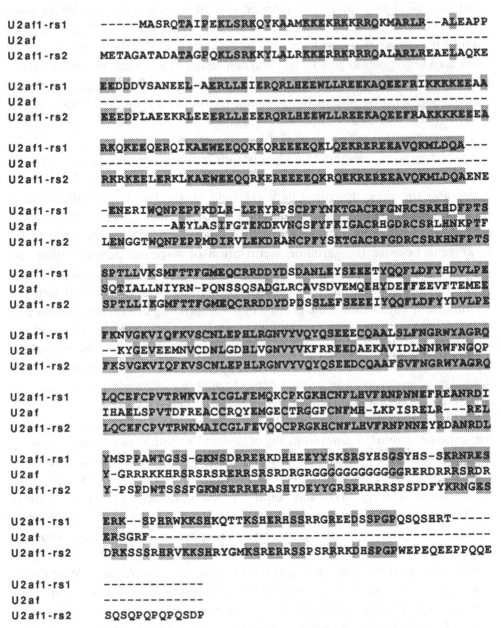

Fig. 23.7. Comparison of amino acid sequences of the putative polypeptide encoded by *U2af1-rs1* and *-rs2* with U2 small nuclear ribonucleoprotein auxiliary factor small subunits (U2AF[35]) (Zhang *et al.*, 1992). Identical amino acids are shaded darkly and homologous amino acids shaded faintly. A dash indicates that there is no amino acid corresponding to this site.

many biological disorders, such as cancer, animal mutations and genetic diseases (Hirotsune *et al.*, 1992; Hayashizaki *et al.*, 1993). In addition, RLGS is also useful for genome mapping because a polymorphic site in the individual land-mark spot segregates as genetic loci that can be used for genetic mapping. Here, we used this method as a genetic tool to detect epigenetic change, such as a methylation-sensitive site in the genome, by use of the methylation-sensitive restriction enzyme as a landmark cleavage.

The functional significance of DNA methylation in genomic imprinting was suggested by recent findings that CpG islands in four imprinted genes, e.g. *Igf2* (Sasaki *et al.*, 1992), *Igf2r* (Bartolomei *et al.*, 1993), *H19* (Ferguson-Smith *et al.*, 1993) and the gene described here (Hatada *et al.*, 1993), are differentially methylated depending upon their parental origin. Furthermore, Barlow and her colleagues showed that methylation might be necessary for the expression of the *Igf2r* gene because the germline methylation of a specific region within the expressed maternal locus is inherited from the female gamete (Stöger *et al.*, 1993). Finally, Jaenisch and his group (Li *et al.*, 1993) showed that methylation is an important key event for the process of the imprinting in a methyltransferase-deficient mouse. These observations strongly support our strategy of searching for differential methylation sites as a method of isolating imprinting genes, although it remains to be proven whether each region of differential methylation is always adjacent to an imprinted gene. In fact, we succeeded in isolating an imprinted gene that is differentially methylated and expressed in a parental-specific manner (Hatada *et al.*, 1993). Thus, this method is generally applicable for isolating imprinted genes from any organism by using a restriction enzyme as landmark cleavage in combination with second and third restriction enzymes.

Four imprinting genes have been so far isolated and mapped on the mouse chromosome. The *Igf2*, *H19* and *Snrpn* genes were mapped on chromosome 7; *Igf2r* was mapped on chromosome 17; the *U2af1-rs1* gene, which was verified as an imprinted gene, is the fifth gene and was mapped on mouse chromosome 11 (Fig. 23.8). Cattanach & Kirk (1985) proved that chromosome 11 has differential activity in maternally and paternally derived chromosome regions. When both chromosome 11s were of maternal origin, the mice were smaller than their littermates; and when both were of paternal origin, such mice were consistently larger. *U2af1-rs1* is the first gene identified as an imprinted gene on chromosome 11. It is possible that this gene is concerned with the regulation of body size. It is necessary to examine further the function of this gene by *in vitro* and *in vivo* gene transfer experiments. We also examined whether the *Rel* gene mapped on the proximal region of chromosome 11 is imprinted, and found that it was not (I. Hatada *et al.*, unpublished result).

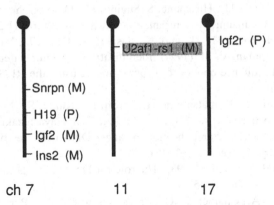

ch 7   11   17

Fig. 23.8. Mapping of imprinting genes in mouse. *Snrpn, H19, Igf2* and *Ins2* genes are mapped on chromosome 7. The orientation of this region including *H19, Igf2* and *Ins2* with respect to the centromere is not known. The *Igf2r* gene is mapped on chromosome 17; *U2af1-rs1* is mapped on chromosome 11. *Ins1* is mapped on chromosome 6 (not listed here). M and P in parenthesis mean maternally and paternally 'imprinted', respectively.

References

Arai, Y., Kajihara, S., Masuda, J., Ohishi, M., Zen, K., Ogata, J. & Mukai, T. (1994). Position-independent, high level, and correct regional expression of the rat aldolase C gene in the central nervous system of transgenic mice. *Eur. J. Biochem.* **221**, 253–60.

Bartolomei, M. S., Webber, A. I., Brunkow, M. E. & Tilghman, S. M. (1993). Epigenetic mechanism underlying the imprinting of the mouse *H19* gene. *Genes Devel.* **7**, 1663–73.

Cattanach, B. M. & Kirk, M. (1985). Differential activity of maternally and paternally derived chromosomal regions in mice. *Nature* **315**, 496–8.

Ferguson-Smith, A. C., Sasaki, H., Cattanach, B. R. & Surani, M. A. (1993). Parental-origin-specific epigenetic modification of the mouse *H19* gene. *Nature* **362**, 751–5.

Hatada, I., Hayashizaki, Y., Hirotsune, S., Komatsubara, H. & Mukai, T. (1991). A genomic scanning method for higher organisms using restriction sites as landmarks. *Proc. Natl. Acad. Sci. USA* **88**, 9523–7.

Hatada, I., Sugama, T. & Mukai, T. (1993). A new imprinted gene cloned by a methylation-sensitive scanning method. *Nucleic Acids Res.* **21**, 5577–82.

Hatada, I., Kitagawa, K., Yamaoka, T., Wang, X., Arai, Y., Hashido, K., Ohishi, S., Masuda, J., Ogata, J. & Mukai, T. (1995) Allele-specific methylation and expression of an imprinted *U2af1-rsl* (SP2) gene. *Nucleic Acids Res.* **23**, 36–41.

Hayashizaki, Y., Hirotsune, S., Okazaki, Y., Hatada, I., Shibata, H., Kawai, J., Hirose, K., Watanabe, S., Fushiki, S., Wada, S., Sigimoto, T., Kobayakawa, K., Kawara, T., Katsuki, M., Shibuya, T. & Mukai, T. (1993). Restriction landmark genomic scanning method and its application. *Electrophoresis* **14**, 251–8.

Hayashizaki, Y., Shibata, H., Hirotsune, S. Sugino, H., Okazaki, Y., Sasaki, N., Hirose, K., Imoto, H., Okuizumi, H., Muramatsu, M., Komatsubara, H., Shiroishi, T., Moriwaki, K., Katsuki, M., Hatano, N., Sasaki, H., Ueda, T., Mise, N., Takagi, N., Plass, C. & Chapman, V. M. (1994). Identification of an imprinted U2af binding protein related sequence on mouse chromosome 11 using the RLGS method. *Nature Genet.* **6**, 33–40.

Hirotsune, S., Hatada, I., Komatsubara, H., Nagai, H., Kuma, K., Kobayakawa, K., Kawara, T., Nakagawara, A., Fujii, K., Mukai, T. & Hayashizaki,Y. (1992). New approach for detection of amplification in cancer DNA using restriction landmark genome scanning. *Cancer Res.* **52**, 3642–7.

Li, E., Beard, C. & Jaenisch, R. (1993). The role for DNA methylation in genomic imprinting. *Nature* **366**, 362–5.

Sasaki, H., Jones, P. A., Chaillet, J. R., Ferguson-Smith, A. C., Barton, S. A., Reik, W. & Surani, M. A. (1992). Parental imprinting: potentially active chromatin of the repressed maternal allele of the mouse insulin-like growth factor II (*Igf2*) gene. *Genes Devel.* **6**, 1843–56.

Stöger, R., Kubicka, P., Liu, C.-G., Kafri, T., Razin, A., Cedar, H. & Barlow, D. P. (1993). Maternal-specific methylation of the imprinted mouse *Igf2r* locus identifies the expressed locus as carrying the imprinting signal. *Cell* **73**, 61–71.

Yamaoka, T., Hatada, I., Kitagawa, K., Wang, X. & Mukai, T. (1995). Cloning and mapping of *U2af1-rs2* gene with a high distortion in interspecific backcross progeny. *Genomics* (in press).

Zhang, M., Zamore, P. D., Carmo-Fonseca, M., Lamond, A. I. & Green, M. R. (1992). Cloning and intracellular localization of the U2 small nuclear ribonucleoprotein auxiliary factor small subunit. *Proc. Natl. Acad. Sci. USA* **89**, 8769–73.

Note added in proof

Since submission of this manuscript, four more genes (*ZNF127*, *PAR1*, *PAR5* and *Mas*) have been reported to be imprinted.

24

The mouse Igf2/MPR gene: a model for all gametic imprinted genes?

DENISE P. BARLOW

What is gametic imprinting?

Mammals inherit one chromosome set from each parent, and are therefore genetically diploid at autosomal loci; however, because of a phenomenon known as gametic imprinting, not all autosomal loci are functionally equivalent. Gametic imprinting is a reversible process in which a gamete-specific modification in the parental generation can sometimes lead to functional differences between the maternal and paternal genome in diploid cells of the offspring. See Appendix for an explanation of some of the terms associated with this phenomenon. One consequence of gametic imprinting is that there is a unique requirement in mammals for both the maternal and the paternal genome to be present for embryogenesis to proceed. Mammals, alone among the vertebrates, do not undergo parthenogenesis, whereby spontaneous activation of the oocyte can lead to a diploid, viable offspring. The primary reason for this is that the expression of some essential embryonic genes is subject to gametic imprinting: some of these genes are exclusively expressed from a maternally inherited chromosome whereas others show exclusive paternal expression. Thus a diploid parthenogenetic embryo will lack essential paternally expressed genes. The *Igf2/ MPR* gene is an example of a gene that shows exclusive maternal expression in the mid-gestation embryo (*Igf2/MPR:* insulin-like growth factor type 2 receptor, also known as the cation-independent mannose 6-phosphate receptor).

Table 24.1 lists all the genes known so far to be subject to parental-specific regulation. Gametic imprinting occurs in eutherian mammals but not in other vertebrates. A functionally similar process has been described in plants, insects (Sciaridae) and fission yeast (reviewed in Monk & Surani, 1990) but it is not so well documented as in mammals. The occurrence of gametic imprinting in mammals has generated the speculation that this process played a particular role in their evolution. Because the key feature distinguishing mammals from other

357

Table 24.1. *Mammalian genes subject to gametic imprinting*

Gene	Expression	Mouse chromosome	Human chromosome	Reference
Igf2/MPR	maternal	17	6[a]	a
Igf2	paternal	7	11	b
H19	maternal	7	11	c
Snrpn	paternal	7	15	d
Sp2(U2afbp-rs)	paternal	11	unmapped (nd)[b]	e
Xist	paternal[c]	X	X	f
Ins2	paternal[c]	7	11 (nd)[b]	g
Ins1	paternal[c]	6	not present	h
Wt1	monoallelic	2	11	i

[a] Biallelic in humans.
[b] Expression orientation not determined.
[c] Paternal-specific expression in some tissues, biallelic or random monoallelic expression in others.
Sources: a, Barlow *et al.* (1991); b, DeChiara *et al.* (1991); c, Bartolomei *et al.* (1991); d, Cattanach *et al.* (1992), Leff *et al.* (1992); e, Hatada *et al.* (1993), Hayashizaki *et al.* (1993); f, Brockdorff *et al.* (1992), Brown *et al.* (1992); g,h, Giddings *et al.* (1994); i, Jinno *et al.* (1994).

vertebrates is intrauterine embryonic development, it is of relevance that genes subject to gametic imprinting appear to be involved in regulating embryonic growth and development.

Gametic imprinting affects other processes in addition to gene expression (see Table 24.2). However, the full range of chromosomal function affected by gametic imprinting is still not clear, nor is it clear, despite some superficially attractive theories (Moore & Haig, 1991; Varmuza & Mann, 1994), why gametic imprinting so profoundly affects the embryonic development of mammals. A full resolution of this enigma awaits the isolation and study of a large number of chromosomal regions, genes and non-expressed sequences that are subject to gametic imprinting. It is with this aim in mind that many laboratories are attempting to identify the molecular machinery that allows a gene to be subject to parental-specific control, and to use this information to isolate other imprinted chromosomal regions from the mammalian genome. This chapter describes my laboratory's recent analysis of the imprinted and maternally expressed *Igf2/MPR* gene and discusses how this analysis has shed light on the molecular mechanisms regulating gametic imprinting.

Table 24.2. *Non-expression phenomena subject to gametic imprinting*

1. Chromosome replication timing
(e.g. maternal chromosome is late replicating in some regions while paternal
replicates early)[a]

2. Chromosome translocations
(e.g. the translocated chromosome 9 in the Philadelphia chromosome is of
paternal origin)[b]

3. Methylation of non-expression transgenes
(e.g. transgenes are methylated on maternal, but not paternal inheritance)[c]

4. Meiotic recombination frequency
(e.g. higher in females than males)[d]

5. Triplet repeat expansion and retreat
(e.g. preferential expansion of Huntington's associated repeat in males)[e]

Sources: [a] Kitsberg *et al.* (1993), Knoll *et al.* (1993); [b] Haas *et al.* (1992); [c] Surani *et al.* (1988); [d] Thomas & Rothstein 1991; [e] Goldberg *et al.* (1993).

Changes in the field of gametic imprinting

The field of mammalian gametic imprinting (reviewed in Solter, 1988; Monk &
Surani, 1990) arose from the pioneering work of the laboratories of Davor
Solter (McGrath & Solter, 1984) and Azim Surani (Surani *et al.*, 1984) who
showed, by experimental manipulation of early embryonic nuclei, that mammalian embryogenesis requires the presence of both parental genomes. This
work demonstrated that, during embryogenesis, the expression of essential
genes is regulated by parental inheritance. Later, the research groups of Bruce
Cattanach and Colin Beechey (Cattanach & Beechey, 1990; Beechey & Cattanach, 1993) used a genetic approach to show that only a small proportion of the
genome, probably representing fewer than a hundred genes, is regulated in this
manner. The field is, however, currently undergoing a quiet revolution (reviewed in Efstratiadis, 1994). The roots of this revolution lie in the recent
identification and characterization of endogenous, imprinted mammalian genes
and the discovery that other processes most likely not involving gene expression
are also subject to gametic imprinting. Endogenous imprinted genes were first
identified in the mouse in 1991, with the simultaneous demonstration that the
receptor *Igf2/MPR* was expressed from a maternally inherited chromosome
while one of its ligands, the growth factor *Igf2*, was expressed from a paternally
inherited chromosome (Barlow *et al.*, 1991; DeChiara *et al.*, 1991). In the past
few years these and other imprinted genes have been analyzed in order to

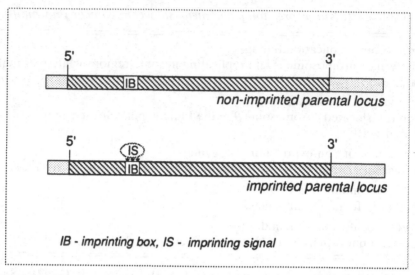

Fig. 24.1. The nature of the imprint. The maternal and paternal alleles of an imprinted gene contain an imprinting box, but only one parental allele inherits an imprinting signal from the gamete and is the 'imprinted' allele. The imprinting box can be located in the gene locus itself or in the vicinity of the gene, and may influence the activity of several genes. Once the imprinting signal is bound to the imprinting box the locus is said to be imprinted even if this does not immediately result in a functional difference between the two parental loci. Functional differences only arise when the diploid cell produces regulatory factors sensitive to the presence or absence of the imprinting signal.

identify elements that control gametic imprinting. The results have proven unexpected and have modified the existing view of the molecular mechanisms involved (reviewed by Barlow, 1994).

Lessons from endogenous gametic imprinted genes

The nature of the imprint

Gametic imprinting can cause the behavior of a chromosomal locus to be dependent on its parent of origin. A model to explain this behavior suggests that imprinted genes contain a recognition sequence called the 'imprinting box' and become imprinted when an 'imprinting signal' is bound to the imprinting box (Fig. 24.1). Two criteria for the imprinting signal are that it should be restricted to one parental chromosome and be inherited from one parental gamete. Functional differences between the two parental loci can then arise when regulatory molecules are produced that are sensitive to the presence or absence of the imprinting signal. My laboratory has previously shown that the mouse *Igf2/MPR* gene is expressed exclusively from the maternally inherited locus at day 14.5 of embryonic development (Barlow *et al.*, 1991). We have more recently attempted to identify the imprinting box by scanning this gene locus for the presence of a parental-specific DNA modification that could act as an imprinting signal. Although mammalian DNA is known to be subject to many modifications, the only one that could fit the criteria of an imprinting signal (as described above) is CpG methylation. We therefore examined the mouse *Igf2/MPR* gene for the presence of DNA methylation. This work (Stöger *et al.*, 1993) identified two separate regions of parental-specific DNA methylation that were present at day 14.5 of embryonic development. However, analysis of earlier embryonic stages showed that only one of these (named region 2) is inherited in a methylated state from the gamete and is thus likely to be the imprinting signal. Other laboratories have also identified parental-specific DNA methylation at the imprinted *Igf2* (Sasaki *et al.*, 1992) and *H19* loci (Ferguson-Smith *et al.*, 1993; Bartolomei *et al.*, 1993); however, because this methylation was not gamete-specific (Brandeis *et al.*, 1993) it most likely represents a secondary somatic imprint arising as a consequence of gene silencing. A similar secondary somatic imprint acquired late in the developing embryo by the silenced paternal locus has been identified in the *Igf2/MPR* gene (region 1; Stöger *et al.*, 1993).

The expressed Igf2/MPR *locus is imprinted*

The identification of the methylation of region 2 as a putative imprinting signal present on the expressed *Igf2/MPR* locus challenges two dogmas: first, that repressed loci are imprinted, and second, that methylation is associated with gene repression. These contentious results from the *Igf2/MPR* gene are, however, experimentally testable. One prediction arising from the proposal that the expressed locus carries a methylation imprint is that the gene would become repressed if methylation were removed. Li *et al.* (1993) have generated mice with a mutated DNA methyltransferase gene. Mice homozygous for this mutation lack significant genomic methylation and expression of *Igf2/MPR* is abolished. Thus this experiment supports the identification of the expressed *Igf2/MPR* locus as the one carrying a methylation imprinting signal. Examination of the *Igf2* and *H19* genes in the same mutant embryos showed that *Igf2*, like the *Igf2/MPR* gene, was repressed, but *H19* was activated from its previously silent locus. This analysis allows a model to be envisaged whereby the methylation imprint simply acts to inhibit factor access to one parental chromosome. In the *Igf2/MPR* and *Igf2* genes, it is proposed that repressor factors are inhibited from binding, allowing these genes to be expressed from the methylated locus. In the case of

H19, it is proposed that transcription-activating factors are inhibited from binding and thus the gene is repressed at the methylated locus.

This model, whereby a single parental locus can be silenced or activated simply by interfering with factor access to a negative or positive regulatory element, although still tentative, has received strong support from the experiments of Li *et al.* (1993) described above.

The onset of functional differences at imprinted loci

The definition of mammalian gametic imprinting used above states that the primary gametic imprint can 'sometimes' lead to functional differences between parental chromosomes. So far, the onset of functional differences has only been studied with respect to gene expression and these results show that imprinted genes need not necessarily be monoallelically expressed at all times in development. In fact, imprinted genes show three types of expression pattern, which vary in a stage- and cell-type-specific manner. Imprinted genes can sometimes be repressed from both chromosomes, or repressed from one chromosome (monoallelic expression), or expressed from both chromosomes (biallelic expression). As an example, *in situ* hybridization analysis of early postimplantation embryos shows that the *Igf2/MPR* gene is expressed in the heart but not in other tissues (Matzner *et al.*, 1992). Thus imprinted genes, like any other gene, can be completely silent in some tissues, presumably because of the absence of specific transcription factors. In addition, analysis of *Igf2/MPR* expression in embryonic stem cells carrying one allele inactivated by gene targeting (D.P.B., in collaboration with Marion Fung and Erwin Wagner, unpublished data) has shown that embryonic stem cells express *Igf2/MPR* from both parental loci although the gametic imprinting signal remains intact at region 2 (Stöger *et al.*, 1993). This suggests that an imprinted gene can be biallelically expressed at some developmental stages despite the continued presence of the imprinting signal. These data can be used to propose a model, shown in Fig. 24.2, of how a gene can retain its imprinting signal yet still show variations in expression from one or both parental loci. This model explains regulation at imprinted gene loci by suggesting the existence of methylation-sensitive regulatory factors that 'read' the imprinting signal, and by proposing that these regulatory factors are themselves expressed in a stage- and cell-type-specific manner. The proposal that the production of 'imprinting signal regulatory factors' is itself regulated in a stage- and cell-type-specific manner is strengthened by the finding that other imprinted genes such as *Igf2*, *Ins1*, *Ins2* and *Wt1* (DeChiara *et al.*, 1991; Giddings *et al.*, 1994; Jinno *et al.*, 1994) also show cell-type-specific variation in monoallelic and biallelic expression.

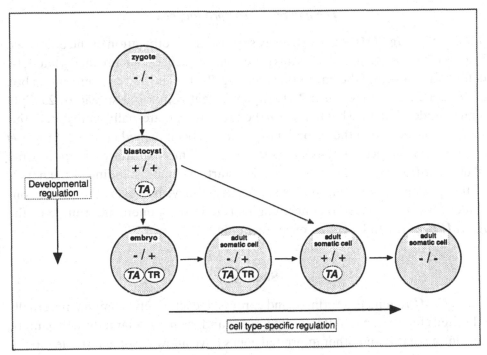

Fig. 24.2. Mono- and biallelic expression at gametic imprinted loci. Imprinted genes whose parental-specific expression is regulated by a transcriptional repressor may have three possible states of expression: $-/-$, repressed from both parental alleles; $-/+$, repressed from one parental allele; $+/+$, expressed from both parental alleles. These states of expression occur as a result of developmental and cell-type-specific variations in the production of transcription activators (TA) that act on both parental loci, and of transcriptional regulators (TR) that are methylation-sensitive and thus act only on the imprinted or non-imprinted parental allele.

Loss of regulation of imprinted genes (LORI) in human disease

It has recently been shown that expression of the *Igf2* gene becomes biallelic in sporadic cases of Wilms' tumor (reviewed by Feinberg, 1993), in some lung carcinomas (Suzuki *et al.*, 1994) and in a mouse oncogene-induced tumor model (Christofori *et al.*, 1994). In each case the non-tumor control tissue retained monoallelic expression. The model presented in Fig. 24.2 could also explain these disease-associated fluctuations between monoallelic and biallelic states by proposing that the expression of the regulatory factor acting on the imprinting signal (depicted as a repressor in Fig. 24.1) is abolished in tumorigenic states. Thus changes in monoallelic and biallelic expression at imprinted gene loci, part of the normal differentiation and development program, could also play a role in tumor progression.

D. P. Barlow

The nature of the imprinting box

Studies of the *Igf2/MPR* gene strongly suggest that methylation of the expressed locus is the imprinting signal for this gene. The sequences that are methylated, by definition, constitute the imprinting box (Fig. 24.1). The putative imprinting box for *Igf2/MPR* is defined as a 2 kb sequence that contains a spread of 29 CpG dinucleotides that have been shown to be exclusively maternally methylated; this sequence is located in the second intron and has been named region 2 (Stöger *et al.*, 1993). Sequence analysis shows that region 2 has features of a typical CpG island (Bird, 1993) but not a transcription start. An understanding of the nature of this putative imprinting box is still in its infancy; however, the predictions made (Stöger *et al.*, 1993) concerning its role in the gametic imprinting of the *Igf2/MPR* gene can be tested experimentally.

Summary

The *Igf2/MPR* gene is imprinted and expressed exclusively from the maternally inherited chromosome. Attempts to understand the molecular nature of gametic imprinting of this and other imprinted genes have allowed some testable models to be proposed, some of which have already been experimentally verified. However, the majority of the models presented here are a long way from being fully tested and at present merely represent the most likely scenario to explain the available data. With this caveat in mind, the recent analysis of endogenous imprinted genes (reviewed by Efstratiadis, 1994) has led to some surprising and slightly heretical results that not only have broad implications for development and disease, but can be used to modify the existing model of the molecular regulation of gametic imprinting. The main surprises are that the results predict that either the expressed or repressed parental locus could carry the imprinting signal, and that the onset of monoallelic expression is not coincident with the acquisition of the imprinting signal but instead can vary in development, differentiation and disease. Taken together, these data suggest that an understanding of the normal transcriptional control of an imprinted gene is crucial to an understanding of the parental-specific regulation of that locus. In the long run, gametic imprinting effects may simply be a consequence of perturbing the normal regulation of a gene by rendering one allele dependent on a methylation-sensitive regulatory factor. The issue of *why* the mammalian embryo should regulate some essential genes in this manner may take somewhat longer to resolve.

References

Barlow, D. P. (1994). Imprinting: a gamete's point of view. *Trends Genet.* **10**, 194–9.

Barlow, D. P., Stöger, R., Herrmann, B. G., Saito, K. & Schweifer, N. (1991). The mouse insulin-like growth factor type 2 receptor is imprinted and closely linked to the *Tme* locus. *Nature* **349**, 84–7.

Bartolomei, M. S., Webber, A. L., Brunkow, M. E. & Tilghman, S. M. (1993). Epigenetic mechanisms underlying the imprinting of the mouse H19 gene. *Genes Devel.* **7**, 1663–73.

Bartolomei, M. S., Zemel, S. & Tilghman, S. M. (1991). Parental imprinting of the mouse H19 gene. *Nature* **351**, 153–5.

Beechey, C. V. & Cattanach, B. M. (1993). Genetic imprinting map. *Mouse Genome* **91**, 102–4.

Bird, A. P. (1993). Imprints on islands. *Curr. Biol.* **3**, 275–7.

Brandeis, M., Kafri, T. Ariel, M., Chaillet, J. R., McCarrey, J., Razin, A. & Cedar, H. (1993). The ontogeny of allele-specific methylation associated with imprinted genes in the mouse. *EMBO J.* **12**, 3669–77.

Brockdorff, N., Ashworth, A., Kay, G. F., Cooper, P., Smith, S., McCabe, V. M., Norris, D. P., Cooper, P. J., Swift, S. & Rastan, S. (1992). The product of the mouse Xist gene is a 15 kb inactive X-specific transcript containing no conserved ORF and located in the nucleus. *Cell* **71**, 515–26.

Brown, C. J., Hendrich, B. D., Rupert, J. L., Lafrenere, R. G., Xing, Y., Lawrence, J. W. & Willard, H. F. (1992). The human Xist gene: analysis of a 17 kb inactive X-specific RNA that contains conserved repeats and is highly localised within the nucleus. *Cell* **71**, 527–42.

Cattanach, B. M., Barr, J. A., Evans, E. P., Burtenshaw, M., Beechey, C. V., Leff, S. E., Brannen, C. I., Copeland, N. G., Jenkins, N. A. & Jones, J. (1992). A candidate mouse model for Prader–Willi syndrome which shows an absence of Snrpn expression. *Nature Genet.* **2**, 270–4.

Cattanach, B. M. & Beechey, C. V. (1990). Autosomal and X-chromosome imprinting. In *Genomic Imprinting (Development,* Suppl.), ed. M. Monk & A. Surani, pp. 63–72. Cambridge: Company of Biologists.

Christofori, G., Naik, P. & Hanahan, D. (1994). Insulin-like growth factor is focally upregulated and functionally involved as a second signal in oncogene-induced tumourigenesis. *Nature* (in press).

DeChiara, T. M., Robertson, E. J. & Efstratiadis, A. (1991). Paternal imprinting of the mouse insulin-like growth factor II gene. *Cell* **64**, 849–59.

Efstratiadis, A. (1994). Parental imprinting of autosomal mammalian genes. *Curr. Opin. Genet. Devel.* **4**, 265–80.

Feinberg, A. P. (1993). Genomic imprinting and gene inactivation in cancer. *Nature Genet.* **4**, 110–13.

Ferguson-Smith, A. C., Sasaki, H., Cattanach, B. M. & Surani, M. A. (1993). Parental-origin-specific epigenetic modification of the mouse H19 gene. *Nature* **362**, 751–5.

Giddings, S. J., King, C. D., Harman, K. W., Flood, J. F. & Carnaghi, L. R. (1994). Allele-specific inactivation of insulin 1 and 2, in the mouse yolk sac indicates imprinting. *Nature Genet.* **6**, 310–13.

Goldberg, Y. P., Kremer, B., Andrew, S. E., Theilman, J., Graham, R. K., Squitieri, F., Telenius, H., Adam, S., Sajoo, A., Starr, E., Heiberg, A., Wolff, G. & Hayden, M. R. (1993). Molecular analysis of new mutations for Huntington's disease: intermediate alleles and sex of origin effects. *Nature Genet.* **5**, 174–9.

Haas, O. A., Argyriou-Tirita, A. & Lion, T. (1992). Parental origin of chromosomes involved in the translocation t(9:22). *Nature* **359**, 414–16.

Hatada, I., Sugama, T. & Mukai, T. (1993). A new imprinted gene cloned by a methylation sensitive genome scanning method. *Nucleic Acids Res.* **21**, 5577–82.

Hayashizaki, Y., Shibata, H., Hirotsune, S., Sugino, H., Okazaki, Y., Sasaki, N., Hirose, K., Imoto, H., Okuizumi, H., Muramatsu, M., Komatsubara, H., Shiroishi, T., Moriwaki, K., Katsuki, M., Hatano, N., Sasaki, H., Ueda, T., Mise, N., Takagi, N., Plass, C. & Chapman, V. N. (1993). Identification of an imprinted U2af binding protein related sequence on mouse chromosome 11 using the RLGS method. *Nature Genet.* **6**, 33–9.

Jinno, Y., Yun, K., Nishiwaki, K., Kuboto, T., Ogawa, O., Reeve, A. E. & Niikawa, N. (1994). Mosaic and polymorphic imprinting of the WT1 gene in humans. *Nature Genet.* **6**, 305–9.

Kitsberg, D., Selig, S., Brandeis, M., Simon, I., Keshet, I., Driscoll, D. J., Nicholls, R. D. & Cedar, H. (1993). Allele-specific replication timing of imprinted gene regions. *Nature* **364**, 459–63.

Knoll, J. H. M., Cheng, S.-D. & Lalande, M. (1993). Allele specificity of DNA replication timing in the Angelman/Prader–Willi syndrome region. *Nature Genet.* **6**, 41–6.

Leff, S. E., Brannan, C. I., Reed, M. L., Ozcelik, T., Francke, U., Copeland, N. G. & Jenkins, N. A. (1992). Maternal imprinting of the mouse Snrpn gene, and conserved linkage homology with the human Prader–Willi syndrome region. *Nature Genet.* **2**, 259–64.

Li, E., Beard, C. & Jaenisch, R. (1993). Role for DNA methylation in genomic imprinting. *Nature* **366**, 362–5.

McGrath, J. & Solter, D. (1984). Completion of mouse embryogenesis requires both the maternal and paternal genomes. *Cell* **37**, 179–83.

Matzner, U., Von Figura, K. & Pohlman, R. (1992). Expression of the two mannose 6-phosphate receptors is spatially and temporally different during mouse embryogenesis. *Development* **114**, 965–72.

Monk, M. & Surani, M. A. (eds) (1990). *Genomic Imprinting. Development* (Suppl.), pp. 63–72. Cambridge: Company of Biologists.

Moore, T. & Haig, D. (1991). Genomic imprinting in mammalian development: a parental tug of war. *Trends Genet.* **7**, 1–4.

Sasaki, H., Jones, P. A., Chaillet, R. J., Ferguson-Smith, A. C., Barton, S. C., Reik, W. & Surani, M. A. (1992). Parental imprinting: potentially active chromatin of the repressed maternal allele of the mouse insulin-like growth factor II (Igf2) gene. *Genes Devel.* **6**, 1843–56.

Solter, D. (1988). Differential imprinting and expression of maternal and paternal genomes. *A. Rev. Genet.* **22**, 127–46.

Stöger, R., Kubicka, P., Liu, C.-G., Kafri, T., Razin, A., Cedar, H. & Barlow, D. P. (1993). Maternal-specific methylation of the imprinted mouse *Igf2r* locus identifies the expressed locus as carrying the imprinting signal. *Cell* **73**, 61–71.

Surani, M. A., Barton, S. C. & Norris, M. L. (1984). Development of reconstituted mouse eggs suggests imprinting of the mouse genome during gametogenesis. *Nature* **308**, 548–50.

Surani, M. A., Reik, W. & Allen, A. (1988). Transgenes as molecular probes for genomic imprinting. *Trends Genet.* **4**, 59–62.

Suzuki, H., Ueda, R., Takahaski, T. & Takahaski, T. (1994). Altered imprinting in lung cancer. *Nature Genet.* **6**, 332–3.

Thomas, B. J. & Rothstein, R. (1991). Sex, maps and imprinting. *Cell* **64**, 1–3.

Varmuza, S. & Mann, M. (1994). Genomic imprinting – defusing the ovarian time bomb. *Trends Genet.* **10**, 118–23.

Appendix: an imprinting lexicon

Gametic imprinting: a reversible process whereby a gamete-specific modification in the parental generation can sometimes lead to functional differences between the maternal and paternal genome in the diploid cells of the offspring. Also known as: genomic, parental, chromosomal, gene, genetic or just imprinting and not to be confused with behavioral, hormonal or molecular imprinting.

Parental-specific expression: gene expression from either the maternal or paternal chromosome but not from both; not to be confused with paternal-specific expression.

Monoallelic or monoparental expression: genes expressed from only one chromosome where the expression orientation is unknown, e.g. genes on the X chromosome in somatic tissues of female mammals, allelic exclusion in the immune system, imprinted genes of unknown orientation.

Biallelic or biparental expression: gene expression from both parental chromosomes, e.g. the majority of mammalian genes, but also imprinted genes in some development stages, in some cell types, and in some disease conditions.

Amnesic chromosomes: diploid chromosomes that are without their parental-specific imprinting signal, e.g. chromosomes in early germ cells.

LORI: loss of regulation of imprinted genes. A term used to indicate the transition, at an imprinted gene locus, from mono- to biallelic expression in a disease condition. Also called LOI, loss of imprinting.

Imprinting signal: the molecular mark, added to one parental chromosome in the gamete, that remains restricted to the same chromosome in the embryo and which subsequently distinguishes the parental chromosomes in the diploid cell. Creates the primary gametic imprint.

Imprinting box: the DNA sequence, located within or close to the gametic imprinted gene, that is modified by the imprinted signal.

Imprinted gene: a gene with an imprinting signal bound to its imprinted box.

Secondary somatic imprint: a parental-specific mark added to one parental chromosome in the somatic cells of the embryo, that most likely is a consequence of a functional difference arising between parental loci.

Index

Note: **Bold** page numbers denote illustrations

ALL-1 gene, 111
allele-specific gene expression
  immunoglobulin locus, 201
  inactivation of X chromosome, 109–17
  marking of parental alleles, 196–7, **197**
  methylation, 112–14
  regional regulation, 195–206
allele-specific gene inactivation, 114–15
allele-specific timing of DNA replication, 157
allelic exclusion
  olfactory receptor, **202**
  model, **202**
allelic methylation
  imprinted modifiers, 157–69
  mechanism of genomic imprinting, 157–69
    structural aspects, 159–61
    tissue-specific control, 161–2
  see also DNA methylation
amnesic chromosomes, defined, 368
androgenetic embryos, 3–5, 135–6
  H19 gene expression, 146–7
  Xist gene expression, 149–50
Angelman syndrome
  clinical findings *(table)*, 296, 310–11
  imprinting center hypothesis, **302**
  imprinting mutations, 300–4
    model, **303**
  PWS/AS locus, **312**
    molecular delineation of minimal deletion
      regions, 311–12
  ZNF127, DNA methylation, 43
  see also Prader–Willi syndrome
aniridia, WAGR, 262

BALB/c modifier genes, 165–7
Beckwith–Wiedemann syndrome, 224–51,
  273–6
  11p15 region, **225–8**
    chromosomal breakpoints, 228–32, **231**
    cloning of BWS-associated breakpoints,
      228–9
    duplication of paternal allele, 214
    summary, **233**
  allelic methylation, 162–4
  autosomal dominant pedigrees, 246–7
  BWSCR1, 228–32, **231**
  clinical findings, 224–5, 273–4
    outcome, 288–9
  etiology, 237–47
  H19 gene expression, 162–4

IGF2 gene expression, 35, 162–4
  index patient, *IGF2* imprinting, **186**
  loss of imprinting (LOI), *INS, IGF2* and
    H19, 229–32, 278–80, **280**
  maternal LOH, **226**
  models, 247–8
  mosaicism, 215
  tracking imprinting, 224–36
  see also Wilms' tumor
biallelic expression, defined, 368
Brachyury gene, expression, 40–1
bromodeoxyuridine, replication time zones, 197

cancer
  domain of abnormal imprinting, 273–92
    gene dosage model, 214–16
    imprinting switch model, 217–19
    Knudson two-hit model, 209–10
    tumor suppressor gene model, 210–14
    Wilkins model, 209–10
  and imprinting, 209, 273
  loss of imprinting (LOI), 229–32, 278–80, **280**
    model of LOI, 285–6
    questions to be answered, 287–9
cellular determination, 71–108
choriocarcinoma, Jeg-3 cells, 187–8
choroid plexus
  allelic methylation, 161–2
  expression of (normally repressed) maternal
    allele *IGF2* gene, 170–1, 184
chromatin, activity vs repression, 56–8
chromatin structures, 47–126
  chromobox genes, 71–108
  inheritance, 49–70
    hypotheses, 59–64
      models for duplication, 63
      S phase, 63–4
      X chromosomes, 64–5
      yeast origin recognition complex, 63
chromobox genes
  and cellular determination, 71–108
  HP1 and *Pc-G*, 91–4
  species and cloning, 91–4
chromodomain proteins
  amino acid sequences, **92**
  HP1, 53–4, 63
  Polycomb, 53–4, 63
  structure, 94
chromosomal translocation, spermatogenetic
  arrest, 41–2

chromosome 2, T1Wa and T28H breakpoints, 329
chromosome 11p15 region, 225–32, **231**
  11p15.5, *H19* gene, 265–8
  additional tumor suppression gene, 286–7
  see also Beckwith–Wiedemann syndrome
chromosome 15q11–13 region
  D15S63 methylation pattern, **298**
  locus order, **287**
  parent-of-origin-specific DNA methylation, 296–9, **298**
    diagnostic applications, 300
chromosome(s)
  chromosome walking, 228–9
  human, gene mapping, 329–30
  mitotic crossing-over, 252–63
    theoretical genetics, 253–8
  position effects, 54
  position-effect variegation, 53–4, 72–108
  rearrangements, use for investigations into imprinting, 327–41
  see also chromatin
cis- and *trans*-acting factors
  mitotic crossing over, 252–4
  in replication, 198
colon cancer, DNA methylation, **283**
CpG dinucleotides
  DNA methylation, **60**, 61, 159–61, 342
  methylation pattern, island, **284**
  search for parental-origin-specific CpG methylation, RLGS, 346–9
  see also DNA methylation
cystic fibrosis gene, 198–9, **199**
cytosine
  methylation, **60**, 61
    role in allele-specific gene expression, 112–14

D15S63 locus, chromosome 15q11–13 region, 298–9
dermoid cysts, derived from parthenogenetic embryos, 13
disomies/duplications, Di/Dp system, 329–41
  Gabrb3 and *GABRB3* genes, 335–6
  Snrpn, 333–4
  U2afbp-rs, 332–3
  Znf127, 334–5
DNA cloning, 344
DNA methylation
  androgenetic embryos, 135–6, 149–50
  colon cancer, **283**
  CpG dinucleotides, **60**, 61, 159–61, 342
  functional significance, 354
  and gene expression, 299
  and genomic imprinting, 121–3
  gynogenetic embryos, 135–6, 148–9, 150–1
  LOI mechanism, 282–3
  mammalian development, 118–26
  marking of parental alleles, 196–7, **197**
  MTase gene, 118–20
  parent-of-origin-specific
    15q11–13 region, 296–9
    imprinted genes, 147

  see also allelic methylation
DNA modifications, and chromatin structure, 47–126
double dose hypothesis, 214–15
Drosophila
  Antp, 86, **88**
  bithorax complex, 86–88, **88**, 99–100
  euchromatic genes
    abo, 81–6
      copies *(ABO)*, 85
  homeobox genes, order, **88**
  parental imprinting, 95–100
  paternally imprinted modifiers, 164–5
  Polycomb chromodomain protein, 53–4
    shared with HP1, 85
  Polycomb-Group genes *(Pc-G)*, 85–91
    Pc-G–trx-G system, 109–11
  position-effect variegation, 72–108
    eye variegation, **74, 75**
    modifiers and mass-action model, 76–8
    parental origin of rearrangement, **96**, 97
    white mottling, 72–5
  protein-1 (HP1) heterochromatin, 79–85
  trithorax-Group genes, 86
    brahma gene, 89
    Pc-G–trx-G system, 109–11

E36 transgene, 165
embryonal tumors
  imprinting switch model, 217–19
  Knudson two-hit model, 209–10, 216
  and overgrowth disorders, 209–23
  see also Wilms' tumor
embryonic stem cells, gene targeting methods, 119–21
EMG *see* Beckwith–Wiedemann syndrome
endoderm, yolk sac, *Xist* gene, 133, **134**
enhancers
  action, 54–6
  competition model, *Igf2* and *H19* genes, **172**
enhancers of PEV (Evars), 76–8, **77, 80**
  (table), 82–3
epigenetic inheritance, 49–70
  gene activity vs repression, 56–8
  hypotheses *see* chromatin structures
  imprinted and inactive X-linked genes, 114–15
  local position effect, 50–53
  long-range position effect, 53–6
  and methylation, 99–100
  nucleosome and transcription complex assembly, 58–9
  parental imprinting, 95–100
  X chromosomes, activity vs inactivity, 64–5
epigenetic marking, reciprocal imprinting, *Igf2* and *H19* genes, 171–3
Erbb gene, 336
eukaryotic genes *see* genes
evolution of imprinting, 17–28
eye, retinal cones, red and green pigments, 203–5

fluorescent *in situ* hybridization, 228

Gabrb3 and *GABRB3* genes, 335–6
β-galactosidase reporter, 174
gametic imprinting, defined, 357, 368
gene regulation, theories of imprinting, 24
genes
  activity vs repression, 56–8, **58**
  imprinted gene, defined, 368
  regulation of expression, **51**
  transcription machinery, 49–70
    RNA polymerase activity, 49–50
    TATA binding protein, 49–50
genome scanning strategies, 345–6
  2D gel electrophoresis, **346**
genomic imprinting
  analysis, assumptions and expectations,
    258–9
  applied genetics, 260–2
  changes in field of, 359–60
  disruption, mitotic crossing over, 252–63
  DNA methylation, 121–3
  embryonal tumors and overgrowth disorders,
    209–23
  list of genes *(table)*, 358
  mechanisms, 129–206
    allele-specific gene expression, 195–206
    allelic methylation, 157–69
    H19 and *Igf2* genes in mouse, 170–81
    H19 and *Xist* genes in uniparental
      embryos, 142–56
    plasticity of imprinting, 182–94
    X chromosome inactivation, 129–41
  model for all imprinted genes, 357–67
  nature of the imprint, 360–1
  non-expression phenomena *(table)*, 359
  onset of functional differences at imprinted
    loci, 362–3
  theoretical genetics, 253–8
GTFs *see* transcription process
gynogenetic embryos, 3–5, 135–6
  Xist gene expression, 148–9

H19 gene
  DNA methylation, 121–3, 142, 157–69,
    171–3
  enhancers, role, 173
  expression, BWS, 245–6
  imprinting, role, 143–7, 174–8, 276–8
  mapping, 354–5
  in mouse, 170–81
  reciprocal imprinting with *Igf2* gene, 170–1,
    173–4
    epigenetic marking, 171–3
  replication, 65
  similarities with *XIST*, 174–8
    (table), 176
  structure, **177**
    conserved stem–loop structures, **178**
  as tumor suppressor gene, 264–72
  tumorigenesis, 218–19
  in uniparental embryos, 142–56
heterochromatin
  action, model, **55**
  action on chromatin structure, 54–6

β-heterochromatin *see* -, protein-1 (HP1)
  formation, molecular characteristics *(table)*,
    76–8, 82–3
  position effects, *cis-* and *trans-*acting factors,
    81
  position-effect variegation, 53–4, 72–108
    modifiers and mass-action model, 76–8
  protein-1 (HP1), 53–4, 63
    distribution pattern, **84**
    Drosophila, 79–85
    isolation from mammals, 79
    and *Pc-G*, 91–4
    PEV modifier, 79–85
    protein subfamilies, amino acid sequences,
      92
    swi-6, 93
histones
  acetylation, 58–9
  displacement from DNA, 56–7
  modification, and protein retention, 57
  position-effect variegation, 53–4
  post-translational modification, nascent vs
    mature chromatin, 58–9
  structural role, 50–1
  transcription process, 51–3
HMG1 and 2, DNA recognition, 52
homeogenes
  characteristics, 85–6
  Pc-G products, 90–1
    assembly, 91
host defense, theories of imprinting, 23–4
housekeeping genes, 197–8
HP1 *see* heterochromatin, protein-1
HRX, 111
HRX/ALL-1 protein, and murine All-1, 111

Igf1r gene, 7
  parthenogenetic and control embryos, 7–11
Igf2/MPR gene as model for all imprinted
    genes, 357–67
Igf2 gene, 6–14, 19–20, 65, 98–9, 170–81
  allelic methylation, 157–69, **158**, **159**
  enhancers, role, 173
  mapping, 354–5
  parthenogenetic and control embryos, 7–11
  reciprocal imprinting with *H19* gene, 170–1
    enhancer competition model, **172**
  reciprocal imprinting with *Igf2* gene,
    epigenetic marking, 171–3
  replication, 65
IGF2 gene (human)
  allelic usage, RNase protection analysis,
    PCR, 184, **185**
  expression, **244**
    in BWS, 242–3
    in human control tissues, 240
    of (normally repressed) maternal allele in
      choroid plexus, 170–1, 184
    in tumors with LOI and LOH, **281**
  loss of imprinting, 276–8
    in liver development, 188–90
  opposite allelic usage, results in tumor cells,
    183–8

IGF2 gene (human) – *cont'd.*
    paternal chromosome expression, 184–5
    promoter-specific allelic usage, 188–90, **189**,
        190
        evaluation, 183–8
    promoters, maps, **243**
    transcription, direct analysis, 240–2
    transcriptional unit, **184**
    tumorigenesis, 217–18
Igf2r gene, 6–14, 19–20, 98–9
    differential DNA methylation, 147
    mapping, 354–5
    model for all imprinted genes, 357–67
    replication, 65
IGF2R gene (human), 6–7, 12
    polymorphism of imprinting, 30, 182–3
immunoglobulin locus, allele-specific gene
        expression, 201
imprint, defined, 100, 368
imprintase, 212, **213**
imprinting
    evolution, 17–28
    theories *see* theories of imprinting
imprinting box, **360**, 364
    defined, 368
imprinting center hypothesis, **302**
imprinting mutation model, AS and PWS, **303**
imprinting signal, **360**
    defined, 368
imprintor, defined, 100
Imprintor genes, 40
in situ hybridization, 344
ins2 gene
    conditional imprinting, 170
    expression in yolk-sac, 182
insulators
    action, model, **55**
    defined, 54
insulin-like growth factor-2 and receptor *see*
        Igf2 and *Igf2r* genes

keratin-promoter–*lacZ* transgene, 161
Knudson two-hit model, cancer, 209–10

leptomeninges
    allelic methylation, 161–2
    expression of (normally repressed) maternal
        allele *IGF2* gene, 170–1, 184
liver development
    IGF2 gene (human), loss of imprinting,
        188–90, 241–2
    mRNA, primer extension analysis, **242**
    tumorigenesis, 188–9
locus control regions (LCRs), action, 54–6, **55**
loss of heterozygosity (LOH), 209–10, 255–6,
        255
    11p15 tumor suppressor gene, 215
    mosaicism, 252–3
    predictions, 259–60
    Wilms' tumor, 212–16
loss of imprinting (LOI), 229–32, 278–80, **280**,
        285–9
    defined, 368

loss of regulation of imprinted genes (LORI)
    defined, 368
    human disease, 363

M31, **84**
mAbs
    C1A9, 79
        see also heterochromatin, protein-1
mammal, *trithorax*-homolog *HRX*, 111–12
mammalian development, 3–16
    DNA methylation, 118–26
    preimplantation, 3–14
Mat/Pat Di and Dp genotypes, 329
methyltransferase (MTase)
    de novo, 120–1
    DNA methylation, 118–26
    ES cell viability, 118–20
mitotic crossing over
    analysis, assumptions and expectations,
        258–9
    intrachromosomal switch over, 256, **257**
    multiple crossing over, 257
    predictions, 259–60
    theoretical genetics, disruption of genomic
        imprinting, 252–63
    triggering factors, 257–8
Mnt gene, 337–8
modifier genes
    paternal imprinting, **166**
    TKZ751 transgenic locus, 165
modulo, 81, 82
monoallelic expression, defined, 368
mosaicism
    and Beckwith–Wiedemann syndrome, 215
    loss of heterozygosity (LOH), 252–3
mouse
    chromosome 17, imprinting on, 29–45
    chromosome 7, mapping, **355**
    chromosome rearrangements, use for
        investigations into imprinting, 327–41
        dosage effects and imprinting, 330–1
        reduction in imprinting region, 329–30
    F₁ hybrid (*M. m. domesticus X M. m.
        castaneus*), 171–3
    imprinted genes, 6–14, 29–45
        chromosome 17, 29–45
        Brachyury gene expression, 40–1
        Tme (T-associated maternal effect)
            locus, 30–40
        see also H19; *Xist*
    imprinting chromosomes, **328**
    Mnt gene, 337–8
    spermatogenetic arrest caused by
        chromosomal translocation, 41–2
    X chromosome, changes in activity, **132**
mus209/Pcna, 83

Neurospora, single-chromosome analysis of
        methylation, 161
new genes, 356
    search, 327–67
nucleosomes
    disruption during replication, 56–8
    transcription machinery, 50–2, **52**

olfactory receptor
  allelic exclusion, **202**
  model, **204**
  gene family, *17* and *M50*, 201, 202–3
ovarian teratoma, derived from
          parthenogenetic embryos, 13

parent-of-origin-specific DNA methylation,
          296–9
  diagnostic applications, 300
  SNRPN gene, 317–18
parent–offspring conflict theory, 12–13
parental imprinting
  defined, 29
  epigenetic inheritance, PEV, 95–100
  parental origin effect, 95
  reversibility, 95–7
  X chromosome, 95–100
parental-specific expression, defined, 368
parthenogenetic embryos, 135–6
paternal imprinting, modifier genes, **166**
Petunia, single-chromosome analysis of
          methylation, 161
PEV *see* position-effect variegation
placentation
  invasive and non-invasive, 22–3
  theory of imprinting, 22–3
Plannococcus citri, parental imprinting, 97–8
plasticity of imprinting, 182–94
Polycomb, chromodomain protein, 53–4
Polycomb-Group genes (*Pc*-G), 85–91
  binding sites, 87
  and HP1, 91–4
  immunostaining of polytene chromosomes,
          86–7
  protein subfamilies, amino acid sequences, **92**
  protein-1 (HP1), protein subfamilies, **92**
position-effect variegation, 53–4, 72–108
  characteristics, 73
  degree of variegation, **96**
  enhancers of PEV (Evar), 76–8
  suppressors of PEV (Suvar), 76–8
  white mottling, 72–5
Prader–Willi syndrome, 295–323
  clinical findings *(table)*, 296, 310
  history, 309
  imprinting center hypothesis, **302**
  imprinting mutations, 300–4
  model, **303**
  parent-of-origin-specific DNA methylation,
          296–9
  PWS/AS locus, **312**
    asynchronous replication, 200
    molecular delineation of minimal deletion
          regions, 311–12
  ZNF127, DNA methylation, 43
preimplantation development, expression of
          imprinted genes, 3–14
proliferating cell nuclear antigen (PCNA), 83
promoter-specific allele usage, **189**, 190
pulsed field gradient electrophoresis, 228

reciprocal imprinting

Igf2 and *H19* genes, 171–3
  BWS, 171–3, 243–5
replication
  cis- and *trans*-acting factors, 198
  time zones, 197–9
  timing
    analysis, 198–9
    asynchronous in *Igf2r*, **200**
replication fork, transcription machinery, 49–70
repressive protein *see* histones; Polycomb
restriction landmark genome scanning (RLGS),
          342–56
  methods, 343–5
  results, 345–52
  summary and discussion, 352–5
retroviruses, LTRs, 297–9
RFLPs, insulin, *IGF2* and tyrosine hydroxylase,
          245
rhabdomyosarcoma, tumor suppressor gene
          model, 210–12
RNA polymerase activity, basal transcription
          machinery, 49–53
RNase protection analysis, PCR, 184, **185**
rRNA gene, replication fork progression, 57
RSVIgMyc imprinted transgene, 196–7
RT–PCR analysis, 344

Sciara coprophila, parental imprinting, 97–8
secondary somatic imprint, defined, 368
silencer sequences, yeast, epigenetic
          modifications, 161
snRNP-associated polypeptide-N, 313
SNRPN gene (human)
  C/T sequence polymorphism, **315**
  CpG sites, parent-of-origin-specific
          methylation, 317–18
  imprinting center hypothesis, **302**
  locus, 297
  mapping, 313
  maternal imprinting, 315–16
  structure, **314**
Snrpn gene
  mapping, **355**
  maternal imprinting, 29
    UPD, 313–15
  paternal/maternal imprinting, Di/Dp system,
          333–4
  replication, 65
Sp2 gene *see U2afbp-rs* gene
spermatogenetic arrest, caused by chromosomal
          translocation, 41–2
stem cells *see* embryonic stem cells
suppressors of PEV (Suvar), 76–8, **77**, **80**
          (table), 82–3
SWI1,2,3,snf5,6 complex, 54, 55

T43H translocation, 41–3
T cell receptor locus, allele-specific gene
          expression, 201
TAFs *see* TATA binding protein,
          (TBP)-associated factors
TATA binding protein, 49–50
  TBP-associated factors (TAFs), 49–50

Tgfa ligand, 336
theories of imprinting, 11–14
  genetic-conflict hypothesis, 17–21
    future tests, 20–1
    Igf2 and *Igf2r* genes, 19–20
    taxonomic distribution, 19
  hypotheses *(table)*, 60
  other hypotheses
    gene regulation, 24
    host defense, 23–4
    placentation, 22–3
    prevention of parthenogenesis, 21–2
  overview, 24–5
  parent–offspring conflict theory, 12–13
TKZ751 transgenic locus, modifier genes, 165,
    166
Tme (T-associated maternal effect) locus,
    30–40
  modification of lethality, mice with null *Igf2*
    mutations, 33–5
  rescue of maternal deletions, 31–3, **34**
    genetic analysis, 35–40, **39**
transcription complexes, maintenance through
    replication, **62**
transcription factors
  hypotheses to explain inheritance of
    chromatin states, 59–64
  sequence-specific, **51**
transcription machinery, 49–53
transcription process
  general transcription factors (GTFs), 51–3
  and imprinting, 190–2
  nascent vs mature chromatin, 58–9
  nucleosomes, potentiation, 50–2, **52**
  replication fork, 49–70
Trithorax-Group genes (*trx*-G), 86, 91
tumor suppressor gene
  11p15, loss of heterozygosity (LOH) gene,
    216
  H19 gene, 264–72
  model of cancer, 210–14
twins, monozygotic (MZ)
  discordance, 260
  X-linked disorders, 239–40, 259–60

U2afbp-rs gene, 29, 332–3, 342–56
U2af1-rs1 and *U2af1-rs2* genes, 344–5
  amino acid sequences, **353**
  cloning and expression in brain, 350–2
  paternal expression, **351**
uniparental disomy (UPD), 237–8, 254, **255**,
    311
  mitotic crossing over, 259–60

WAGR, aniridia, 262
Wilkins model, 209–10, **211**
Wilms' tumor, 182–3
  H19 gene as tumor suppressor gene, 264–72
  imprinting switch model, **219**

LOH and *IGF2*, 217–19
  biallelic transcription, 217
  molecular study, 260–2
  Wilkins model, 209–10, **211**
  see also Beckwith–Wiedemann syndrome
Wilms' tumor gene, *WT1*
  zinc finger, 261–2

X chromosome
  changes in activity, mouse, **132**
  chromatin structure inheritance, 64–5
  counting mechanism, 138
  Drosophila, *white* variegation, **74**
  hypotheses of inheritance, 64–5
  inactivation, 129–41
    allele-specific gene expression, 109–17
    embryonic and extraembryonic lineages,
      152–3
    evolution, 138–9
    mechanism, 129–37
    method of spreading, 137
    and parental imprinting, evidence, 137–9
    see also Xist gene
  inactivation center, 130
    see also Xist gene
  parental imprinting, 95–100
  paternal
    early replication, 199
    inactivation, 98–9
  spermatogenetic arrest caused by
    chromosomal translocation, 41–2
U2af1-rs2 gene, 352
Xist gene, 29
  changes in activity, mouse, **132**
  cloning, 130
  control of expression, **152**
  DNA methylation, 121–3, 133–7, 142
  first expression, paternal allele, 186–7
  imprinting, 133–7, 146–50, **146**
  regulation, 150–3
  role, evidence, 131–3
  short tandem repeats, 176–7
  similarities with *H19*, 174–8
    (table), 176
  structure of *XIST*, **177**
    conserved stem–loop structures, **178**
  in uniparental embryos, 142–56

yeast
  replication and transcription, linkage,
    63–4
  silencer sequences, epigenetic modifications,
    161
yeast artificial chromosomes, 229

Znf127 gene, 334–5
  BWS, hemihypertrophy, 232–4
  DNA methylation, 42